OXFORD MEDICAL PUBLICATIONS

PRINCIPLES OF SURVEILLANCE

Illustrated by plague surveillance in London in the 17th century

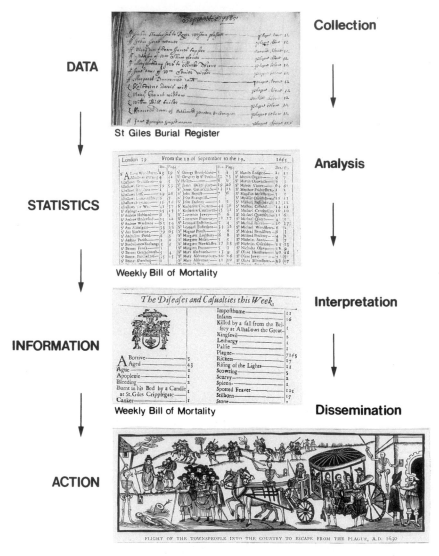

DATA — Collection

St Giles Burial Register

STATISTICS — Analysis

Weekly Bill of Mortality

INFORMATION — Interpretation

Weekly Bill of Mortality

ACTION — Dissemination

From 'Recent Advances in Community Medicine, No.2.' Churchill Livingstone. London 1982

Surveillance in Health and Disease

Edited by

W. J. EYLENBOSCH

Professor of Epidemiology and Community Medicine, University of Antwerp

and

N. D. NOAH

Consultant Epidemiologist, PHLS Communicable Disease Surveillance Centre, London

Published on behalf of
the Commission of the European Communities
by Oxford University Press

OXFORD NEW YORK TOKYO
OXFORD UNIVERSITY PRESS
1988

Oxford University Press, Walton Street, Oxford OX2 6DP
Oxford New York Toronto
Delhi Bombay Calcutta Madras Karachi
Petaling Jaya Singapore Hong Kong Tokyo
Nairobi Dar es Salaam Cape Town
Melbourne Auckland
and associated companies in
Berlin Ibadan

Oxford is a trade mark of Oxford University Press

Published in the United States
by Oxford University Press, New York

Publication No. EUR 10856 of the
Commission of the European Communities,
Directorate-General Telecommunications, Information
Industries and Innovation, Luxembourg

British Library Cataloguing in Publication Data
Surveillance in health and disease.—
(Oxford medical publications).
1. Health survey
I. Eylenbosch, W. J.   II. Noah, Norman D.
613   RA407
ISBN 0-19-261611-0

Library of Congress Cataloguing in Publication Data
Surveillance in health and disease.
(Oxford medical publications)
Includes bibliographies and indexes.
1. Diseases—Reporting.   2. Diseases—Reporting—
Europe.   3. Public health—Information services—Europe.
I. Eylenbosch, W. J. (Willy J.)   II. Noah, N. D.
(Norman D.)   III. Series. [DNLM: 1. Disease Outbreaks—
occurrence—Europe.   2. Disease outbreaks—prevention &
control—Europe.   3. Epidemiologic Methods—Europe.
WA 950 S963]
RA404.A1S87   1988   616.4'24   87-24731
ISBN 0-19-261611-0

Typeset by Eta Services (Typesetters) Ltd, Beccles, Suffolk
Printed in Great Britain by
The Alden Press, Oxford

Foreword

A. E. BENNETT

Director, Health and Safety Directorate,
Commission of the European Communities, Luxembourg

This book is about concepts and methods of surveillance in health care. It complements two earlier texts which described the methods of epidemiology in relation to health care and the relevant techniques of evaluation.

The Commission of the European Communities commissioned the Panel for Epidemiology and Social Medicine to prepare these three volumes in order to promote better communication, understanding, and exchange between health-care policy-makers and health administrators, clinicians, and epidemiologists. They are intended for use at the interface between health administration, clinical care, and medical research.

These three books provide the basic tools for comparative, cross cultural, and international analyses in the development of health care.

Bibliography

Holland, W. W. and Karhausen, L. (ed.), *Health care and epidemiology*. Henry Kimpton, London (1978).

Holland, W. W. (ed.), *Evaluation of health care*. Oxford University Press (1983).

Acknowledgements

The Editorial Board members are grateful to Mrs Barbara Boeynaems and Mrs Tessa Dunscombe for typing and final revision of the text. We are also grateful to Dr N. S. Galbraith for permission to reproduce the frontispiece.

The authors made extensive use of *A dictionary of epidemiology* by John Last (Oxford University Press, New York, 1983) when compiling the Glossary.

Contents

Contributors

MALCOLM BARROW
Head of Safety Research Section (from August 1986), Consumer Safety Unit, Department of Trade and Industry, Millbank Tower, Millbank, London SW1P 4PU, United Kingdom

GUY DE BACKER MD
Senior Research Associate, National Fund for Scientific Research, Belgium, Department of Hygiene and Social Medicine, Academisch Ziekenhuis, De Pintelaan 185, Ghent, Belgium

ARNOLD DE BOCK Ir
Civil Engineer in Chemistry and Nuclear Sciences.
Director of the Central Service for Safety and Radioprotection at the Flemish Catholic University of Leuven, de Croylaan 58, B-3030 Leuven-Heverlee, Belgium

WILLY J. EYLENBOSCH MD
Professor of Epidemiology and Social Medicine and Dean of the Faculty of Medicine, University of Antwerp, Universiteitsplein 1, B-2610 Antwerpen, Belgium

ANDERS FOLDSPANG MD
Associate Professor, Institute of Social Medicine, University of Aarhus, Vesterbro Torv 1–3, 6, 8000 Aarhus C, Denmark

GEOFFREY FRANCE
Head of Safety Research Section (1976–1986), Consumer Safety Unit, Department of Trade and Industry, Millbank Tower, Millbank, London SW1P 4PU, United Kingdom

CATHERINE GOUJON MD
Responsable du Service des Vaccinations, Institut Pasteur, Hôpital, Service des Vaccinations, 211 Rue du Vaugirard, 75015 Paris, France

LUCIEN KARHAUSEN MD
Medical Research Officer, Commission of the European Communities, Jean Monnet Building, Plateau de Kirchberg, L-2920 Luxembourg

VASSILIOS KATSOUYANNOPOULOS MD
Professor of Public Health, Director of the Laboratory of Hygiene, Medical School, University of Ioannina, Greece

ALLAN KELLY

Manager, Nutritional Surveillance Programme, University of Dublin, Department of Statistics, Trinity College, Dublin 2, Eire

KARL H. KIMBEL MD

Wullnerstrasse 139, 5 Köln 41, Federal Republic of Germany

U. LAASER MD

Deutsches Institut zur Bekämpfung des hohen Blutdruckes, Postfach 101449, 6900 Heidelberg 1, Federal Republic of Germany

HENK LAMBERTS MD

Professor, Department of General Practice, University of Amsterdam, Meibergdreef 15, 1105 AZ Amsterdam, The Netherlands

ELSEBETH LYNGE

Danish Cancer Registry, Institute of Cancer Epidemiology, Danish Cancer Society, Landskronagade 66, 2100 Copenhagen Ø, Denmark

LOUIS MASSE MD

Professeur, Ecole Nationale de la Santé Publique, Avenue du Professeur Léon Bernard, 35043 Rennes Cedex, France

ANNA McCORMICK MB, FFCM

Consultant Epidemiologist, PHLS Communicable Disease Surveillance Centre, 61 Colindale Avenue, London NW9 5EQ, United Kingdom

MARIA LUISA MORO MD

Istituto Superiore di Sanità, Laboratorio di Epidemiologia e Biostatistica, Viale Regina Elena, 299, 00161 Roma-Nomentano, Italia

NORMAN D. NOAH MB, MRCP, FFCM

Consultant Epidemiologist, PHLS Communicable Disease Surveillance Centre, 61 Colindale Avenue, London NW9 5EQ, United Kingdom

D. M. PARKIN MD

Chief, Unit of Descriptive Epidemiology, Division of Epidemiology and Biostatistics, International Agency for Research on Cancer, 150 Cours Albert Thomas, Lyon, France

J. GORDON PATERSON MD

Community Medicine Specialist, Grampian Health Board, P.O. Box 119, 1–7 Albyn Place, Aberdeen, AB9 8QP, United Kingdom

BERT SCHADE MD

Department of General Practice, University of Amsterdam, Meibergdreef 15, 1105 AZ Amsterdam, The Netherlands

ANDRE STROOBANT MD
Head, Institute of Hygiene and Epidemiology, 14 Juliette Wijtsmanstraat, 1050 Brussels, Belgium

GODFRIED THIERS MD
Director, Institute of Hygiene and Epidemiology, 14 Juliette Wijtsmanstraat, 1050 Brussels, Belgium

DIMITRIS TRICHOPOULOS MD
Professor of Hygiene and Epidemiology, School of Medicine, University of Athens, Athens (609) Goudi, Greece

YANNIS TOUNTAS MD
Assistant Professor of Social Medicine, School of Medicine, University of Athens, Athens (609) Goudi, Greece

VIVIANE VAN CASTEREN MD
Institute of Hygiene and Epidemiology, 14 Juilette Wijtsmanstraat, 1050 Brussels, Belgium

HANS P. VERBRUGGE MD
Medical Officer of Maternal and Child Health, Chief Medical Officer of Health, Ministry of Welfare, Health and Culture, Sir Winston Churchillaan 362, P.O. 5406, 2280 HK Rijswijk, The Netherlands

GLYN N. VOLANS MD, FRCP
Director, The Poisons Unit, Guy's Hospital, London SE1 9RT, United Kingdom

DERMOT WALSH MD
The Medico Social Research Board, 73, Lr. Baggot Street, Dublin 2, Eire

JOSEPHINE A. C. WEATHERALL MD
Willows, Church Lane, Charlbury, Oxford 0X7 3PX, United Kingdom

H. WENZEL MD
Deutsches Institut zur Bekämpfung des hohen Blutdruckes, Postfach 10 14 49, 6900 Heidelberg 1, Federal Republic of Germany

HEATHER M. WISEMAN MSc
Information Officer, The Poisons Unit, Guy's Hospital, London SE1 9RT, United Kingdom

M. WOHLERT MD
Institute of Social Medicine, University of Aarhus, Vesterbro Torv 1–3, 6, 8000 Aarhus C, Denmark

Introduction

Disease surveillance (the continuing scrutiny of all aspects of occurrence and spread of disease that are pertinent to effective control) plays a critical role in the implementation of health-care policy. This holds for primary as well as other forms of health care.

One could even ask whether any health-care system can afford not to have some form of surveillance system for the control of disease. How could one select the most imperative health problems to be handled in a nation or its regions without some basic knowledge of their frequency? How could one set priorities concerning preventive or curative programmes? How could one evaluate whether goals were reached in the target groups—or, in other words, whether efforts were worth the resources spent in the programmes?

In describing basic principles of surveillance as well as selected health fields suitable for surveillance and examples of ways of organizing surveillance systems, the purpose of this book is to stress the need and to raise demands for the establishment of proper surveillance. Even if the need for surveillance seems rather clear-cut, surveillance is still not an obligatory decision tool in health policy-making. It should be.

As the text of the book shows, the concept of surveillance is not a new one but, on the contrary, rather ancient. Still there is some confusion concerning what surveillance actually is. In the WHO *Glossary of health care terminology*[1] the word is not listed, but the content of the concept is found under 'Monitoring', i.e. 'first, the making of routine measurements on health and environmental indices and the recording and transmission of the data and, second, the collation and interpretation of such data with a view to detecting changes in the health status of populations and their environment'. In the French version[2] of this Glossary the same definition appears under the word 'surveillance'. These linguistic peculiarities lead to some confusion. In Part 1 an attempt has been made to clarify the differences between both concepts.

Surveillance was considered already more than ten years ago as 'part of the cooperative venture between the epidemiologist and all sectors of the health system and should therefore contribute to total economic development of which health is a vital part'.[3] Health being a crucial dimension of life conditions, health fields with high priority concerning surveillance are dissimilar in different regions. Third-world countries are still struggling primarily with communicable and nutrition-related diseases. On the European scene the diseases of affluence constitute a major obstacle to good health. Within the European region there are differences between countries, too. Moreover, health and health threats change over time, now and then in unsuspected ways: the occurrence of the AIDS epidemic constitutes an imperative health problem that has to be given high priority in the European region also. Not being in possession of effective preventive or curative tools at present, some sort of surveillance is imperative if we want to control this new communicable disease. The AIDS problem being so new, specific recommendations for surveillance are not mentioned in this book—but the book does give basic principles and examples from related fields, that may be easily adapted to surveillance of AIDS and hopefully almost any other health-related topic.

The type of data collected obviously depends on the data needs of the users and producers, the purposes for which the data will be used and the resources available.[4] Surveillance may be limited to the reporting of cases in terms of presenting signs and symptoms and is expressed in numbers. Besides morbidity, mortality data may also be utilized in surveillance for more detailed analysis and study of long-term trends, especially of diseases with high case fatality. Other data needed for surveillance include demographic data (population by age, sex, occupation, etc.) and vital statistics (births and deaths). Data on health resources and service data, such as hospital-activity analysis data can also be of use. As these data are usually available from other sources (such as the census or from health services research) and not included in regular surveillance reports they are not primarily dealt with in this volume.

There is great variation in the quality of surveillance systems and in the accuracy of surveillance data. This causes great concern especially as all international comparisons depend on good quality data at national, regional, and local level. Moreover, data needs for surveillance may not be the same at the various levels of the health system. Data providers will not be permanently motivated to collect and report data that satisfy only the needs of higher levels. Problems of lack of enthusiasm and motivation of individual doctors and difficulties in setting up an adequate feedback system are also dealt with in Part 1 of the book. On the other hand one should not aim at a perfect—but unrealistic—surveillance system. As also discussed in Part 1 a less than perfect system can produce considerable benefit if used in the most efficient way. It is more important that surveillance should be part of a continuing system in order to allow comparisons of variations in disease patterns with time. Causal inferences can then be made. This also means that surveillance has to be limited as far as possible to preventable and/or curable diseases. Not all 'target' diseases will be equally conveniently monitored.

Part 1 of the book, written by the members of the editorial board, goes through the basic features of surveillance: roots and history; selection of indicators of health and environment; the planning and organization of the flow of information; action and benefit; ethical issues. Surprisingly little published scientific work is available on these general aspects of the topic of this book. We feel that this part constitutes an important section of the book for which a general need is present amongst health care workers dealing with current health statistics.

Part 2 describes the ways and means of surveillance in selected health fields, whether defined by disease, by environment, or by the age of the population. The list of topics for surveillance is, however, not exhaustive. For example, the surveillance of important modern risk factors such as smoking and illicit drug use is not part of the text. Concerning smoking, several sources on surveillance are already available, among them a summary document by the EEC commission.[5] Concerning the surveillance of the consumption of illegal drugs, this is, of course, for obvious reasons complicated by the non-existence of sales and consumption data.[6] Thus this problem has to be handled by the use of more indirect and less sufficient tools, such as data on treatment of patients in the primary health system, in hospitals, or in specialized clinical centres.[7]

Part 2 does, however, deal with most of the major diseases and health problems in the European region. In addition it describes examples of the use of data from primary health care and hospital sources. All the chapters of Part 2 have been written by invited contributors involved in the development and practice of the surveillance of specific health problems.

The book is clearly intended to guide all those who are in charge of working with routine health statistics and who try to improve the use of existing data. It includes medical doctors working in public health, epidemiology, and interested clinicians and non-medical professionals involved in the various aspects of health care and public health.

Finally, it is hoped that the book will stimulate especially the EEC countries to make a joint effort in order to improve the use of existing data sources and the development of effective surveillance systems.

Bibliography

1. Hogarth, J. (1975). *Glossary of health care terminology*. Public Health in Europe No. 4, WHO, Copenhagen.
2. Hogarth, J. (1977). *Vocabulaire de la santé publique*. La Santé Publique en Europe No. 4. OMS, Copenhagen.
3. Editorial. (1976). Epidemiological surveillance. *Int. J. Epidemiol.* **5,** 4–6.
4. Ludovice, Z. O. (1983). Data needs and gaps in disease surveillance to support primary health care. In *Disease surveillance in primary health care* (ed. J. C. Azurin). Proceedings of the 10th SEAMIC Seminar. Tokyo.
5. Todd, G. (1986). *Statistics of smoking in the member states of the European Community*. CEE, Luxemburg.
6. Walsh, D. Personal correspondence.
7. Ghodse, A. H., Sheehan, M., Taylor, L., and Edwards, G. (1985). Deaths of drug addicts in the United Kingdom, 1967–1981. *Br. med. J.* **290,** 425–8.

In conclusion, it seems to me that the most powerful, effective and under-rated tool in communicable disease control is the technique of surveillance. In essence, it represents organically the brain and the nervous system in a management process.

D. A. Henderson. *Int. J. Epidemiol.* **5,** 19–28 (1976).

Part 1
General aspects

1
Historical aspects

Interest in relating environmental factors to health goes back to Hippocrates and Herodotus but one has to wait until the eighteenth century to see the development of the first health surveys.

The idea of observing, recording, and collecting facts and analysing them to direct courses of action stems from Hippocrates. However, the development of surveys and their use for health care was impossible without: (i) an organized health-care system of some sort which in itself presupposes the existence of a strong and stable government, such as was provided by the Romans, (ii) some sort of reproducible and widely acknowledged classificatory system for entities such as symptoms, syndromes, and diseases as initiated by Sydenham, and (iii) a more sophisticated approach to measuring, counting, and summing events which only started in the seventeenth century.

In fact, censuses and surveys were made by the Romans and again during the Renaissance, in Florence and Sienna, for example, and they usually covered various aspects of the problems of urban life such as sanitation and food supply. Sydenham's (1624–89) studies on the natural history of various diseases and his efforts to define clinical entities based on the observation of signs and symptoms laid the foundations for developments in clinical science and the possibility of health surveillance.

One has to wait until the seventeenth century for the concept of surveillance to take shape. Gottfried Wilhelm von Leibnitz (1647–1716), the famous philosopher and mathematician, suggested setting up a Health Council and in the 1680s was one of the first to stress the need for appropriate numerical analyses and mortality statistics.

Although surveys were first initiated for political reasons (such as the *Domesday Book*, which in 1066 reviewed all the resources of the kingdom conquered by the Normans), records of vital events were preserved in numerous European towns from the sixteenth century on. The first London Bills of Mortality were prepared by an unknown person in 1532 although their use for health care and scientific purposes did not begin until a hundred years later.

The publication of the first Bill of Mortality in London was the consequence of the fear of a plague epidemic. It led to the pioneering work of Captain John Graunt (1620–74), whose book *Natural and Political Observations made upon the Bills of Mortality* was published in 1662 and was presented at the Royal Academy. He attempted to define the basic laws of natality and mortality and discovered some of the fundamental principles.

He was the first to estimate the population of London and to count the number that died from specific causes. He was also the first to conceptualize and quantitate the patterns of disease and to understand that numerical data on a population could be used to study the causes of disease.

In France, Colbert introduced the practice of demographic statistics though full coverage of the whole of the French population was not achieved till the end of the seventeenth century. At the same time the Great Elector did likewise in Prussian cities and villages. During this period came publication of William Petty's *Political Arithmetick* and the discussion subsequent to its printing. William Petty (1623–87) was a physician economist and a scientist and his book was published posthumously. He made use of statistical reports made on the cities of Britain as well as on Leyden and Utrecht where he received his medical education. He also drew up a plan for a teaching hospital or 'Nosocomium Academicum' in his first publication *The Advice of W. P. to Mr Samuel Harilib* (1648). Among other things the hospital administrator was expected to help the medical and nursing staff by providing them with information on medical statistics and meteorology.

He clearly felt this was a new empirical approach to medical care which was based on the Hippocratic tradition rather than on the medieval or Renaissance metaphysical and conceptual approach to health care. He wrote,

As for Physicians . . . it is not hard by the help of the observations which have been lately made upon the Bills of Mortality, to know how many are sick in London by the number of them that dye, and by the proportions of the City to find out the same of the Country; and by both by the advice of the Learned Colledge of that Faculty to calculate how many Physicans were requisite for the whole Nation; and consequently, how many students in that art to permit and encourage; and lastly, having calculated these numbers, to adoptate a proportion of Chyrurgeons, Apothecaries, and Nurses to them, and so by the whole to cut off and estinguish that infinite swarm of vain pretenders unto, and abusers of that God-like Faculty, which of alle Secular Employments our Saviour himself after he began to preach engaged himself upon.

Like Theophraste Renaudot (1586–1653), who was a physician in France, Samuel Harilib's *Further Discovery of the Office of Address* (1648) suggested the setting up of a central office which would keep numerous registers of information on various topics, such as trade and employment, in addition to demographic and medical information. Special reports were to be published concerning the sick and poor which would be circulated to physicians and thus help them to diagnose and treat illnesses. Moreover, they would provide basic material for describing the natural history of disease as suggested by Sydenham. Samuel Harilib studied at Cambridge in 1625 and 1626 and became a leading activist of the puritan movement.

However, these systems of information were still limited to communal or regional use or to mere models of what a health-care system ought to be.

There was no national health-care policy although the ideas were born early in the seventeenth century.

Ludwig von Seckendorff developed one of the first systematic doctrines of health care. He worked for the ducal Court of Gotha for whom the aim of government was to ensure the welfare of the people. But the main spur for considering health care in terms of the population at large was the economic philosophy of mercantilism. The Quaker cloth merchant and philanthropist John Bellers (1654–1725) claimed in his *Essay towards the Improvement of Physick* (1714) that deaths and diseases were a waste of human resources— they ought to be approached at the level of the community and not left to mere individual initiative. So political arithmetic became a means to the end of national prosperity and power, with the intermediate objective of maintaining and augmenting a healthy population which was seen as the foundation of political and economic strength. The German Sociologist George Simmel wrote that 'the cash economy first brought into life the ideal of numerical calculability'.

In 1749, the journalist and statistician Gottfried Achenwall (1719–72) introduced the term 'Statistics' which replaced the old expression of 'political arithmetic'. Though the Enlightenment came late to medicine, vital statistics were widely used in the second half of the eighteenth century. What was probably the first national census was initiated in Sweden in 1748. The United States followed suit together with France and then Britain and the German States. Hospital statistics were collected enabling results of treatment to be monitored.

This was particularly the case for mental hospitals early in the sixteenth and seventeenth centuries. John Graunt himself in his *Natural and political observations made upon the Bills of Mortality*, gave morbidity and mortality rates for insanity and suicide in London from figures covering a period of twenty years.

Black (1749–1829), a physician and historian who graduated from Leyden and became a physician in London, wrote a *Dissertation on insanity illustrated with tables, and extracted from between two and three thousand cases in Bedlam*, published in London in 1810. The first extensive mental health statistics were published by the Aberdeen physician John Thurnam (1810–73) in London in 1845: *Observations and essays on the statistics of insantiy, and on establishments for the insane, to which are added the statistics of the Retreat, near York*.

Similarly, following up the earlier leads of Bernadino Ramazzini (1633–1717) of Modena, concern for the health of specified groups of population led to the systematic observation and description of conditions linked to the work environment in Britain, Germany, and France.

Finally, geographical pathology and medical topography developed in Central Europe. Numerous German cities in the second half of the eighteenth century published reports dealing with health conditions, life-style of inhabitants, meteorological and hydrographic data.

The spread of the use of the statistical methods to matters related to health was clearly associated with the development of a systematic concept of health-care policy. The German physician Johann Peter Frank's (1745–1821) great work *System einer vollstaendigen medizinischen Polizey* (1779–1827) suggested that health policy should be legally enforced thereby causing what Sigerist called 'Hygiene from above'. Six successive volumes described a complete health-care and welfare system; they appeared at the turn of the century and were followed by three more volumes at the beginning of the nineteenth century which, among other topics, described the use of vital statistics within a comprehensive health-care system.

Surveillance as a means of collection and interpretation of data related to environmental and health monitoring processes for the definition of appropriate action, for prevention and health care, became a reality in the nineteenth century. Sir Edwin Chadwick (1800–90), a pupil of Jeremy Bentham and Secretary of the Poor Law Commission, was the first health administrator to demonstrate that poverty and disease were closely related. He launched investigations into the living conditions of the past in some of the most destitute areas of London, and pointed out that the prevention of disease was a matter of economy as well as of humanity. In 1842, Chadwick published *The Sanitary Conditions of the Labouring Population of Great Britain*, which investigated the relationship between environmental conditions and disease. This is usually considered a landmark in medical history, though similar but more limited surveys were being made and reported at the same time in various other countries.

Louis René Villerme analysed the relationship between poverty and mortality in Paris in *Mémoires sur la mortalité 1828*, and the same was done in Manchester (1832) and New York (1865). However, the most important report after Chadwick's was probably Lemuel Shattuck's *Report of the Massachussetts Sanitary Commission* (1850) which related deaths, infant and maternal mortality, and communicable diseases (scarlet fever, typhus, typhoid fever, diphtheria, tuberculosis) with living conditions. Shattuck (1793–1859) was an American publisher and bookseller. He recommended decennial censuses, standardization of nomenclature of cause of disease and deaths, and the collection of health data by age, sex, occupation, socio-economic level, and locality. The relationship between health information and policy was clearly demonstrated by Shattuck in various areas such as vaccination, child and school health, mental health, health education related to smoking, and alcohol abuse, and he introduced this concept into the teaching of preventive medicine. Chadwick did stress sanitary aspects but with Shattuck and John Simon, surveillance turned to medical knowledge and activity. John C. Griscom, a physician and inspector of the New York

Board of Health, published in 1848 a study in depth of the health problems of the city of New York 'where he developed by a statistical approach the concept of preventable deaths'.

In 1837, the interrupted work of J. Graunt was taken up again and the office of the Registrar General was established to collect information on births and deaths in England.

Early in 1838 came the statistical returns and reports of the Registrar General and they provided strong support for the public health reform movement. In addition, the English physician William Farr (1807–83) appended reports to those of the Registrar General which dealt with infectious diseases, hazardous work conditions and occupational diseases or accidents. His statistical analyses provided invaluable information and aid to the public health reformers and officers, to the physicians and to the scientists. The United States did not develop a comparable information system until 1900 and only reached full national coverage in 1933.

In 1842 a Committee of the council of the Statistical Society published the first statistics about patients treated in six general hospitals in London. This was the beginning of a succession of reports and analyses which ended with a full-scale national system in 1929.

John Simon, who became the first Medical Officer of Health of the City of London in 1848 and later a medical officer to the general Board of Health, was well known for his descriptions of the gloomy picture of community health in Victorian England.

The Medical Department had to develop a scientific basis for the progress of sanitary law and administration; and we had to aim at stamping on public health a character of greater exactitude than it had hitherto had. Confident that if the knowledge were got, its utilisation would speedily follow, we had to endeavour that all considerable phenomena of disease-prevalence in the country should be seen and measured with precision in respect of their causes and mode of origin.

The twentieth century saw the expansion and the development of surveillance systems. It has been characterized by the diversification of methods of collection, analysis, and dissemination of data and the particular emphasis put on methodological issues.

The following list shows some of the salient dates related to the development of surveillance in the last century.

1893 International list of causes of death (International Statistical Institute)
1899 Compulsory Notification of Infectious Diseases (GB)
1911 Surveillance data resulting from the National Health Insurance (GB)
1935 National Health Survey (US)
1943 Danish Cancer Registry (DK)
      Sickness Survey (UK)

1950   US Framingham Study
1967   General practitioners' Sentinel Systems (UK/NL)

Bibliography

1. Deruffe, L., *Essai historique de la statistique sanitaire en France.* Services des Statistiques, des Etudes et de Systèmes d'Information. Ministère des Affaires Sociales et de la Solidarité Nationale, Paris (1986).
2. Hunter, R. and Macalpine, I., *Three hundred years of psychiatry 1535–1860.* Oxford University Press (1963).
3. Parry-Jones, W. L., *The trade of lunacy: A study of private madhouses in England in the eighteenth and nineteenth centuries.* Routledge & Kegan Paul, London (1972).
4. Rosen, G., *From medical policy to social medicine. Essays on the history of health care.* Science History Publications, New York (1974).
5. Rosen, G., *A history of public health.* MD Publications, New York (1958).
6. Rosen, G., Madness in society. In *The historical sociology of mental illness.* University of Chicago Press (1969).
7. Schryock, R. H., *The development of modern medicine.* Hafner Publishing Company, New York (1969).
8. Webster, C., *The great instauration: science, medicine and reform 1626–1660.* Holmes & Meier, New York (1976).
9. Wain, H., *History of preventive medicine.* Charles C. Thomas, Springfield, Illinois (1970).

2

The surveillance of disease

Definitions: Surveillance and Monitoring

The French word 'surveillance' was introduced into English at the time of the Napoleonic wars and meant: keeping a close watch over an individual or group of individuals in order to detect any subversive tendencies. The modern dictionary definition of surveillance still has a sinister overtone: 'vigilant supervision; spy-like watching' (*Chambers Twentieth Century Dictionary*) 'watch or guard, especially over a suspected person' (*Oxford English Dictionary*). In accepting that disease is undesirable, this sense of the sinister is apt for the attachment of the word surveillance to disease. Indeed, the term 'police medicine' was applied to the form of public health surveillance evolved by Johann Frank in Germany in 1766 (see p. 000), and an earlier use of surveillance was in relation to contacts of dangerous infections.[2]

Thus the present conception of epidemiological surveillance originated from personal surveillance and sanitary control; the objective was to identify persons ill with a communicable disease, to isolate them, and to take action to protect their entourage. It led to compulsory notification. The word, however, is no longer confined to communicable disease. A more modern concept of the term surveillance is 'ongoing scrutiny, generally using methods distinguished by their practicability, uniformity and, frequently, their rapidity, rather than by complete accuracy. Its main purpose is to detect changes in trends or distribution in order to facilitate investigative or control measures'.[1] The World Health Organization definition is substantially the same:

1. Systematic measurement of health and environment parameters, recording, and transmission of data.
2. Comparison and interpretation of data in order to detect possible changes in the health and environmental status of populations.[15]

Thus surveillance in the context of health may relate not only to specific disorders but also to the factors influencing disease and its occurrence.

The definitions do not include the older, and original, use of the term surveillance, that of personal surveillance, as with contacts of a person with an infectious disease or of an infectious carrier. Personal surveillance is the practice of close medical or other supervision of contacts, or of carriers of disease, which involves making systematic observations in order to promote prompt recognition of infection or illness, but without restricting their movements (at least until an illness is recognized). Personal surveillance is an important tool in the management of diseases. This form of surveillance will not be considered further in this book.

Surveillance and Monitoring

The terms 'surveillance' and 'monitoring' are often used interchangeably, but are in fact distinct. Surveillance has already been defined and is one form of the ongoing measurement of data. The term monitoring should be confined in its use to the dynamics of intervention. It is applicable to the continuous assessment of an *intervention–change* relationship. Monitoring evaluates intervention, or action. One of the three definitions of monitoring by Last[1] approaches this concept: 'ongoing measurement of performance of a health service or a health professional'.

Surveillance and monitoring have in common the routine and ongoing collection of data, and the methods for both tend to be pragmatic and rapid. Surrogate or proxy measures (or indicators—see below) may be used to identify the underlying changes.

Doll[3] included the evaluation of health services within the scope of health surveillance, although this should more correctly be termed monitoring. Measuring urban air- and blood-lead levels before and after the introduction of lead-free petrol would require the techniques of surveillance in the collection and assessment of data, but the total process is one of monitoring. Similarly, surveillance would be used to assess say, the impact of an infectious disease on a population, and again following the introduction of a vaccine, and the extent of its usage, whereas monitoring would describe the process of measuring the effect of the vaccine on the disease. Monitoring also implies a constant adjustment of performance in relation to results, and is an important management tool. It can also be applied to quality control.

In this book only the surveillance of factors relating to health and disease or to the occurrence and spread of disease, will be considered.

Surveillance, Surveys, and Screening

Surveys are finite rather than ongoing, unlike surveillance. A series of surveys may be adapted to form a surveillance system. The terms should be used specifically, and should not be interchanged. Screening should also be clearly distinguished from surveillance and these words should not be used as synonyms. Screening may be ongoing, though usually short-term, and is generally applied to a population at risk to identify persons at risk. Results of screening or mass surveys can, however, be used for surveillance.

Scope of Surveillance

As the surveillance of disease is the ongoing scrutiny of *all* aspects of occurrence and spread of disease that are pertinent to effective control,[1] its scope is broad. Jenicek and Cleroux's conception of surveillance[16] was the study of disease as a dynamic process which includes the ecology of the pathogen, host, reservoir, vectors, and the environment as well as the mechanism of transmission of the disease and the degree and the extent of its spread. Retrospective or prospective data may be sought. Examples of various factors that can be placed under surveillance follow. More specific examples are described in Part 2 of this book.

Disease

Mortality   The routine collection and analysis of death certificates is a form of surveillance that is practised fairly universally in the industrial world. The coding of death according to the WHO International Classification of Diseases (ICD) ensures a degree of uniformity both within and between countries, and facilitates international comparisons. Nevertheless, while the counting of deaths is fairly accurate, the notification of the causes is often imprecise, owing to the fact that the diagnosis made by the certifying physician may be wrong or restricted to the direct cause, without taking into account the underlying pathology. There can also be mistakes in coding. In some countries more detailed information, on occupation, for example, is routinely collected. Death can be viewed as the end-point of severity of illness and mortality data alone will give only a biased, albeit essential, picture of the disease experience of a population. When the case fatality is high, and particularly when the interval between onset and death is short, (as in AIDS and some cancers) mortality approximates to morbidity and surveillance of mortality is likely to provide a fair approximation of the disease burden. In the case of curable or mild diseases, mortality surveillance alone is likely to be unhelpful. In diseases with a high case-fatality rate but a long interval between onset and death, trends in mortality may prove to be insufficiently sensitive (in that they will respond late) for the purposes of surveillance, especially if effects of treatment are being monitored. Some of the limitations of surveillance using mortality have been expressed by Doll[3] and by Wynne Griffith.[23]

Morbidity   Morbidity reports can be obtained from various sources and it may be useful to consider these at various levels of severity of illness. Hospitals can provide data on the severest stages and types of illness. In many countries hospital-based diagnostic statistics are fairly well developed and freely available, e.g. Hospital In Patient Enquiry (HIPE) in England and Wales (see also Chapter 6). Less severe illness, albeit enough to warrant medical attention, can be surveilled through general practice reports. These, a step further down the ladder of severity from hospital data, are more difficult to organize than hospital data, but will provide a broader perspective on the illness experience of a population. Again, many countries, (Belgium, The Netherlands, the UK) have organized systems based on general practice[4] (see Chapter 7). As laboratory data may operate at several different levels, surveillance of these data may provide information on mortality, hospital morbidity, and general morbidity. There are several well-developed surveillance systems based on laboratory data in the EEC. Laboratory data are objective, comparable, and reproducible,[19] and they need not only be available in well-developed countries or only in sophisticated surveillance programmes; a worthwhile surveillance programme can be implemented using laboratory data without morbidity data recording. Surveillance of sickness certificates for social security purposes are a crude but useful indicator of hospital and general practice morbidity, and school absence data can be similarly used.

Surveillance systems designed to provide information on perceived but unreported morbidity are perhaps the most sophisticated of all. Such information is usually obtained by special surveys rather than surveillance, although the General Household Survey in England and Wales provides one example of this.[9] Other sources of data on morbidity which may be used for surveillance include child-health clinics and drug-sales data.[17]

Outbreaks

Surveillance of outbreaks, in reality a special example of morbidity and mortality surveillance, can provide useful information not only on disease experience within a population, but also on the environment (physical, chemical, and biological). Outbreak surveillance provides a fruitful and relatively cheap source of preventive action. On the other hand surveillance of outbreaks without surveillance of any of the basic disease problems, although important as a 'fire-fighting' exercise, remains an essentially crude indicator of the disease experience of a population. A more sophisticated surveillance system will perhaps uncover the possibility of the occurrence of an outbreak at an early stage, making prevention feasible.[8]

Vaccine and drug utilization

Vaccines, drugs, and any other therapeutic, diagnostic, or prophylactic procedure may be placed under surveillance. Surveillance of vaccine use is essential to any organized vaccination programme. Both vaccine uptake and efficacy, as well as side effects from a vaccine, need to be closely surveilled, especially in the early stages of a programme or after the introduction of a new vaccine. Batch numbers of vaccines need to be recorded to detect problems with particular vaccine lots but it may be difficult to decide, with rare events, whether an association with vaccine was real or coincidental. Regular serological surveys (see below) may be needed to assess population immunity. Both the number of cases of the disease and any relevant characteristics of the agent (especially organisms like the influenza virus that may change antigenically) need to be included in the surveillance programme. For selective vaccination, such as yellow fever vaccine for travellers from EEC countries to endemic areas, the need for surveillance is less urgent. Extensive and ethically performed trials of any new drug or vaccine may not show up rare serious side effects which may only become apparent after prolonged use, and a system of reporting any serious—or especially unusual—illness associated with a new drug or vaccine may be of some value in uncovering rare side-effects, or suspicious associations that need to be further pursued by a more penetrating analytical epidemiological study. In England and Wales the Committee on Safety of Medicines fulfils this function (see Chapter 22). Record linkage studies may also be used in this way. Surveillance of usage of certain drugs may also be useful indicators of morbidity.[17]

Disease determinants

Surveillance can be carried out on biological functions in man and external determinants of disease. Surveillance of growth, development and nutritional status of children for example[5,6,21] may detect early changes in population health—this is arguably even more important than surveillance of disease because the conditions responsible for ill health are under observation. Similarly, surveillance of biological changes in infectious agents, whether 'natural' as with the influenza virus, or 'acquired' as with antibiotic resistance in bacteria, may provide early warning of a need to change vaccine or drug policies.

The WHO, through collaborating centres for influenza, which provide information on influenza strains isolated in outbreaks and sporadic cases, makes recommendations yearly on the composition of influenza vaccine for the forthcoming season. Hospitals formulate antibiotic policies depending on resistance patterns of pathogenic bacteria isolated from patients. These are planned to provide not only effective treatment for patients but also to minimize the emergence of further resistance to antibiotics used. For malaria, constant vigilance (surveillance) is required to determine areas where *Plasmodium falciparum* is resistant to chloroquine, so that the best available treatment or prophylaxis may be given.

Examples of several environmental and occupational factors related to pollution—toxic or radioactive substances and smoking—that may need surveillance in certain situations, spring readily to mind (see Chapters 15 and 19). Reservoirs of infection, such as tularaemia in hedgehogs (see Chapter 14) or rabies in wildlife, or vectors of transmission of infection may also be included in surveillance programmes. Social disease determinants, including social network (family composition and employment) are becoming increasingly important for surveillance, as is unemployment and associated changes in health status.

Factors Reflecting Susceptibility

These include regular antibody surveys, or skin testing (as for tuberculosis), to ascertain the extent of and to follow trends in susceptibility to certain infections in a community. Objective international comparisons and assessments can be made using serum banks.[19] In a selective rubella vaccination programme which does not affect the overall incidence of rubella, non-immune women of childbearing age will be regularly exposed to the infection and regular serum antibody surveys in this target population are important both from the patient's point of view (so that non-immunes can be vaccinated) and from the point of view of assessing the success or failure of the vaccination programme.[26] Serum banks can also be used for many infections for retrospective data on the natural history of the infection, or to provide baseline information. Moreover, one advantage of serological surveys is that sophisticated tests may be done on sera outside the country of origin if the laboratory services within that country are not able to do so.[19]

Other factors that may affect susceptibility to disease may also be placed under surveillance. Tobacco smoking and alcohol consumption are good examples of this. Pharmacogenetic surveillance; for example, G-6-PD deficiency or specific dietary deficiences can also be included.[25]

Objectives and Purposes of Surveillance

Before a surveillance system is set up objectives must be clear. What is it for? Do we need to do it all the time or can it be done by one survey or periodical surveys? An important purpose of surveillance is to detect changes, and to detect them early on, so that action can be taken on control or prevention. A sustained increase in the numbers of reports of a rare salmonella[8] clearly implies that an outbreak may be imminent, and observance of such phenomena demands investigation. An increase in deaths from asthma[11] in UK in the 1960s was found to coincide with the use of metered isoprenaline or orciprenaline aerosols, and limitation of the use of these aerosols brought about a decrease in the number of deaths.[12] Although the outcome of asthma attacks was not part of an organized surveillance scheme, the trend was noticed[13] because death, which is certifiable, was the outcome; a serious, though not life-threatening side-effect of treatment, might not have been picked up, except possibly by an astute clinician, and dependence on clinical observation alone is not systematic or reliable enough. Surveillance can also detect important changes in the life-style, environment, or vectors that may lead to change in human disease patterns; or may identify changes in population susceptibility, as with serological or biochemical studies.

Other important purposes of surveillance are to measure the extent and limits of a disease in a population by establishing its incidence and prevalence, to determine the population at risk, so that vulnerable groups or areas can be identified, and to determine the natural history of the disease, its severity, and complications. The data obtained may enable forecasting of trends, and highlight priorities. Such data may be used either for assessing the benefits of an intervention (e.g. fluoridation) or for planning health services. The intervention can be monitored. Surveillance or monitoring may provide the basis for studies of cost–benefit or for comparisons of cost–benefit, and in this way help to determine priorities and evaluate the effectiveness of different interventions. Occasionally surveillance of disease may provide clues as to its aetiology.

A special and especially intensive type of surveillance has been necessary after smallpox eradication to discover isolated cases. Rewards may be offered to encourage reporting of rare occurrences.

Elements of Surveillance

'Surveillance is part of a co-operative venture between the epidemiologist and all sectors of the health system and contributes therefore to total economic development of which health is a vital part'.[10] Any surveillance scheme must be tailor-made to the country in which it is operating. Nevertheless, the three fundamental elements of any surveillance programme are the *ongoing collection*, *analysis*, and *feedback* or *dissemination* of data (Fig. 2.1). Surveillance ultimately implies action. However, it is worth quoting Inman[20] 'No scheme is likely to succeed that does not have two vital ingredients—independence from political or commercial pressures and a totally committed person or group of people at its core'.

Before we consider the elements of surveillance it is important to establish the denominators of the target population. Basic demographic data may be sufficient, enabling some calculations of rates. Even in the absence of these data, provided the population covered by the surveillance is unchanged, surveillance may allow some comparisons of trends. The whole of the target population may not, however, be reached by the surveillance unit. Several factors may affect this—for instance, distance from a medical facility affects use of that facility, as does the belief of the consumer about what the facility can accomplish.[22]

Data Collection

Collecting the data is the most costly and difficult element of a surveillance

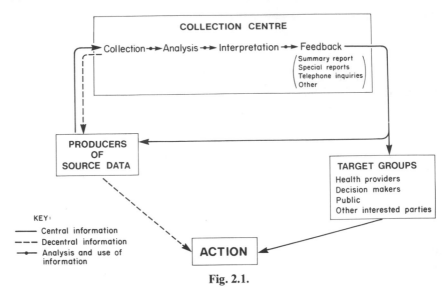

Fig. 2.1.

system.[22] The collection of data has to be systematic and uniform. The producers of the data have to be trained, or at least provided with clear and strict guidelines for reporting, and encouraged to provide the information regularly. It helps if they are interested in the results of surveillance and are sufficiently motivated to provide the information. The producer of raw data is not necessarily the person who fills in the forms. This person needs even more to be motivated and trained to complete the forms accurately and objectively.

Ideally, reports should be made on standard forms. From the point of view of the providers, characteristics of a well-designed form which will encourage accuracy, regularity, and completeness include:

(a) clarity of design, so that the information requested flows in as rational a manner as possible;
(b) simplicity, with as little provision made for writing as possible, and most of the information provided by tick boxed, or one word answers;
(c) only important and essential information available to the provider should be requested;
(d) there should be no ambiguity in the questions on the form.

Definitions, where required, should also be clear. Surveillance based on the telephone system should still require information in a standard format. Reporters should be required to complete forms at regular intervals; for example, daily, weekly, monthly. These principles should ensure uniformity and reliability of reporting so that any biases in the surveillance system would then be inherent within the reporting system, and would be consistent. Such biases can be more easily interpreted and allowed for at the analysis stage. Irregular, patchy, or selective reporting as, for example, when the data provider reports only on interesting or severe cases, leads to inconsistent biases which may be difficult or impossible to interpret in the analysis. It is often necessary, and may be worthwhile, to sacrifice a measure of completeness to ensure regular and systematic reporting.

A distinction can be made between *passive surveillance, active surveillance,* and *sentinel disease surveillance.* In a passive surveillance system, the recipient may have initiated the system, but essentially waits for the provider to report. Sometimes the provider is required by law to produce the information, as in a notification system, or otherwise has some obligation to do so. With many forms of surveillance, passive or routine reporting is expedient: routine data already provided for other reasons in the health services of the country are channelled centrally for analysis. Although this covers, and requires the co-operation of, all health-care facilities in the country, the inconsistency and slowness of reporting are common defects (see Chapter 14). In certain circumstances a specific surveillance system needs to be organized and data are obtained specially by searching and, perhaps, periodic contact with the providers: this is known as active surveillance. Active surveillance procedures are well exemplified by Henderson in his account of smallpox surveillance.[14] In certain, usually rare, diseases (where completeness becomes more important), a more active surveillance system over and above the basic routine reporting framework is necessary so that cases that may be missed without actively seeking them are sought using whatever source, including the media. For this type of surveillance, routine reminders may have to be sent to possible providers of information. Because of the large amount of effort and low return, active surveillance tends to be expensive in terms of cost–benefit.

With sentinel disease surveillance, completeness is sacrificed to greater reliability, speed, and sometimes cheapness. In this system a selected sample of health sources is used—the sample should include as wide a geographical and demographic spread as possible (see Chapters 7 and 8). This type of surveillance is usually only worthwhile for common diseases, which also tend to be public-health problems. It can be used both for the active or passive forms of surveillance. A form of sentinel disease surveillance based on political polling techniques has been advocated by Foege *et al.*[22]

The choice of type of data provider clearly depends on the disease or factor to be surveilled: child-health clinics for child-nutritional surveillance, general practitioners for common infectious diseases, hospitals for cancer, etc. Rarely is it possible to choose providers on grounds of reliability—this may be possible for sentinel disease surveillance, but choice here is usually based on demographic or geographical criteria.

The Collection or Surveillance Unit

Usually the collection, analysis and feedback are performed in one centre, where it is important to have some epidemiological expertise. Sophisticated collection centres are not always necessary, especially in Third World countries where a remarkable amount of useful information gathering and feedback can be obtained from a rudimentary but well-organized system. Langmuir has stated[18]

The one essential requirement for a surveillance system is a reasonably sophisticated epidemiologist who is located in a central position in the health structure, who has access to information on the occurrence of communicable disease, who has power to inquire into and verify his facts and who has the ear and confidence of his chief medical officer of health.

An existing health facility may be used as the surveillance centre, and the existing health framework can often be adapted to staff it. Medical auxiliaries may be used as reporters, as is done for gastroenteritis and malnutrition in many developing countries. Countries of the European Community, however, can usually afford more sophisticated central units and the basic needs of such a unit will be described briefly. One or more epidemiologists should be in post and provide guidance for the unit. Other essential staff should include trained clerks to organize the sorting of incoming data and preparation of tables ready for analysis, and supporting secretarial and other staff to ensure regular feedback. Statistical help is usually invaluable. In the most simple types of surveillance, data can be collected, analysed, and stored by hand, but some form of mechanical assistance is usually necessary—a punch card and counter sorter at the very least, or, at best, a computer. Systems for transferring data from the source directly on to computer tape or disc, or directly to a control computer held at the central collection centre are being explored in England and Wales for infectious disease data from laboratories. If successful, this will obviate the need for forms to be filled in at source, or to be handled in the central collection unit. The potential advantages of such a system are more accurate and systematic reporting. Computers may be found to be more useful for the storage, linkage, and analysis of data than in assisting in the rapid feedback of information—the weekly *Communicable Disease Report* of the PHLS Communicable Disease Surveillance Centre in England and Wales, where the turnaround time is seven days, is still produced mainly by hand. National routine mortality and other statistics are often many years late, although produced with the help of computers.

It seems hardly necessary to point out the importance of good organization in a collection unit. This is essential at all levels of the unit—in collection, storage, and retrieval of data; the ready availability, or ability to obtain rapidly, pertinent data or requests for data; in the systematic collection and analysis of data from other sources and linking these with the surveillance data; and in the provision of regular feedback.

Registers

A form of surveillance that cuts across the different levels of severity of illness is the disease register. The principal objective of a register is to collate information about defined groups over periods of time. Routine health-registers can be described as extensions in time of the *ad hoc* study. In addition they form a fundamental partial data base for more penetrating *ad hoc* studies. Cancer registries are the best known, but any definable chronic, genetic, or infectious disease may be included, such as diabetes mellitus, phenylketonuria, or Reye's syndrome. These registers may show up important changes in trends, whether of overall occurrence or of specific age, sex, or geographical factors, and about the natural history of the disease. A register need not be solely disease specific. It is also used[24] in preventive medicine, as in immunization and screening programmes for children, or in genetic registers which record families at high risk of having a child with a serious hereditary disorder. Registers may also be used for evaluation of treatment (e.g. radiotherapy or iatrogenic thyroid disease); or for after-care, as with the handicapped or disabled. At-risk registers containing, for example, names of problem families, occupational or medical hazards, are becoming increasingly common. Registers may also be used for skills and resources as, for example, with blood or organ banks. The main features of a register[24] are that it should be population-based, detailed, and complete; should include outcome, and can be used to identify persons, families at risk, or to plan services, to judge the effects of treatment or other intervention, or act purely as an information centre. For success a register has to be accurate, restricted to essentials, and meet a need that cannot be satisfied in any other way. An example of a register used to good effect for surveillance is given in Chapter 4.

Costs

Few detailed studies of cost of surveillance have been made. Surveillance is not necessarily an expensive operation, as it makes use of data already available. The diagnostic information or laboratory confirmation on which surveillance depends is not obtained primarily for surveillance purposes, but for clinical reasons. Disease surveillance usually makes use of, and is dependent on, data already available, but the relationship is essentially a saprophytic rather than a parasitic one. Occasionally, for example, in serological surveys, the information is obtained primarily for surveillance. The costs of surveillance lie in collecting, analysing, and disseminating information, but benefits may be considerable—see below.

Analysis and Interpretation

It is not proposed to describe in detail the analytical, epidemiological and statistical techniques that can be used to analyse surveillance data, because the methods are similar to those used in the analysis of any epidemiological problem, and are described in most textbooks. Only some general comments will be made.

Completeness of reporting is often considered so important that considerable cost, time, and energy are expended in attaining this goal. The problem of incompleteness in itself is inevitable with a common disease, but trends shown even by incompletely reported cases may be adequate for meaningful epidemiological interpretation. Indeed, in these situations completeness of reporting may be expensive and a waste of time, with little extra gain. However, with most passive surveillance systems completeness is not a feature, and indeed the need for completeness should be carefully considered before it should be attempted. For very uncommon diseases, e.g. Reye's syndrome, completeness requiring active surveillance clearly becomes a more important consideration. Occasionally, as a control measure progresses and a common disease becomes rarer, completeness also becomes necessary, e.g. paralytic poliomyelitis in most EEC countries and measles in the USA. In the USA every ascertained case of measles puts into operation an intensive and costly local control programme.[27] For most diseases, however, incomplete reporting may provide just as accurate a picture of the occurrence and distribution of the disease.

More important perhaps than completeness are any biases in reporting, first by the reporting unit and second by the actual identification system. Biases by the reporting unit—for example, reporting only the more severe or interesting cases—should be avoided by instituting a routine system of reporting so that no cases fulfilling the reporting criteria are missed. Biases in the identification of cases cannot usually be avoided—for example, children may be more likely to be investigated than adults, or severe illness more than mild ones. The only way to resolve these biases is by conducting a special study on a sample of the population. Details of outcome can be particularly difficult to obtain, as when death occurs after a case has been reported or notified.

The basic epidemiological parameters of time, place, and person are most often used in analysing surveillance data. Denominator data are usually but not always necessary to detect changes. Changes in categorization of disease or other factors may affect the result of the analysis. Variations in time may be seasonal, may indicate an outbreak, or may be an artifact caused by changes in reporting habits or a change in method by the reporting source. Geographical variation may indicate a local outbreak, or again may be an artifact. Variations in person may signify a change in the existing pattern of the disease, the effect of an outbreak affecting a particular group or age of person, or the effect of an intervention. It can also be affected by differing diagnostic procedures or ease of diagnosis (for example, gonorrhoea in males compared with females); or the finding that the disease is particularly import-ant or can be prevented in certain groups (for example, rubella in women of childbearing age) or by a change in the levels of ascertainment (for example, less among older people). In many instances it may be difficult to decide if the change detected is real or artificial, but this question must be answered before action can be contemplated. For these reasons analysis and interpretation are best done by the staff in the collection unit, and requests for information to the unit should ideally be answered with an analytical commentary on the significance of the data requested. Computerization of records and a pro-gramme that will provide the data in an easily assimilable form, enabling the most frequently requested types of information to be easily extracted, are usually invaluable, though not essential.

Analysis of records will include relevant statistics from other sources—although simple duplication may occur, data from other sources often augment rather than supplant. The analytical duties of the surveillance unit will include in addition, evaluation and interpretation of these other sources of data.

The analytical processes in a surveillance unit will also include the regular evaluation of existing statistical material to estimate completeness and reli-ability. It should be possible to detect changes in reporting habits that occur from time to time, and these should be verified and any problems rectified.

Finally, and most important of all, the staff of the surveillance unit should acquire a feel for their data—and so understand the information that inter-pretations made on the results neither overestimate nor underestimate its sig-nificance.

Feedback

Feedback should be regular, relevant, and reliable. '. . . the understanding by the health authorities and politicians of the information provided requires education, patience and presentation in an intelligible and useful manner'.[10] 'The key is an open communication system, free of bureaucratic restraints . . .'.[18] The most usual and practical form of feedback is the summary report. The optimum time intervals between reports depend on the nature of the sur-veillance system; for example, possibly weekly for infectious diseases, monthly, quarterly, or even yearly for chronic diseases. Flexibility should however be built into the system for special circumstances; for example, for urgent dissemination of information such as outbreak, letters, telephone, telex, or television (Prestel) could be used.

Content and presentation

The content should be readily assimilable, and should be current and relevant. The reproduction of raw data should in general be avoided. Complicated and indigestible tables should be as few as possible, and in any case should be accompanied by a commentary, preferably one with a clear message. Apropos Farr, 'His weekly return was no archive for stale data but with his facile pen became a literate weapon for effecting change'[2] A summary of the current situation, appropriate analysis, and presentation of data, with an accompanying and meaningful commentary discussing the trends or other important features, are the basic elements of a feedback text. Comparisons with previous years or other countries may be useful. Review articles arising out of the data presented provide an important educational function. Reports of special experiences submitted by participants for publication, for example accounts of infectious disease outbreaks, add further to the educational value and interest of the surveillance report. A successful report will educate and provide current scientific information for planning, prevention, or change; it will also stimulate the providers to continue reporting, especially if their contribution is acknowledged.

The power of appropriate feedback was apparent to William Farr more than a hundred years ago

... from early in his career he gained complete access to and substantial control of the basic sources of epidemiological and demographic information for England and Wales. He proceeded to exploit these with consummate imagination and talent and by means of weekly, annual, decennial and special reports he brought to official and public attention the results of his keen analysis. Unique as a civil servant he did not cleave to the neutrality that his office could have afforded. He presented his analysis with objectivity but then stated his own interpretation forcefully and argued fearlessly for his recommended changes regardless of what vested interests might be involved.[2]

Ad hoc *enquiry*

A successful surveillance system should also offer an information service for research studies and planning exercises. Adequate trained staff and a system that facilitates extraction of data in an appropriate form (computerization) are valuable features of a surveillance system.

Other forms of communication will be necessary, particularly in emergencies. Of these the most important by far is the telephone. The telephone may be used for the routine reporting of data, but it is of primary importance during emergencies or when following up a problem or a lead. Moreover, its importance as a personal link between the surveillance unit and the providers of information should not be underestimated. If the surveillance unit can be so organized as to deal with *ad hoc* inquiries or requests for advice by telephone, this also helps considerably to build up the successful personal relationships on which the success of a surveillance unit ultimately depends.

Telex and Fax are useful from time to time especially for international communication. At other times of emergency letters may have to be sent to all contributors or special subgroups of them.

Target Groups

The groups of individuals to whom the regular surveillance reports need to be addressed are the data providers, decision-makers and appropriate research workers. Sometimes it may be possible to 'tailor' the surveillance report to the audience; for example, in England and Wales the Communicable Disease Report is sent to a selected group of data providers and other specialists and interested health personnel on a confidential basis, but certain reports of more general relevance are reproduced in the *British Medical Journal*.

Members of the public and media may be included as part of the target groups. Indeed it could be considered that the population under surveillance—in a country, region, occupation group, or special 'at-risk' group—constitutes the core target group for communication of surveillance results. Traditionally reports on, for instance, deaths and births are public though usually too technical from the lay point of view. Attempts could be made to further develop ways of communication that favour public understanding of health problems. In accordance with WHO ideals, 'health profiles' of local populations in Denmark (such as municipalities and counties) are being developed, stimulating public discussion about health, disease prevention, and priorities in the health-care system.

Bibliography

1. Last J. M., (ed.) *Dictionary of epidemiology*. International Epidemiological Association, Oxford University Press, Oxford (1983).
2. Langmuir, A. D., William Farr: Founder of modern concepts of surveillance. *Int. J. Epidemiol.* **5,** 13–18 (1976).
3. Doll, R., Surveillance and monitoring. *Int. J. Epidemiol.* **3,** 305–14 (1974).
4. Fleming, D. M. and Crombie, D. L., The incidence of common infectious diseases: The weekly returns service of the Royal College of General Practitioners. *Hlth Trends* **17,** 13–17 (1985).
5. Irwig, L. M., Surveillance in developed countries with particular reference to child growth. *Int. J. Epidemiol.* **5,** 57–61, (1976).
6. Morley, D., Nutritional surveillance of young children in developing countries. *Int. J. Epidemiol.* **5, 51**–5 (1975).
7. Dondero, T., Target disease surveillance and disease reduction targets. WHO, EPI/GEN/84/6 (1984).
8. Gill, O. N., Bartlett, C. L. R., Sockett, P. N., Vaile, M. S. D. B., and Rowe, B. *et al.*, Outbreak of *Salmonella napoli* infection caused by contaminated chocolate bars. *Lancet* **i,** 574–577 (1983).

9. Office of Population Censuses and Surveys, *General Household Survey*. Series GHS, No. 11 (1981). HMSO, London. 1983.
10. Anonymous, Epidemiological surveillance, *Int. J. Epidemiol.* **5**, 4–7 (1976).
11. McManis, A. G., Adrenaline and Isoprenaline: A warning. *Med. J. Aust.* **2**, 76 (1964).
12. Inman, W. H. W. and Adelstein, A., Rise and fall of asthma mortality in England and Wales in relation to use of pressurised aerosols. *Lancet* **2**, 279–85 (1969).
13. Smith, J. M., Death from asthma. *Lancet* **1**, 1042 (1966).
14. Henderson, D. A., Surveillance of smallpox. *Int. J. Epidemiol.* **5**, 19–28 (1976).
15. Organisation Mondiale de la Santé, Série de rapports tecniques No. 535. Surveillance de l'environnement et de la Santé en médecine du travail: Rapport d'un comité d'experts, p. 7, Geneva (1973).
16. Jenicek, M. and Cleroux, R., *Epidémiologie: Principes, techniques, applications.* Maloine, Paris (1984).
17. Fontbonne, A., Papoz, L., and Eschwoge, E. Drug sales data and prevalence of diabetes in France. *Rev. d'Epidém. et Santé Publique* **34**, 100–5 (1986).
18. Langmuir, A. D., Evolution of the concept of surveillance in the United States. *Proc. R. Soc. Med.* **64**, 681–4 (1971).
19. Raska, K., Epidemiological surveillance with particular reference to the use of immunological surveys. *Proc. R. Soc. Med.* **64**, 681–8 (1971).
20. Inman, W. H. W., Prescription event monitoring. *Lancet* **1**, 443 (1986).
21. Carne, S., Place of development surveillance in general practice. *J. R. Soc. Med.* **77**, 819–20 (1984).
22. Foege, W. H., Hogan, R. C., and Newton, L. H., Surveillance projects for selected diseases. *Int. J. Epidemiol.* **5**, 29–37 (1976).
23. Wynne Griffith, G., Cancer surveillance with particular reference to the uses of mortality data. *Int. J. Epidemiol.* **5**, 69–76 (1976).
24. Weddell, J. M., Registers and registries: A review. *Int. J. Epidemiol.* **2** (1973).
25. McIntire, M. S. and Angle, C. R. Air-lead relation to lead in blood in black schoolchildren deficient in G-6-P-D. *Science* **177**, 520–6 (1972).
26. Clarke, M., Schild, G. C., Miller, C., *et al.* Survey of rubella antibodies in young adults. *Lancet*, **1**, 667–9 (1983).
27. Noah, N. D. What can we do about measles? *British Medical Journal* **289**, 1476 (1984).

3
Indicators

An indicator is a device that records or registers something, such as the movements of a lift, or that shows information, such as arrival and departure times of trains.[1] In the health field, variables measuring changes in health status are used. Indicators measure the extent to which set targets are achieved. Thus surveillance of health, disease, and causes of death is not possible without the use of relevant indicators.

Why Should One Use Indicators

The question of why we need indicators can be answered briefly by stating that health and disease are such complex entities that observable measures, simplifying reality, are needed. Moreover, indicators play an important role in making explicit what would otherwise remain vague statements or judgements. The ultimate aim is to develop strategies for improving the health of population groups. These strategies have to be evaluated by observable measurements.

Types and Characteristics of Indicators

Although the World Health Organization[2] proposes four broad categories of indicators, the examples in this volume are mainly those concerned with one of these categories: the health status of population groups and the related quality of life. Indicators that measure the provision of health care will only be discussed briefly and the two other types, i.e. health policy indicators and social and economic indicators, although of great importance in the evaluation of the health status and of provision of health care, will only be mentioned when considered relevant.

The perfect indicator—the one that measures exactly what we want to measure—does not, of course, exist. In other words it should be completely *valid*, but a perfectly valid measure is one that correlates completely with 'God's opinion' concerning the attribute.[3]

In real life for an indicator to be valid it has to be reasonably sensitive and specific. Sensitive in this context means that a good indicator should reflect correctly changes occurring in a given situation. An indicator should also be specific enough to avoid the measurement of changes arising from external factors not related to the objectives and targets.

Apart from validity a good indicator should also have a number of other characteristics. One is *objectivity*. This means that different observers under the same or similar circumstances produce the same results or values for a given indicator. It will be clear that objectivity can only be reached when the indicator is constructed so as to minimize possible subjectivity on the part of the researcher. This means that the use of indicators in objectively measurable terms is crucial in scientific work.

Another aspect relates to the *feasibility* of an indicator. Problems in terms of money, manpower, and material (the 3 Ms) and also of timing may be constraints. Thus one has to be sure that the proposed measurements, as well as the analyses, are realistic and feasible. Moreover, a good indicator should also be *relevant*: it should be able to reflect the health policy and the broader socio-economic and cultural context of the setting where the indicator is used. The relevance (in French 'la pertinence') of an indicator is often improved by involving very closely all those in charge of the health problem under consideration. Relevance so relates to local circumstances that indicators need to be adapted in this way. Another important point is whether a value for the indicator can be reliably estimated from the available information.

It will be clear that it is not easy to find indicators that meet all these requirements. Compromises will have to be made in order to meet the constraints of real life. Adaptation to actual local conditions has on each occasion to be considered, and there is no standard list of indicators that can be used in all circumstances.

The Optimal Number of Indicators

Apart from the qualitative aspect of indicators one has to select an adequate number. Ideally the minimum number of indicators necessary to meet the set targets should be the rule. This is also important in order not to overload workers with unnecessary data collection and analysis.

As one indicator does not usually suffice to characterize the situation, the only solution is to collect and analyse combinations of indicators so that finally a balanced picture emerges.

Attempts have been made to construct complex indicators making use of several single indicators. This has been done, for example, in the field of quality of life.[4,5] It remains a difficult task and the validity of such complex indicators may be doubtful and the results difficult to interpret.

Data Sources

Before tackling the problem of which indicators to select when using routine health data, it should be clear that routinely collected statistics have one big advantage over all other sources. Routine statistics are part of an ongoing system that enables us to follow up and evaluate these data without too much extra effort: 'before looking for information sources other than health service data, ways of improving this information should be found and this can often be done with relatively limited resources'.[2] The principal sources of health indicator data include: vital events registers, disease registers, routine health service data, epidemiological surveillance data, and sample surveys.

One of the main data sources lies in *vital events statistics*. In European countries these data are reasonably complete and useful for deriving demographic indicators based on births and deaths. Together with population data usually collected at ten-yearly censuses they form the basis for information on the actual population structure and for projections.

Routinely collected disease data can also be found in *disease registers*. These are usually developed for one or more specific conditions such as cancer, tuberculosis, cardiovascular diseases, or mental disorders. Registers have already been described. Nevertheless, it is worth repeating that it is not an easy task to set up an adequate disease register and many less than successful attempts have been made.

When concentrating on the use of *routine health service records* it appears that there is a wealth of data from this source. Unfortunately most of these records are kept for administrative rather than for surveillance purposes so that they are neither readily available nor exploitable for surveillance. One of the more serious problems with routine health-service data relates to the absence of a firm population denominator. The population at risk is not clearly defined, a common problem in non-population-based epidemiological research.

Another problem concerns the poor accessibility of data both because of the need to maintain privacy and for bureaucratic reasons. WHO recommends trying to improve routine health-service information rather than to look for other information sources, as it can often be done with limited resources.

Disease occurrence can also be derived from epidemiological *surveillance information* mainly on communicable diseases and especially related to outbreaks of acute disease and certain endemic diseases.

Information on health and disease is also frequently sought by conducting special *surveys*.

Categories of Indicators

Although health and disease are influenced by many forces outside the more narrow health field, this discussion will be limited to indicators of the health status of population groups, and not to health-policy indicators, social and economic indicators related to health or indicators of the provision of health.

The kinds of indicators found to be useful will vary from country to country.[5,6] Even within EEC countries priorities are dissimilar.

One should first make the distinction between positive and negative health indicators. It is appealing to try to make use as much as possible of indicators describing (positive) health rather than disease or death. Although several attempts have been made, no consensus exists on what might be the acceptable indices of good health. Social indicators have been developed mainly in the field of geriatrics in order to describe, for example, the degree of independence of individuals in performing activities of daily living (i.e. self-care, communication, ambulation, travelling, and non-specific manual activities). In fact there are few examples of positive health indicators in routine surveillance systems. Physical growth in children measured by indicators of the nutritional status (for example, birth weight and anthropometrical indices) and psychosocial development of children should be examples of this, although surveillance systems may not exist for the latter (see also Chapter 12 on nutritional surveillance). To a great extent we have to rely on so-called negative indicators of health, i.e. death and disease measurement.

One of the traditional indicators of poor health in a community is the *infant mortality rate*. On the one hand collection of data for deriving this indicator is straightforward at least in developed countries, but on the other this index is less useful when the rates are low, as in many European countries. The discriminatory power of the indicators then becomes too small to be of any real value.

To a certain extent in EEC countries the same reasoning applies to other (negative) health status indicators based on mortality figures, such as the *child mortality rate*, the *under-five mortality rate*, to *life expectancy* at birth and at a given age and to the *maternal mortality rate*.

Apart from general mortality figures routine mortality data can also indicate *disease-specific* mortality. In EEC countries the non-communicable mortality rates are now of major importance, the leading causes of death being cardiovascular diseases, cancer, accidents, suicides, and other mental disorders.

Morbidity data are more difficult to obtain than mortality data. Each country will have to select its own priorities. These are likely to include cardiovascular diseases, cancer, suicide, accidents, alcohol abuse, drug addiction, and dental health. In the second part of this book chapters have been devoted to these conditions.

Information Requirements

For each health status indicator there are certain information requirements. This means that we are looking for methods of data collection and analysis currently used to establish indicators that are likely to be useful for monitoring purposes.[2] Standard sources and techniques to obtain these data for selected diseases and health services are discussed elsewhere in the book.

Bibliography

1. Collins, *Dictionary of the English language*, 2nd edn., Collins, London (1986).
2. WHO, Targets for health for all. WHO Regional Office for Europe, Copenhagen (1985).
3. A concept ascribed to Cochrane, A. L., quoted in *Survey methods in community medicine* (ed. J. H. Abramson). Churchill Livingstone, London (1974).
4. Ruch, L. O., A multidimensional analysis of the concept of life change. *J. Hlth. Soc. Behav.* **18**, 1, 77–83 (1977).
5. Holland, W. W. *et al.*, *Measurement of levels of health*. WHO Regional Publications, European Series No. 7, Copenhagen (1979).
6. Azurin, J. C., (ed.) *Disease surveillance in primary health care*. South Asian Medical Information Centre, Proceedings of the 10th Seamic Seminar (1983).

4

Action and benefit

Systematic Health and Disease Information: The Rational Basis for Goal-Oriented Action

The collection of systematic health and disease information forms the basis for the description of the health dynamics of populations. This is in turn the basis for setting priorities concerning health improvement and disease control and prevention. This holds for the *ad hoc* study as well as for the continuous collection of data for surveillance systems.

The basis for surveillance is the acceptance of a continuous responsibility for the health of a population. The main reason for the establishment of epidemiological surveillance systems lies in their ability to help fulfil this responsibility in the possibilities they present in terms of health improvement and reduction of morbidity and mortality. Consequently, the types and amounts of data in a surveillance system, as well as the way the information is handled, must balance the need to know against the need to act.

Many surveillance systems contain information concerning individuals. Because of the continuity of function they not only offer possibilities for action at population level but also possibilities for action directed towards individuals, taking their specific characteristics (disease status) into account.

Surveillance systems are units in larger health-oriented systems. These units are meant to produce information necessary for the function of the system, whether national, regional, or local. Ideally this means that before the establishment of a surveillance system, the need for specific information that the register may yield should be outlined together with the different types of action needed: what are the necessary categories of information and how much of it is needed in order for a health-care system to act according to its purpose?

Systematic information forms the basis for rational goal attainment and thus for strategy formulation. Surveillance systems are necessary and integrated components of goal-seeking health-care systems. This calls for principles concerning problem-solving and categories of information needed, as well as for the choice of action and evaluation of outcome. What is to be gained from surveillance? Is it really necessary? Or, in fact, can we afford not to have surveillance?

Targets and Planned Problem Solving

The World Health Organization has in its programme 'Health for All by the

Year 2000'[1] proposed a set of health and health-related targets for populations. The targets involve most sectors of modern society, because they are based on the concept of health being a process resulting from the interaction of a variety of factors affecting human beings and the environment. Consequently, steps taken to improve health must integrate action in different fields. Public sectors whose activities have health consequences should be health-orientated, i.e. rational planning aimed at improving the population's health should also be instituted in sectors in which health is not a primary responsibility. This calls for systematic information concerning health consequences in a wide variety of settings and activities. Thus there is a great need for continuous, systematic research concerning actual health status and its determinants in populations.[2] The natural backbone of this necessary production of information would be epidemiological surveillance systems.

Growing knowledge concerning systematic variations in morbidity and mortality according to biological, social, psychological, physical, chemical, and other factors, offers the possibility of setting goals and targets in health questions. In addition, the development of scientific research methods suggests that, provided that the resources are available, we can plan scientific research activities so that gaps in our knowledge can be filled within scheduled time-limits. In this respect surveillance systems play a dominant role, producing information themselves and forming the basis for more penetrating studies. The development of prevention against caries is an example. Even with the knowledge available today we can decide to aim at certain defined levels of health-'targets' in populations within scheduled time-limits.

In common every-day activities as well as in health work, the process of problem-solving may be divided into stages. Together these stages form a chain: if one link is missed or weakened, the whole chain will be influenced or fail to function as a whole. The chain may be linked as follows:

(1) definition of problems;
(2) definition of targets;
(3) consideration of theoretical and practical possibilities to reach defined goals;
(4) decision and action or implementation;
(5) evaluation of outcome (monitoring)—return to stage (1).

Each individual chain is but one element in a spiral, aiming at still higher levels of problem solution. If this spiral-shaped process stops, problems will not be solved or will be only partially solved—or will be left to chance.

Problem-Solving and Goal Attainment in Health Work

In the formation of health strategies in populations, the problem-solving chain may take the following form:

1. *Definition, identification, and description of disease or other health-related phenomenon*:
   Nature, severity, frequency, and distribution. Determinants of variations of occurrence and consequences.
2. *Definition of targets and target groups*:
   What dimension of the disease or health-related phenomenon should be changed?
   How much should it be changed?
   For whom and how much should it be changed within scheduled time limits?
3. *Setting of priorities*:
   Alternative tools for goal attainment: relevance and appropriateness, acceptability, effect (positive and negative benefits), resource consumption, etc.
4. *Decision and action*:
   Decision.
   Resource allocation.
   Implementation.
   Process control monitoring: process surveillance, evaluation, and adjustment.
5. *Evaluation*:
   Overall evaluation (monitoring) of the process and its outcome: to what degree were goals reached by the intervention?
   Evaluation of present health status of the target population and its subgroups—return to stage (1).

Elements of this process may, of course, be found in planning and management of health in today's society. The accomplishment of vaccination programmes is one example, where surveillance for communicable diseases has been present. In addition, the results of surveillance of communicable diseases may serve as the information base on which a decision not to act is made.

Other examples of comprehensive, integrated decision and implementation processes might be quoted, but, generally speaking, they represent exceptions rather than the rule in health care. The crucial problem is that historically we inherited health systems built on the experience of scarcity of resources—i.e. doing something, at least, to perceived existing health problems, was the guiding factor in making a choice in most instances. But we are now in possession of the means to do more than just cure an illness.

We can do more than just 'mop up the water from the floor while the tap is still running'—we can stop the source or at least slow it down. We have the technology and, to a large extent, the knowledge necessary for action. What is missing is the systematic implementation of knowledge and technology to promote health, to prevent disease, and to refine curative methods in order to be cost-effective.

So the problem-solving chain should be an indispensable, integrated part of the planning and accomplishment of health work, although it is not so today, either in developing countries or in the industrialized countries of Western Europe. This holds true in spite of the fact that the process must be a *sine qua non* if we are to change health status not by leaving it to chance but by rational, planned, goal-oriented human activity.

Where Information is Needed in the Process: The Role of Surveillance

Information concerning the health of populations is needed in all stages of the problem-solving process. First, epidemiological data must be readily available to describe the burden of disease, its causes, and its consequences. Second, this will establish the necessary platform for priority setting concerning targets and for the choice of target groups.

Output from the surveillance system will also be necessary for the estimation of possibilities of reaching target groups, budgeting, and for other planning and priority setting. General epidemiological knowledge—i.e. originating from sources other than the surveillance system, for instance from scientific research reports—as well as clinical, economic, and administrative know-how must of course play an important role. But the crucial information concerning the health of the defined target population has to come from a defined source: the surveillance system.

Surveillance of the intervention itself (monitoring) is, too, indispensable to the effective adjustment of the planned health work process. Finally the achievement of goals cannot be evaluated without systematic registration of health status (health indicators) in the target groups.

It follows that, without adequate relevant information, one would not accurately know the kinds of problems that had actually been treated, to what extent they were treated, or whether the effect of the intervention (health promotion, prevention, curative activities, care) was beneficial, neutral, or negative. Had it been worthwhile? One would not know the answer without an existing surveillance procedure.

Nevertheless, it is true that considerable time and resources are spent on health work by the population, the professionals, by decision-makers, by others, etc.

As mentioned earlier, the amount of relevant information in a surveillance system must balance the need for information with the need to act. Consequently, a surveillance system should only collect information sufficient for rational goal-seeking and problem-solving. Other sources of information are published scientific *ad hoc* studies, as well as more penetrating *ad hoc* research which may originate from the output of surveillance.

The selection of data collected on each item placed under surveillance is, however, crucial to the practical functioning of the surveillance system. If the information from the surveillance is not used purposefully—as the relevant basis for decisions to act, for implementation, and for evaluation— experience shows that the quality of the reporting will diminish. This might even make the information useless. Only data that are intended for use in practical health work should be reported, and the mere publication of another statistical year-book would not comply with the meaning of the phrase 'useful in practical health work'. Surveillance systems should be fully *integrated* into health-care systems.

There are exceptions to these rules, as the production and publication of information on the population's health status may in itself create a demand that something should be planned to be done. In this sense, the surveillance of basic health indicators will serve a purpose similar to that of a scientific epidemiologic study: open our eyes to the fact that there is a problem that we have to deal with.

Types of Action on the Basis of Surveillance Information

A considerable proportion of health work in Western Europe is concerned with individuals and their diseases rather than with populations. So the most common and popular form of action is curative and care-oriented. This is because, among other things, disease is a here-and-now phenomenon, usually easy to recognize and impossible to let alone for ethical reasons.

Health promotion and disease prevention are activities related to much more complex and theoretical concepts, especially as they are based on the idea that something beneficial might occur if some activity is carried out in a normal every-day healthy existence or that something negative might happen if not. Disease prevention is concerned with phenomena not yet in existence. The concepts of health promotion and disease prevention are, consequently, based on such theoretical concepts as probabilities and prognoses, all concerning the future.

Surveillance systems forge links between the level of the individual and the more theoretical population level, as those individuals who collectively have formed the basis for computing the population probabilities are themselves members of target groups for action. In addition, action can be applied to 'risk groups'—i.e. groups of individuals thought to have a high risk of developing disease—as well as to individuals already ill. Rationally, both types of action should be planned and controlled both at the population and the individual level. Consequently, the idea is that of an interactive process between the observation, treatment, and follow-up of individuals and the observation of, intervention in, and follow-up of population groups, as seen in Fig. 4.1.

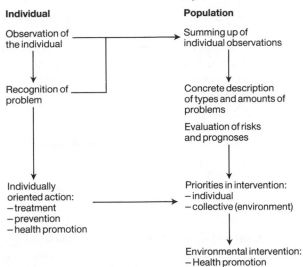

Fig. 4.1. Interaction between observation and action on the individual and the population level.

For the decision-makers and planners, the surveillance and monitoring systems will be tools for controlling what happens to the population's health. So the results are to be considered by planners in making strategies: setting priorities, controlling resource consumption in relation to need as well as relevance and effect of intervention. It is worth noting that the mere surveillance of the intervention itself by describing those involved in it, the patients or clients (see item 4, p. 32)—in a screening programme, a clinic, or a primary health care centre—is insufficient for the evaluation of goal attainment in the population, though it is often thought to be sufficient. The whole picture of course, involves the population or its target groups at large, as well as those who actually receive the service. In Danish rehabilitation services, for instance, it has been a problem to define the target groups in the population. The actual client group consists of persons who need rehabilitative services as well as those who attend for other reasons. However, some members of the target group who could benefit do not become members of the client group. This is a result of poor target definition and poor empirical tools for identifying candidates for the service—a problem inherent in health and social service systems which do not integrate population surveillance.[3]

Responsibilities

The task of changing a population's health is not limited to experts.[1] There are several necessary parties in the process. These include the population, the decision-makers in the political and administrative system, professional health workers and other experts.

There are numerous ethical and other problems in storing personal data and avoiding their misuse (see Chapter 5). So, if the population is not actively and effectively involved in the use of a surveillance system, it may become a tool for social control rather than one for the improvement of the population's health.

That means, in practical terms, that the principles of the integration process, outlined earlier, should involve the population and its organizations effectively, not only in the implementation of the health plans (which is, of course, a must) but also in the decision and planning processes. It is worth remembering that no expert and no technical equipment can ensure that data are not used for purposes other than those originally intended. Thus the establishment of surveillance systems should be the responsibility of the population to which each system refers. However, organized systems where the local population is an integral part of the planning and management of health care are still developments for the future in Europe.

In this process experts and decision-makers in the political and administrative system will, of course, play a vital role. Looking at the problem-solving chain, the population should be involved in all phases: the discussion of health problems and their possible causes and consequences in the region, setting the priorities in relation to resource consumption, mapping out of possibilities—theoretical and practical —for intervention, the decision process, the implementation of plans, and the evaluation and resulting discussion about future action. It should be the responsibility of the population itself to decide what to do about health problems and to implement plans. The surveillance expert (the epidemiologist) and other experts have the responsibility for mapping out realities, whether expressed in concrete examples or in theoretical information such as probabilities and prognoses. The interaction between the epidemiologist and the population will sometimes cause the epidemiologist to reconsider his value judgements when discussing important preventive issues with the population.

Organizational Structure and the Planning Process

In order to collect and interpret data, to communicate the information, to implement consequent actions, to allocate resources, to evaluate benefits and drawbacks of intervention, and to communicate with the national, regional, or local population, the organizational structure must be of an integrated and intersectorial nature. Thus it will vary from country to country and from region to region as well, depending also on the size of the target population.

One example will be mentioned here: oral health in Danish school children. Since the beginning of the 1970s the dental status of all Danish schoolchildren has been recorded and the information stored in a nationwide register.[7,8,9,10] National, regional, and local surveillance reports from the register have formed the basis for the assessment of the problem (i.e. frequency of caries and its geographical distribution), further scientific research (determinants of caries incidence, effectiveness of fluoride intervention, and other types of intervention)—in combination with laboratory and clinical research,[11] programme planning (i.e. whether services should be public or private), and evaluation.

Figure 4.2 shows the integrated flow of register data as well as evaluation reports and suggestions for planning from the clinics to higher administrative and political levels and the flow of surveillance reports and resource plans back to counties, municipalities, and clinics. Strategies as well as plans for everyday preventive and curative interventions are worked out at each level. Figure 4.3 shows the annual caries increment in Danish schoolchildren 1972–

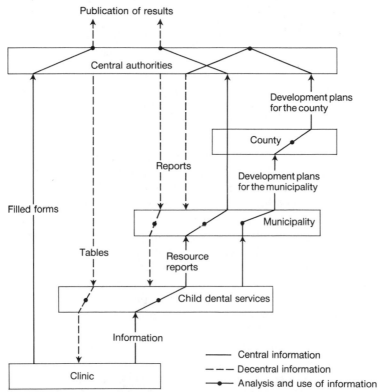

Fig. 4.2. The flow and treatment of information concerning child dental services. [Source: Heidemann, J. (1983) Organisation af børnetandplejen (The organization of the child dental services). The Royal Dental College, Aarhus.]

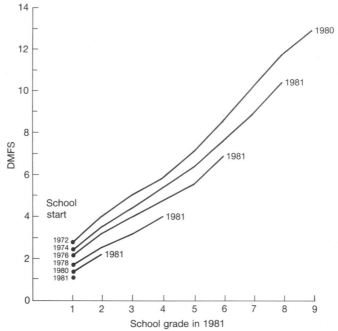

Fig. 4.3. Annual caries increment (permanent teeth) in Danish schoolchildren start-ing school in 1972–81. Each cohort demonstrates lower DMFS-levels than the pre-vious cohort. DMFS = Decayed-Missing-Filled-Score. (Source: Schwarz[9].)

1981, based on information from the registry. The general conclusion is that the dental status of the schoolchildren has improved over the years. This has led to consequences for the planning of the local school dental services in that projections of the number of dentists needed can be made (Fig. 4.4). The lower number required has been determined mainly by the decrease in caries, although decreasing fertility and a decrease in the number of dentists qualify-ing has also contributed. This change in planning would not have been pos-sible had the surveillance register not been in existence.

Based on the information from the register, public school dental services seem to have a better cost-effectiveness than private ones. The results from the register have influenced recent legislation on the organization of school dental services.

Thus the register has had a great impact on the choice of appropriate target groups, the choice of preventive and curative interventions, and the de-velopment of a proper organizational framework. The consequences con-cerning planning and resource allocation have also been significant.

Concerning broader health questions, problems are usually more complex. In many health problems we have some indicators for future preventive and

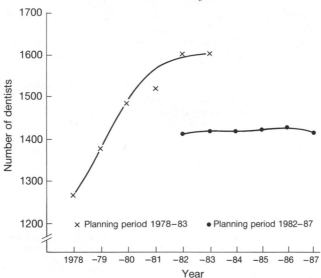

Fig. 4.4. Number of dentists in the children's dental service as planned for 1978–83 and for 1982–87. From the first to the second plan the numbers have been reduced drastically. (Source: Schwarz[9].)

curative action, and in some we know what to do but do not have the information on the local appropriate target groups. So, future developments should be concentrated on how to make national, regional, and local registers interact. National registers might, for instance, contain aggregated person-linked indicators of environment, illness and intervention. Regional and local registers should be more detailed. The delegation of tasks between national, regional, and local registers will, of course, also depend on resources, i.e. for data processing and concerning the availability of skilled epidemiologists, computer professionals, and others. The aim is to make an integrated, flexible, and potent system in local communities, where the population itself has the greatest ability to contribute relevant information. They can then devise appropriate measures to implement health interventions.

Bibliography

1. Targets for Health for All, Targets in support of the European regional strategy for health for all. WHO, Regional Office for Europe, Copenhagen (1984).
2. Taylor, C. E., The uses of health systems research. WHO, Geneva (1984).
3. Foldspang, A., Nogle studier over revalidering: Tilgang og afgang. (A few studies on rehabilitation: Intake and discharge. With a summary in English). Social-medicinsk Institut, Publication No. 28, Aarhus (1982).
4. Kleczkowski, B. M., Romer, M. I., and Van Der Werf, A., National health sys-

tems and their reorientation towards health for all: Guidance for policy-making. WHO Public Health Papers, No. 77. WHO, Geneva (1984).

5. Meulengracht, A. and Madsen, M., Registre inden for sundhedsomradet (Registers concerning health). Dansk Institut for Klinisk Epidemiologi, Copenhagen (1983).
6. Lynge, E., Dødelighed og erhverv 1970–75 (Mortality and occupation). Statistisk undersøgelse no. 37. Danmarks Statistik, Copenhagen (1979).
7. Helm, S., Recording system for the Danish child dental health services. *Community Dent. Oral Epidemiol.* **1,** 3–8 (1973).
8. Schwarz, E. and Hansens, E. R., Caries experience of Danish children evaluated by the child dental health recording system. *Community Dent. Oral Epidemiol.* **7,** 107–14 (1979).
9. Schwarz, E., The Danish oral health service for children: Its achievements. *Int. Dental J.* **3,** 221–30 (1983).
10. Schwarz, E., Dental programmes for children and young adults in Denmark in a social perspective. *Scand. J. primary Hlth. Care* **3,** 113–20 (1985).
11. Foldspang, A. and Hvidman, L., Danish primary health care research 1950–1980. Organisation, content, methods. *Scand. J. primary Hlth. Care* **3,** 183–8 (1985).

5

Ethical dilemmas behind surveillance

Medical Information and the Preservation of Confidentiality

Successful surveillance of any kind is based on adequate and correct records. Medical information available through methods and processes described in the special chapters of this book is the foundation of various surveillance systems.

It is widely agreed that socio-medical information about health and disease is required not only for diagnosis and treatment, but also for medical research purposes, the evaluation of the effectiveness and efficiency of health-care services, and for epidemiological surveillance. All these activities require medical information and communication, and also demand access to medical records and to registries used for surveillance.

Adequate and accurate reporting is important in a surveillance system and of benefit to the surveillance itself, to the public health authorities, the doctor, and the whole community. Medical data have to be correctly used for this purpose, first in recording and then in communication of information. In return for their cooperation doctors are supplied with summaries of the community's total experience and with periodic analyses of trends of the reported cases.

The sharing of medical information must, however, be done with care if it is to promote the general good and be of help and value to other patients and to the whole community.[1] Whilst our chief purpose should be to facilitate the objectives of surveillance, at the same time the confidentiality of the information on which surveillance is based needs to be protected.

Although the medical profession has a clear duty to cooperate in supplying any necessary data for effective surveillance, the issues of personal liberty of the patient and his right to confidentiality are often raised at this point, and they may affect greatly the completeness and accuracy of data.

Surveillance and the Traditional Medical Deontology on Secrecy

Traditionally the doctor–patient relationship has been regarded as a contract between two persons. Doctors are bound by the Hippocratic Oath or Hippocratic Tradition, and in modern times by the obligations of confidence laid down in their professional code of ethics, not to use the information they acquire for any purpose other than the continuing care of the patient, and not to release it without his or her consent to anyone who is not directly involved in the patient's care. Medical confidentiality, a prima facie duty of any doctor, is a legal requirement as well as an ethical necessity in all EEC countries. It can be said that secrecy between patient and doctor is elevated to a fundamental right for the individual human being.

The Hippocratic Oath expresses an old, long-standing and widely acceptable tradition of medical deontology, 'to respect the trust of the patient at all times and to preserve confidentiality'. The survival of the Oath throughout recorded history reflects the fundamental and unchanging requirements of sick people for the preservation of secrecy entrusted to medical persons. In the Oath it is stated that 'what I may see or hear in the course of the treatment or even outside of the treatment in regard to the life of men, which on no account one must spread abroad, I will keep to myself holding such things shameful to be spoken about'. It is worth noting that even the death of the patient does not absolve the doctor from the obligation to maintain secrecy.[2] Moreover, the Hippocratic Oath and the traditional medical deontology do not generally limit secrecy to what is seen or heard in professional practice. The Oath is almost universally accepted despite the social changes over the past centuries.

The general principles of the Hippocratic tradition, however, have been reformulated on several occasions; for example, in the 'Declaration of Geneva' of 1948. They have also been substantially incorporated into the legal codes of most countries, so that tradition and the law operate in concert.

At the same time, the conventions and requirements of secrecy have seldom been regarded as absolute. There is common recognition that the public interest may on certain occasions justify a breach of this principle. The rightful objective is to protect the health of the public. This happens in the case of medical surveillance.

Violation of the rule of confidentiality may be justified on grounds of prevention of harm to others from a disease's negative effect. The most obvious example both in the past and present is the duty to inform public officials of cases of a dangerous contagious disease which poses a threat to the general public.

Surveillance and the Rational Use of Health Information

It is true that in the case of release of information for surveillance and research purposes the physician faces a conflict between his duty to respect the principles of confidentiality and his general social responsibility. On the other hand, it has been suggested that the principle of medical confidentiality described in medical codes of ethics has become old, worn-out, and useless; that it is a decrepit concept.[3] It seems reasonable that in the real world the rule of confidentiality is not absolute. In fact, it may be possible to specify several conditions under which confidentiality should not be maintained.

Other people, authorities and organizations occupying official positions within our society, also have a concern for the health of patients, but a concern which goes beyond the health of the individual. Health authorities, for example, are anxious that infectious diseases should cease to exist within the area for which they are responsible. They are deeply concerned about endemic and even more about the epidemic appearance of infectious diseases in the community. In order to take preventive measures they have to be well informed, and this means release of medical information and notification of the cases. Moreover, it may also mean interference with other rights of an affected patient, for example by isolation in hospital, ward, or by quarantine.

Here we face a real problem. A doctor who has obtained confidential information from a patient is entitled to disclose it to the health officials for the benefit of the public. The justification for the violation of doctor–patient confidentiality in this instance is that society at large must be protected.[4] The right to break medical confidentiality under some circumstances indicates that the medical role may sometimes have to yield to one's role as citizen and as protector of the interest of others.

The medical profession in the EEC countries largely accepts the following exceptions for release of information:[1]

(a) when there is a clear overriding duty to society;
(b) when the information is required by law;
(c) when information is required for purposes of medical research and it is impractical or undesirable to seek explicit consent;
(d) when the patient gives full, free, and informed consent.

In most countries the law may demand from medical persons information gained in the course of a professional relationship. Sometimes the law may punish doctors for refusing to provide information. The notification of infectious diseases, the registration of births, and the certification of deaths and the causes of death are examples of routine health and vital statistics legally required. On those occasions, therefore, the law has intervened to break the bond of secrecy between the doctor and the patient. Moreover, in special instances the law requires a physician to yield information to health officials and may punish those who fail to do so.

The professional ethical responsibility has two sides; one is the obligation of confidentiality, the other is responsibility and communication within the doctor's commitment to the service of society as a whole.[5]

Surveillance, Confidentiality, and the Social Responsibility of the Medical Profession

The ongoing dynamic mechanism of any kind of surveillance should be seen as constituting a fundamental part and activity of preventive medicine and of public-health services, closely tied to actions of control and prevention. By instituting epidemiological surveillance mechanisms medical persons, public-health services and health authorities look forward to the maximization of the good of the society in general. Disease monitoring and control services are brought into immediate action through surveillance mechanisms. Surveillance also contributes greatly to our knowledge and understanding of disease, and its effects on communities. Medical information and communication are required for this activity. Just as the interest of the patient normally dictates confidentiality, so it implies the development of the health services and their mobilization on his behalf. One can imagine the outcry which would have occurred if the detection of the thalidomide catastrophe or cases of AIDS had been delayed through a strict adherence to the principles of secrecy.

Most countries have enacted legislation appropriate to the release of information for surveillance and for processes concerned with the protection of the public at large. For persons working in surveillance units it may be necessary to sign a statement to ensure that data are treated in confidence. Names should preferably not be used and raw data must be kept secure. It is important to ensure that the patient's identity cannot be traced from the surveillance report.

In the promotion of health and prevention of disease, the effectiveness of modern public health measures is ultimately dependent on the health consciousness both of legislators and citizens. Law and medicine have to work together to assure legitimate use of medical records for surveillance.

The most sincere concern of medical persons must be with the human rights and dignity of the patient, and the respect of his or her privacy. Legal and ethical duties of doctors towards their patients dictate preservation of medical secrecy, unless the doctor is required by law to disclose information or unless it becomes necessary in order to protect the welfare of the community at large.

It is argued, however, that better legal definitions of the respective rights and duties of the interested persons should contribute to a better relationship between doctors and patients, and at the same time help surveillance processes and medical research.

Law and medicine must work together to assure what both desire to achieve; the maintenance of the highest standards of altruistic practice in the profession of medicine. Law and medicine have to work together to assure legitimate use of medical records for surveillance and also to preserve confidentiality as is explicitly stated in the Hippocratic Oath, in several formulations of medical ethics, the 'European Convention of Human Rights', promulgated by the Council of Europe, and the 'Declaration of Geneva'.

Bibliography

1. Knox, E. G., The confidentiality of medical records. Report of working party of the Advisory Panel for Social Medicine and Epidemiology in the European Economic Community, Luxembourg (1984).
2. Macara, A. W., Confidentiality—a decrepit concept? *J. R. Soc. Med.* **77**, 577–84 (1984).
3. Siegler, M., Confidentiality in medicine—a decrepit concept. *New Engl. J. Med.* **307**, 24, 1518–21 (1982).
4. Sieghart, P., Medical confidence, the law, and computers. *J. R. Soc. Med.* **77**, 8, 656–62 (1984).
5. Gillon, R., Confidentiality. *Br. med. J.* **291**, 1634–6 (1985).

Part 2
Practical applications of surveillance

6
Surveillance systems from hospital data
J. GORDON PATERSON

Introduction

The following description of hospital-based surveillance systems takes as its model the arrangements which operate in the United Kingdom with particular reference to Scotland. The basic principles on which these have been established are applicable to any country and underly the range of systems to be found in various stages of development throughout the EEC countries.

Information used for surveillance purposes also has potential applicability for service planning, management, and resource allocation, particularly when supplemented by additional data collected specifically for these purposes. These activities and information uses are outside the remit of this publication. Surveillance systems within hospitals—for example antibiotic resistance in bacteria—are similarly not considered here.

Hospital Medical Records for Surveillance

Hospital medical records are compiled by those whose primary motivation and interests are directed to the investigation, diagnosis, treatment, and rehabilitation of individual patients. The functions of these records are therefore to serve as an *aide-mémoire* to the clinical team, both now and in the future, as a means of communication with others authorized to consult the records, research, and, in an increasingly litiginous age, to provide a medicolegal account of clinical management. The variability of structure and content of these records reflects both their evolution, from simple ward registers to sophisticated case folders, and the particular interests and preferences of successive cohorts of clinicians.

Historical Background

The volume and complexity of the individual case record have increased progressively with the introduction of a vast range of investigative procedures, a parallel increase in the number of conditions which are amenable to clinical intervention and the diversity of sophisticated therapeutic regimes. As a result, the retrieval of information from a case record may present considerable difficulty and, in recognition of this, standardization of hospital medical records was recommended by the central health departments of England[1] and Scotland[2] in 1965 and 1967 respectively. The adoption of standard recording procedures was seen to offer clinical and administrative benefits at patient, ward, and hospital level, while creating opportunities for epidemiological research by facilitating the extraction of summary information for each episode of care with which to build up some appreciation of the patterns of morbidity in the relevant population. Thus, the comprehensive use of records designed for easy retrieval of diagnostic information, with periodic analysis of the collected data, would create a form of inbuilt surveillance which should be an integral part of a highly structured national health service.

In Scotland, returns relating to patients treated in mental hospitals and mental deficiency hospitals have been completed since the beginning of the present century, but for legal rather than epidemiological purposes. For other patient groups attempts to collect information on a national basis began in 1936 when the National Radium Commission introduced a system aimed at facilitating the follow-up of patients treated by radium therapy. This formed the basis of the present Cancer Registration scheme which is used predominantly for epidemiological and research purposes, including the calculation of survival times.[3] Registration data are derived mainly from hospital in-patient sources, supplemented by information from out-patient departments, pathology laboratories, and the death registration procedures operated by the Registrar General for Scotland. Registers are considered in greater detail in Part 1 of the book.

In the 1940s the Nuffield Provincial Hospital Trust sponsored studies[4,5] into hospital treated illness in the Scottish counties of Stirlingshire and Ayrshire. Agreement was reached in 1950 between the Scottish Home and Health Department and the five regional hospital boards for the introduction of a system for the routine collection of information, including disease classification, throughout the whole of Scotland. The objectives of this arrangement were twofold:

1. *Administrative*: to assist in the administration of the hospital service by the provision of information to central and local agencies for use in planning and management of health services.
2. *Epidemiological*: to obtain comprehensive statistical information about the conditions for which patients are treated in hospital and the demographic characteristics of those treated.

A pilot scheme was launched, in 1951, in the Northern region, centred in Inverness, but technical and financial restrictions delayed the extension of the scheme to the whole of Scotland until 1961. A similar development in England had begun in 1949 and reached full coverage of the country by 1958. However, unlike the Scottish scheme which provided morbidity recording for

100 per cent of patient episodes, the English system, which covers a much larger population, captured information on only a 10 per cent sample of discharges.

Hospital Data Recording

The Scottish Morbidity Recording System

The Scottish Morbidity Recording system, introduced initially to general hospital only (SMR1), was extended to mental illness and mental handicap hospitals (SMR4) in 1963 and maternity hospitals in 1969 (SMR2), in each case with recording of information on 100 per cent of in-patient episodes.

Inclusion of a neonatal record (SMR11) within the system took place in 1973 following pilot studies led by clinicians in two teaching centres.

With only one minor partial omission, the thirteen items which comprise the minimum basic data set (MBDS) recommended for recording of hospital morbidity in the European Community[6] are included in or can be derived from, the Scottish Morbidity Records in current use. These are:

1. hospital identification
2. patient's number
3. sex
4. age
5. marital status
6. area of residence
7. month and year of admission
8. duration of stay
9. discharge status
10. main diagnosis
11. other diagnosis
12. surgical and obstetric procedures
13. other significant procedures

In the case of item 13, it appears that many of the procedures such as cardiac catheterization and liver biopsy intended for this category are already recorded in the operative treatment section. As codes become available for new techniques, such as interventional radiology, they will be similarly recorded.

Collection of information

The arrangements for capture of information are broadly similar for each of these records schemes. For each patient discharged from or dying within a Scottish hospital a standard form (Scottish Morbidity Record—SMR) appropriate to the type of hospital is completed and the information transferred to a central agency—the Information Services Division of the Scottish

Health Service Common Services Agency—for processing, analysis, and publication of statistical output. The Scottish Morbidity Record for general hospitals in Scotland (form SMR1) is shown in Fig. 6.1. For in-patient episodes in mental illness and mental handicap hospitals, a preliminary return is submitted on admission to avoid the delay which would result if the length of stay was prolonged and no information was collected until discharge.

Completion of the relevant morbidity returns is usually undertaken by trained clerical staff associated with hospital records departments. Although the representatives of the British medical profession have acknowledged that recording of diagnostic information should be the responsibility of medical staff, because of its fundamental importance for the accuracy of morbidity surveillance, in practice this rarely happens. As a result, the identification of the principal condition treated or precipitating admission to hospital is undertaken by the non-medical morbidity-coding staff who rely heavily on the standard structure of the case record and episode summary documents to retrieve this information. It is relevant to note the emphasis which is placed on the principal presenting diagnosis or treated condition, rather than on the underlying cause which forms the basis of death certification and is of greater significance in assessing the aetiology of population morbidity.

Accuracy of recording

Studies of the accuracy with which these morbidity returns are completed have yielded encouraging results. Demographic and administrative information contains few errors and 95 per cent accuracy in the recording of the principal diagnosis has been reported by Lockwood[7] who found that the main errors and omissions related to the recording of occupation, which has now been abandoned on the Scottish general hospitals (SMR1) scheme. Estimates of the completeness of coverage of the morbidity recording system may be obtained by comparison of the numbers of SMR returns with the number of discharges in the relevant statistical recording system for hospital utilization.

Data processing

Transfer of information from individual hospitals to the national processing centre may be by submission of completed forms or by the creation of a local (health authority) computer file with tape extracts forwarded to national level. Computer processing, whether undertaken centrally or locally, must incorporate preliminary scrutiny of the data, involving a complex series of validity and feasibility checks, before acceptance for inclusion in the master file of morbidity records. Each year, when all data relating to the various morbidity schemes have been vetted and added to the national files, standard analyses are carried out to produce a series of published[8,9] and 'unpublished' tabulations, together with hospital and national diagnostic and operation

Scotland In-Patient and Day-Case Records Summary Sheet

SMR1 — MEDICAL — IN CONFIDENCE

HOSPITAL ....

TIME OF ADMISSION/TRANSFER WARD (WARD) 73-75

PREVIOUSLY ATTENDED THIS HOSPITAL YES/NO

IF YES STATE YEAR

ADDRESS (ADDR) 76-135

TEL. No. POSTCODE → POSTCODE (PC) 106-112

RELIGION

NEXT OF KIN (RELATIONSHIP) ....

NAME ....

ADDRESS ....

TEL. No. POSTCODE

FAMILY DOCTOR

NAME ....

ADDRESS ....

TEL. No. POSTCODE

GP CODE (GP) 136-142

PROVISIONAL DIAGNOSIS ON ADMISSION

HOSPITAL CODE (HOSP) 1-5

HOSPITAL CASE REFERENCE No. (CRN) 6-15

SURNAME .... (SN) 16-35

FIRST FORENAME (FN1) 36-50

SECOND FORENAME (FN2) 51-65

MAIDEN NAME (MN) 66-85

ALTERNATIVE CASE REFERENCE No. (ACRN) 86-95

AGE.................. DATE OF BIRTH (DOB) 96-103

SEX (SEX) 104 MARITAL STATE (MRST) 105

OCCUPATION (OCC) (OCCC) 113-175

HUSBAND'S/PARENT'S OCCUPATION (HPO) (HPOC) 176-238

ADMITTED/TRANSFERRED FROM (ADTF) 239 TYPE OF ADMISSION (TADM) 240

DATE PLACED ON WAITING LIST (DWL) 1-6

DATE OF ADMISSION (DOA) 7-12

DATE OF DISCHARGE (DOD) 13-18

TIME OF DISCHARGE .... DISCHARGE CODE (DISC) 19

CATEGORY OF PATIENT (CAT) 20 TYPE OF FACILITY (TOF) 21

SPECIALTY (SPEC) 22-25

CONSULTANT'S SURNAME (CONS) + 26-45

CONSULTANT'S INITIALS 46-47 CONSULTANT CODE (CONC) 48-54

TO BE COMPLETED BY DOCTOR ON DISCHARGE OF PATIENT

(1) MAIN CONDITION (DG1) (DG1C) 55-120

(2) OTHER CONDITIONS (DG2) (DG2C) 121-186

(3) (DG3) (DG3C) 1-66

(4) (DG4) (DG4C) 67-132

(5) (DG5) (DG5C) 133-198

(6) (DG6) (DG6C) 1-66

(1) PRINCIPAL OPERATION (OP1) (OP1C) 67-131

(2) OTHER OPERATION (OP2) (OP2C) 132-196

DATE OF PRINCIPAL OPERATION (DOP1) → DATE OF PRINCIPAL OPERATION (DOP1) 197-202

ERROR REPORT COMMENT: Data items specified in boxes below are correct (COM)

Enter field abbreviations

Additional notes: 1-60

LOCAL USE (LUSE) 61-66

NATIONAL USE (NUSE) 67-72

Fig. 6.1. The Scottish Morbidity Record.

indexes. (The term 'unpublished' refers to the limited distribution of this material within the health service and government adjustments.)

In addition, this material provides a data source for other routine statistical publications.[10] The nationally held data files are also available for *ad hoc* analyses and tabulations on request from central health departments, health boards, or bona fide researchers. Unfortunately, the availability of this valuable national data set, with its 100 per cent coverage of all in-patient episodes, is invariably delayed by late submission of information from one or more health boards. This in turn presents completion of the relevant national file, publication of routine output and processing of *ad hoc* requests. In this respect, those health boards who have devised local computing arrangements for capture of morbidity data have the benefit of early access to their own information independently of the national processing timetable.

Surveillance and monitoring applications

The availability of a long-established collection of hospital morbidity data containing demographic and diagnostic information of 100 per cent of hospital in-patient episodes experienced by a population of five million creates great potential for monitoring and surveillance applications. Answers to the traditional basic epidemiological questions can therefore be sought from this source: which patients are admitted to hospital (WHO) suffering from what diseases (WHY) how frequently (HOW MANY) and over what time-period (WHEN). The additional geographical consideration (WHERE) relates not only to the patient's usual residence but also to the hospital providing treatment.

Posing such questions may highlight variation in the frequency and distribution of disease which prompts further investigation. Such investigations usually require more detailed information than is contained within the standard morbidity record but, as a minimum, the case population for such studies can be identified from this source and, if required, an appropriately matched control population.

The usefulness of the standard Scottish data set for the surveillance of morbidity is clearly restricted to those conditions which require hospital admission. Those individuals and diseases which can be managed within the community and those who die without referral or before transfer to hospital are excluded. A decision to admit to in-patient care is the result of a complex interaction between a number of related factors:

1. The *condition*: its nature and severity, the nature of the treatment required and whether that treatment is best provided in hospital.
2. The *individual*: age, social environment, and attitude to hospitalization.
3. *Hospital services*: availability and accessibility.
4. *Medical practice*: including the attitudes of the referring general practi-

tioner, the admission criteria, and management policy of the relevant hospital clinician.

Variation of one or more of these factors over time or in different localities will have a direct and possibly marked effect on hospital morbidity patterns even when the true global incidence of a particular disease has remained relatively unchanged. Awareness of such a possibility is, therefore, essential in interpreting such information. The virtual absence of in-patients currently being treated for respiratory tuberculosis is largely due to the dramatic fall in the prevalence of this disease but is also related to the management in the community made possible by the availability of effective chemotherapeutic agents.

Record linkage

For those conditions where admission is deemed appropriate, the simple summation of all known episodes of in-patient care over a given time period cannot be used as an accurate measure of incidence, since multiple episodes may be attributable to the same individual. These circumstances would arise, for example, in the treatment of bladder and haematological malignancies or in staged plastic surgical procedures. Even in the management of acute surgical conditions, such as orthopaedic trauma, initial management may routinely be followed by early transfer to convalescent facilities—thus creating two in-patient episode summaries for each individual and the obvious risk of double counting in epidemiological studies. The frequency with which such transfer occurs will vary from area to area and over different time periods. Thus, recognition of this possibility is essential if false conclusions are not to be drawn from hospital morbidity data.

True figures on case frequency and on first presentation, an essential requirement for studies of disease incidence, necessitate linkage of records of all episodes relating to the same individual. The techniques involved in such linkage are complex and based on matching records by comparison of key data fields within the identifying section of the record. As a minimum these are the surname (birth surname in the case of females), sex, and date of birth. To allow for minor errors in the spelling of the surname it is usually converted to a Soundex or similar code for linkage purposes. In most record systems, some form of numbering system in the form of a master patient or population index is adopted, with a unique reference number allocated to each individual at birth of on first contact with health-care or hospital services and used on all manual and computer records thereafter. In some areas this same numbering system extends to community-health and primary-care records within an area. Currently, however, none of the various record numbering systems in use in Scotland extends beyond a single health authority and in some instances, may cover only one large hospital. Any future implementation of a national numbering system for the whole country could increase the value and usefulness of morbidity data and facilitate the linkage of records at national level. However, the existing National Health Service number is of little value outside primary health care administration as it is rarely recorded in hospital information systems.

The linkage of records is usually undertaken to satisfy the information requirements for specific studies. However, in the Grampian Area of Scotland routine linkage of in-patient records has been undertaken for the past fifteen years. All general hospital (SMR1) morbidity records relating to 80 000 in-patient episodes in North-east Scotland, Orkney, and Shetland are added to a locally-held master file annually with routine linkage to records of previous episodes where these exist. Thus this progressively expanding master file contains a series of cumulative linked records for each individual and not a series of unrelated collections of records for the discharges during each calendar year.

This approach to morbidity file architecture is unique within Scotland and, while currently limited in content to general hospital (SMR1) episodes only, the potential exists to link with episode summaries from the other morbidity schemes (maternity, neonatal, mental illness, mental handicap, and cancer registration).

Linkage is most frequently employed to bring together the morbidity experience of one individual but on some occasions the technique is employed to isolate the records of groups of individuals, such as members of the same family as part of a genetic research study.

Confidentiality

While these impressive feats of information manipulation, made possible by modern computer technology, offer great benefits to those engaged in the investigation of morbidity, due regard must be paid to the preservation of security and confidentiality of data. Local codes of practice have now assumed new legal significance with the implementation in the United Kingdom of the Data Protection Act.

Use of Hospital Data for Surveillance

Accuracy and standardization

When hospital morbidity data are used in the context of disease surveillance, the diagnostic section of the episode summary is the one most frequently examined. The use of the International Classification of Diseases[11] allows local, national and international comparisons to be made. Apart from the requirements for accuracy in transcription and coding of diagnoses, there is also a requirement of identification of specific criteria for the assignment of a diagnosis to complex conditions such as pre-eclamptic toxaemia. Agreement to these criteria should be at national and preferably international level if comparisons of morbidity record collections are to be meaningful.

Occupational data

The omission of occupation data from the MBDS may seem surprising when some of the classical examples of occupational disease spring readily to mind—respiratory diseases in coal miners and asbestos workers, malignant diseases in dye and rubber workers. However, reference has already been made to the errors and omission observed in the recording of this information from which socio-economic group and social class are derived. In view of the poor quality of this information and the relative infrequency with which it has been used in the recent past, recording has now been discontinued in the general hospital (SMR1) morbidity scheme in Scotand. In times of economic recession the recording of unemployment and its duration might be of greater relevance in the light of the growing volume of evidence associating this form of social disability with increased levels of other types of morbidity.

Geographical surveillance

The recording of area of residence in the form of a structured postal-code permits accurate identification of the geographical distribution of disease. Population census data are also produced for post-code areas allowing the derivation of local age and sex specific rates, subject to the usual caution with regard to calculations based on small numbers of cases. The availability of a national post-code directory cross-referencing post-codes with health and local government administrative areas allows monitoring of the movement of patients between their usual residence and hospital of treatment, this being of particular interest where patients move between health authority areas. The inclusion in this directory of a link between post-code and grid reference has made possible the development of sophisticated computer mapping techniques which allow the graphical presentation of morbidity data.[12] This procedure is of value in highlighting any unusual clustering of cases, and, when used in conjunction with similar maps showing levels of environmental pollution, radiation, trace elements, etc., may provide some pointers to possible causal associations.

Special studies

The collection of additional information as an extension of the routine data set, for either short- or long-term studies, offers considerable potential. Short-term studies may include examination of the morbidity patterns and demands on hospital services associated with a particular occupational group and their dependants (e.g. oil-related workers and their families).[13]

One well established long-term study is the routine collection of information on medicines prescribed during each in-patient episode and on discharge to the community.[14] This enhanced morbidity record, when held in a linked file, may be used to identify patients who have received a specified drug or drug combination and to follow-up their subsequent hospital morbidity. In this way the incidence of suspected adverse reactions likely to result in hospitalization can be quantified and its significance assessed by comparison with the morbidity experience of a matched control group drawn from the same linked file, who did not receive the medicines in question. This type of drug monitoring or medicines evaluation activity has been undertaken in two Scottish centres for many years and is, in effect, a surveillance system for iatrogenic diseases. Examples of use include investigation of the association between methyldopa and haemolytic anaemia[15] and between amitriptyline and cardiac disease.[16]

Out-patient morbidity surveillance

Although the major investment in hospital morbidity recording has been directed to patients admitted for treatment, attempts have been made to identify the contribution of out-patient care to the management of specific diseases. Most out-patient activity returns contain only statistical information on the numbers of clinic sessions and attenders. However, some out-patient and laboratory departments do produce more detailed information on patient and disease categories which gives some indication of morbidity patterns. Examples of such returns are those produced by cervical cytology laboratories and sexually transmitted diseases clinics.

Trials have been carried out to collect demographic and diagnostic information on patients referred for consultant opinion. While in theory this should provide valuable information for surveillance purposes, the logistics of information collection present many problems. The data capture and processing associated with 100 per cent recording of new attendances is considerable, given the average ratio of three new out-patients to one in-patient episode for most acute medical and surgical specialties. In an attempt to reduce the resource requirements to an acceptable level, the use of sampling techniques has been advocated.[17] However, the very small proportions sampled may well yield results which are of limited value at local level unless information collection is concentrated on individual specialties in rotation.

An additional problem relates to the certainty with which a diagnosis can be established at the first consultation. This may be particularly relevant in those specialties which require extensive investigations to confirm clinical impressions. For these reasons, in particular the major resource implications, the routine application of such recording procedures has not been pursued. *Ad hoc* surveys of limited duration may, however, be appropriate for individual areas of investigation.

In the field of mental illness and mental handicap, where care is increasingly provided in the community, case registers containing demographic and diagnostic information on all patient contacts with these services are well established in a number of centres in the United Kingdom.[18]

Special arrangements are required for the long-term follow-up and management of patients afflicted by chronic conditions. To be effective surveillance of this type demands careful recording of identifying, clinical, and biochemical data; easy access to such information and excellent two-way communications between hospital specialists and primary care physicians. In an attempt to achieve these objectives various computer-based patient record[19] and follow-up systems have been developed. These have found application in the surveillance of hypertension,[20] diabetes, asthma, and in certain forms of rheumatic and thyroid disease.[21]

The availability of such systems assists clinical management in a variety of ways including the prompting of follow-up review and biochemical measurement, production of computer-generated patient profiles, identification of defaulters, and more efficient communication with general practitioners. Additional benefits include the potential to monitor for complications of particular diseases[22] and audit the effectiveness of therapy.

Summary

In the fairly recent past, it was assumed that those conditions which had the greatest relevance to the health of the population would require admission for in-patient care. This belief provided the necessary impetus to seek standardization of recording procedures and the collection of summary information for all in-patient episodes to be used as a means of disease surveillance. The established hospital morbidity recording systems have great potential for use in epidemiology and surveillance but seldom provide more than general pointers to areas, issues, and changes which require more detailed enquiry.

An appreciation of the complex network of factors which determine whether an individual will be referred for hospitalization and the subtle variation in these factors is an essential prerequisite to the appropriate use of these data. Attempts to extend morbidity recording to surveillance of out-patients have, with some limited exceptions, been frustrated by the resource implications. However, as computers will be used increasingly in the future for the administration of all hospital in-patient and out-patient services, opportunities may present to add supplementary morbidity recording to information systems which are established primarily for administrative purposes.

Bibliography

1. Ministry of Health, *The standardisation of hospital medical records*. HMSO, London (1965).
2. Scottish Home and Health Department, *Hospital medical records in Scotland*. HMSO, Edinburgh (1967).
3. Information Services Division, Common Services Agency for the Scottish Health Service, *Cancer registration and survival statistics—Scotland 1963*. ISD, Edinburgh (1981).
4. Nuffield Provincial Hospital Trust, *Hospital and community: Hospital treated sickness amongst the people of Stirlingshire*. London (1948).
5. Nuffield Provincial Hospital Trust, *Hospital and community: Hospital treated sickness amongst the people of Ayrshire*. London (1949)
6. Roger, F. H., *The minimum basic data set for hospital statistics in the EEC*. Office for Official Publications of the European Communities, Luxembourg (1981).
7. Lockwood, E., The accuracy of Scottish hospital morbidity data. *Br. J. prevent. Social Med.* **25,** 76–83 (1971).
8. Information Services Division, Common Services Agency for the Scottish Health Service, Scottish hospital in-patient statistics. Edinburgh (annually).
9. Information Services Division, Common Services Agency for the Scottish Health Service, *Scottish mental health statistics*. Edinburgh (annually).
10. Information Services Division, Common Services Agency for the Scottish Health Service, *Scottish health statistics*. HMSO, Edinburgh.
11. WHO, *Manual for the international statistical classification of diseases, injuries, and causes of death*. WHO, Geneva (1978).
12. Nimmo, A. W., Alexander, E., Innes, G., and Paterson, J. G., Computerised mapping of health data. *Hlth Bull.* (Edinburgh) **42,** 4, 199–208 (1984).
13. Nimmo, A. W., and Innes, G., A survey of in-patients from the oil related industries in north-east Scotland. *Hlth Bull.* **37.1,** 20–3 (1979).
14. Moir, D. C., Alexander, E. R., Barnett, J. W., and Christopher, L. J., A hospital-based drug information system. *Hlth Bull.* **33,** 82–8 (1975).
15. Coull, D. C., Crooks, J., Davidson, J. F., Gallon, S. C., and Weir, R. D., A method for monitoring drugs for adverse reactions: I. Methyldopa in haemolytic anaemia. *Eur. J. clin. Pharmacol.* **3,** 46–50 (1970).
16. Coull, D. C., Crooks, J., Dingwall-Fordyce, I., Scott, A. M., and Weir, R. D., A method of monitoring drugs for adverse reactions: II. Amitriptyline and cardiac disease. *Eur. J. clin. Pharmacol.* **3,** 51–5 (1970).
17. Information Services Division, Common Services Agency for the Scottish Health Service, *Out-patient information systems—a feasibility study*. ISD, Edinburgh (1983).
18. Baldwin, J. A., Innes, G., Millar, W. M., Sharp, G. A., and Dorricott, N., A psychiatric case register in north-east Scotland. *Br. J. Prevent. social Med.* **19,** 38–42 (1965).
19. Petrie, J. C. *et al.*, A computer assisted patient record system. Lecture notes in medical informatics. *Proc. Med. Informatics Europe* **82,** pp. 41–7. Springer-Verlag, New York (1982).
20. Petrie, J. C., Robb, O. J., Webster, J., Scott, A. K., Jeffers, T. A., and Park, M. D., Computer assisted shared care in hypertension. *Br. med. J.* **290,** 1960–1962 (1985).

21. Hedley, A. J., Scott, A. M., and Debenham, G., A computer-assisted follow-up register. *Meth. Inform. Med.* **8,** 67 (1969).
22. Hedley, A. J. *et al.*, Breast cancer in thyroid disease: Fact or fallacy. *Lancet* **1,** 131–133 (1981).

7

Surveillance systems from primary-care data: surveillance through a network of sentinel general practitioners

A. STROOBANT, V. VAN CASTEREN, AND G. THIERS

Introduction

The continuous gathering of data from general practitioners has been successfully organized in the United Kingdom and The Netherlands by means of a sentinel-network.[1,2,3] A similar system was introduced in Belgium in 1978.[4] From 1979 till 1985 there have been four successive registration programmes. Some health problems, such as measles and mumps, are being studied continuously because of their vulnerability through vaccination. In fact, only continuous registration allows confirmation of the trends of the disease and verification of the impact of the vaccination. Other health problems for which no changes are predicted in the short-term are included only in an annual programme. The aim is to determine the level of incidence and the most important characteristics, which can then be compared at regular intervals. The present chapter aims to describe the organisation of the sentinel-network and to analyse the functioning of the Belgian sentinel-general practitioner-network in its present form.

Materials and Methods

Principles of registration

The development of the registration-network is based upon five principles:

1. The participation of the sentinel general practitioners (SGP) is voluntary;
2. the participants are representative of Belgian general practitioners (BGP) and their geographic distribution ensures a homogeneous coverage of the country;
3. the registration is continuous, with weekly reporting, and is of limited duration, generally a period of one year;
4. the identity of the patient is unknown;
5. the results are sent to the participants in quarterly reports.

Criteria for sampling GPs

The voluntary participation of 150 GPs is needed to cover a sufficient cross-section of the population ($\pm$ 150 000), so that statistical data can be obtained. For that purpose a large number of GPs of both sexes ($\pm$ 1500) of all ages and from all over the country were contacted.

At the end of the programme the sample of practitioners will be structured according to three criteria:

– participation for more than 26 of the 52 weeks of the registration period. It appears that above this limit the number of participating practitioners hardly varies (criterion of regularity);
– aged over 29 (criterion of medical practice). According to the most recent surveys,[5] medical practice amongst young general practitioners is strongly reduced. Therefore young GPs should not be considered as representative;
– otherwise representative of Belgian general practitioners according to age and sex.

Choice of administrative entities

Through the application of two hierarchical clustering procedures, the initial number of 43 districts in the country (the smallest administrative entities for which relevant statistical data of epidemiology are available) was reduced to 15 homogeneous district clusters.[6] Each administrative entity was characterized by a well-defined profile based on a relatively compact set of criteria. The purpose of the cluster-analysis was to compare these profiles and to place entities into groups or clusters in such way that entities in a given cluster were similar to each other, and those in different clusters dissimilar.[7] These 15 homogeneous district clusters represented the new geographical framework for analysis purposes.

The criteria for defining the socio-demographical profile of an administrative entity were: rate of urbanization, population of children under 14, population over 65, female population, percentage of immigrants, percentage of unemployed workers registered with social security, number of yearly patient-contacts per GP and per paediatrician, total amount of income, number of doctors between 30 and 39, number of GPs per 1000 inhabitants.

Denominator population

In Belgium there is no list of patients per practitioner, and each individual can choose whichever doctor he likes. Moreover, the participants could not be asked to keep a patient register, as has been done elsewhere,[8] for the workload was unacceptable; in Belgium most GPs work without a secretary. Because of these conditions the denominator population was estimated on the basis of the annual number of consultations and housecalls derived from the practice of the participating doctors. The population covered by an administrative entity was obtained by dividing the annual number of contacts of the SGPs of this entity by the average number of patient contacts per inhabitant and per year in the same entity. This last parameter was obtained on basis of the data collected by 'l'Institut National d'Assurance Maladie Invalidité', which collects the statistics of all health insurance organizations.

List of health problems

The list of health problems was established on the basis of these selective criteria:

1. They must belong to that category of problem for which the diagnosis or treatment is usually the responsibility of the GP.
2. They must be clinically identifiable without the intervention of a laboratory.
3. It must be possible to define the health problem in a clear and standardized way.
4. It must be judged an important health problem not otherwise under surveillance or notified.
5. It must be reasonably common so that the results remained statistically acceptable without representing too much administrative work.

The registration form consisted of a single sheet of paper printed recto–verso. The recto-side of the form contained the different items to be registered, together with some questions in relation to the identification and the activities of the doctor. The definitions for reference were given on the reverse.

A specific list of items was established for each health problem. It took into account the data essential for a satisfactory epidemiological description of the different problems. The items were arranged in a dichotomical way or according to multiple choice; the open items were reduced to the very minimum (Fig. 7.1). In this way the doctor could answer clearly and quickly by filling in the spaces corresponding to the items. These measures also facilitated the introduction of data. The nature of the problem and its supposed frequency determined the number of rows reserved for each health problem. The doctor used a second form if the weekly number was higher.

There was no item related to the patient's identity, thus guaranteeing the anonymity of the registration. The second part, which consisted of the registration of the doctor's activities, aimed to establish the total number of patient contacts during the registration-period. The distribution on the basis of days of the week and type of activity was exclusively intended to facilitate the registration of contacts by the doctor and its use was facultative (Fig. 7.2).

Tent. de suicide	1	2
âge		
sexe		
Situation professionnelle		
étudiant		
indépendant		
employé		
chômeur		
autre		
Etat civil		
célibataire		
marié		
veuf		
divorcé		
autre		
inconnu		

Moyen employé		
Issue fatale?		
oui		
non		
inconnue		
Hospitalization		
non		
Récidive		
oui		
non		
inconnue		
Remarques (se rapportant éventuellement aux semaines précédentes):		

Fig. 7.1. Example of a registration form. The nature of the problem and its supposed frequency determine the number of rows reserved for each health problem. For example, *tent. de suicide*: there is space for two cases (1 and 2). If the weekly number of cases is higher, the doctor uses a second form.

There was a space for the doctor's seal; a code-number given to each participant was also printed on the forms. There was one form for each week. It had the number and dates of the corresponding week to be registered. It was systematically sent back by the doctor, even if no case had occurred. The participants had sufficient forms for three months.

At the beginning of the programme, each doctor received instructions concerning the use of the form and the definition criteria for each registered health problem. Each doctor registered all health problems. From past experience we also knew that it was useful to put the instructions, namely the reference-definitions, on the reverse of the registration-form.

Morbidity was expressed as the number of cases per 1000 contacts and in terms of incidence. The rate of incidence per 10 000 inhabitants in each group was calculated using the distribution by age of the national population established by the National Institute of Statistics.[10]

No. Sem.	Lundi	Dimanche		Cachet Médecin
	Consultations	Visites à domicile	Total	
Lundi				
Mardi				
Mercredi				
Jeudi				
Vendredi				
Samedi				Pas d'enregistrement cette semaine en raison de:
Dimanche				
Total				

Fig. 7.2.   Registration form: data concerning practitioner activities.

Results

1. Doctor's participation

In 1983 the network consisted of 167 GPs at any given moment. 34 of these 167 GPs left during the first semester after less than 15 weeks of participation, a withdrawal rate of 18 per cent. Of the 133 participants remaining, 100 were selected according to criteria 2 and 3.

2. Representativity of the SGPs

Because their participation was voluntary, it was important to determine whether the SGPs had a particular profile and to what degree they were representative of the Belgian GPs. A set of questions was sent to the 100 participants to categorize them according to age, sex, year of graduation, and university. These data are also available for all Belgian doctors.

The average age of the SGPs (42.23 ± 11.57) was significantly different from the average age of the BGPs ($p < 0.05$). The difference between the age distribution of the SGPs and the BGPs over 29 was not statistically significant.[11] The sex distribution of the two groups likewise was not significantly different. The average number of weekly patient-contacts of the SGPs (123·77) was slightly less than that of the BGPs (133·20), taking into account holidays and non-attendances. The difference was most significant in Flanders.

The distribution of SGPs graduating from Dutch-speaking universities did not differ very much from that of BGPs graduating from these universities ($\chi^2_3 = 5.08$; $0.10 < p < 0.20$). On the other hand, the difference between SGPs

Table 7.1 Regional distribution of the total and network populations (at 30 June 1984) and population covered per region

Region	Total population	Network population	Population covered	
	(Proportional distribution)	(Proportional distribution)	(Absolute number)	(Percentage of region)
Flanders	57.55	56.67	60.905	1.1
Wallonia	32.60	32.45	35.257	1.1
Brussels	9.85	10.88	11.829	1.2

and BGPs was statistically significant for the French-speaking universities $\chi^2_2 = 11\cdot5; p < 0\cdot01$).

3. Geographical distribution of the SGPs

The 43 administrative entities were reduced to 15 district clusters and the percentage of population covered ranged from 0 to 20 per cent. 14 of the 15 clusters were covered by SGPs. In 10 clusters 1 per cent or more of the population was covered.

4. Population in the surveillance

The population covered by the network in 1984 was 107 991 persons, which equalled 1·11 per cent of the population of the Kingdom (based on the forecasts of the national statistical bureau (INS)).[12] The population covered in each Community was as shown in Table 7.1.

5. Programmes of registration

5.1. Studied Problems   On the basis of the selection criteria mentioned previously, a list of problems likely to be studied by the network of GPs was established (Table 7.2).

5.2. Work-load   In 1982–83, 7023 episodes were recorded by the SGPs, which represented 12 registrations per 1000 contacts, or 1·57 registrations per week and per GP.

5.3 Completeness of the Forms   Omission rates were calculated for certain general items: the age was not mentioned in 6 cases per 1000, sex in 3 per 1000 and civil status in 2 per 1000. More specific items had higher omission rates, varying from 3 to 12 per cent.

5.4 Continuity of Participation   A doctor who did not actively take part in

Table 7.2 List of problems selected according to the years, during which the programmes have been executed

Health problems	Years					
	1979	1980	1982	1983	1984	1985
Infectious diseases						
Gonorrhea	x	x				
Infectious mononucleosis					x	
Mumps			x	x	x	x
Measles	x	x	x	x	x	x
Herpes zoster					x	
Acute conjunctivitis	x	x				
Acute gastroenteritis	x	x				
Infectious hepatitis	x	x	x	x		
Urinary tract infections			x	x		
Acute respiratory infections						x
Meningitis	x	x				
Otitis media						
Pneumonia			x	x		
Infectious syphilis	x	x				
Urethritis			x	x		
Non-infectious diseases						
Cerebrovascular accident					x	
New cases of cancer						x
Asthma					x	
Chronic bronchitis						x
Cancer of the breast						x
Gastric/duodenal ulcer					x	
Acute myocardial infarction						x
Acute allergic manifestation						x
Diabetes mellitus						x
Behaviour-related problems						
Domestic accident					x	
Alcoholism					x	
Abortion			x	x		
Drug abuse					x	
'Morning-after' pill			x	x		
Attempted suicide			x	x		
Sports accidents					x	

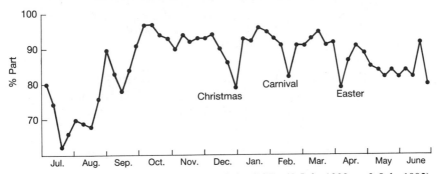

Fig. 7.3. Variation in the participation of the SGPs (5 July 1982 to 3 July 1983). (Source: Instituut voor Hygiëne en Epidemiologie, 1984.)

the registration for one or more weeks could indicate the reason on the registration form. In this way, it was possible to determine the actual number of weeks for which the doctor participated in the registration, whether or not there were cases reported. For a maximum of 5200 active weeks (100 doctors × 52 weeks) the 100 SGPs registered during 4467 weeks, 85·9 per cent of the period. The regularity of the participation can also be seen in Fig. 7.3 which shows that the percentage of participants outside the summer period always varied between 80 and 90 per cent.

The drop in participation of the SGPs coincides with the school holidays and other holiday periods. Figure 7.4 shows the same phenomenon occurring with the consultation rate of the patients.

5.5. Duration The average duration of a programme is 15 months. Usually the first 3 months of a registration present an opportunity for testing the

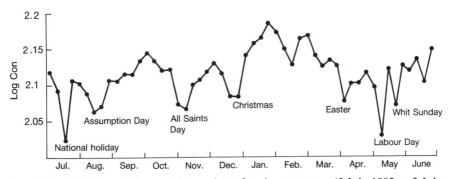

Fig. 7.4. Variation of the weekly number of patient contacts (5 July 1982 to 3 July 1983). (Source: Instituut voor Hygiëne en Epidemiologie, 1984.)

form and introducing any changes. It is also during this period that most withdrawals of participants occur. Only the data obtained in the 12 months following this trial period are analysed.

5.6. Cost The amount of data for analysis corresponds to the capacity of a microcomputer, the annual cost of which can be estimated at approximately £950, over 5 years. The other recurrent costs are stationery and postage, which equals £1250 per year. The personnel working on the programme have been calculated on the basis of full-time activity:

> Epidemiologist (doctor) :1
> Programmer :1/4
> Secretary-typist :1/2

6. Publication of the results

6.1. Quarterly Reports The quarterly report informs the participating doctors on the running of the surveillance network. It consists of two parts: the first part shows the results of the surveillance, namely the number of participating doctors, the absolute number of cases and their frequency per 100 contacts (Table 7.2). In the second part, each problem is discussed separately with concise presentation of the most significant results based on the raw data (Fig. 7.5).

These reports are sent not only to the participants but also to other interested parties, such as the Ministries of Public Health, Faculties of Medicine, professional organizations and medical press.

6.2. Synthesis Reports At the end of each annual programme the data are treated according to the criteria of representativity and the results are expressed in terms of incidence per 10 000 inhabitants. A detailed report is made for each health-problem and widely distributed.[13-20]

Discussion

A continuous morbidity registration by sentinel general practitioners has been working in Belgium since 1978. The use of such a system based on voluntary and selective reporting is unique in a country with a liberal organization of medical practice. This type of organization raises peculiar problems at the level of the choice and representativity of the participants and at the level of the population covered by the registration. Thus, one of the essential conditions for the quality and the continuity of the surveillance network is the voluntary character of the participation.[1] This condition precludes the randomized choice, as an appeal for volunteers inevitably attracts the most motivated GPs. This bias can be reduced by preserving the other cri-

Table 7.3 Quarterly results (Instituut voor Hygiëne en Epidemiologie, 1983, Report No. 1)

	Frequency of registered health problems		
	Total number	Per 100 contacts	Per 100 registered cases
1. Urinary infections	1095	0.73	57.8
2. Measles	198	0.13	10.5
3. Pneumonia	135	0.09	7.1
4. Urethritis	111	0.07	5.9
5. Mumps	106	0.07	5.6
6. Suicide	78	0.05	4.1
7. Abortion	71	0.03	3.7
8. Hepatitis	52	0.03	2.7
9. Morning after pill	48	0.03	2.5
	1894	1.27	100

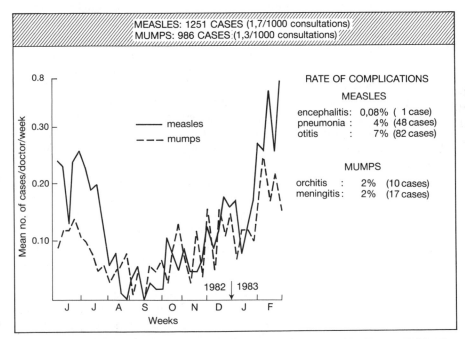

Fig. 7.5 Specific results of the network. (Source: Instituut voor Hygiëne en Epidemiologie, 1983, Report No. 4.)

teria of representativity of the practitioners such as geographical distribution, age, number of patient contacts, medical school, and by a wider distribution of requests for participation.[21]

Statistically, the group of SGPs appears to be comparable to the group of BGPs in all chosen criteria, except for the amount of work which is less with SGPs. But this difference, although statistically significant, is small and makes plausible the argument that only doctors with a reduced workload are willing to participate and fill in the forms.

Another guarantee for the representativity of the network is the homogeneous geographical distribution across the country. This has been readily realized by reconstructing on the basis of the 43 administrative entities of the country 15 clusters, representing each a homogeneous geographical unit according to a certain number of criteria, including the rate of urbanization. The network covers all the clusters and in 10 of them, 1 per cent or more of the population is represented, which guarantees a balance between the different regions. The aim to cover 1.5 per cent of the population has not yet been achieved, but this should be possible by improving publicity for the results.

Another difficulty is the estimate of the population observed by the SGPs. In the United Kingdom and The Netherlands each GP registers his patient population and this allows direct calculation of the population at risk and the incidence rate. When there is no list of patients, the most satisfactory alternative seems to be the number of patient contacts.[22] In this case the rate of contacts per 1000 inhabitants and per administrative entity during a year have been used. The chosen entity represents an interesting observation-unit for the analysis of the data for medical care in Belgium because the GP's practice is generally localized within the limits of this entity and the medicalization of the latter is homogeneous.[23] Obviously this method does not allow the representative nature of the covered population to be checked, but Crombie[24] has demonstrated that if the proportion of participating practitioners is sufficiently high, then their population is more closely related to the general population.

The quality of the participation of the SGPs was measured by the degree of completeness of the form and the continuity of the registration. Everything indicated an excellent level of participation. The forms had been carefully filled in and all of them could be used for processing the data. The omission rates for the different parameters were low and even more so where they formed part of the therapeutic and diagnostic approach. On the other hand, the SGPs registered for an average of 44 out of 52 weeks, or 85·9 per cent of the period taken into consideration. These 44 weeks corresponded with an effective surveillance period and did not include non-attendances because of holiday, illness, or omission. In The Netherlands, during the period 1975–82, the continuity rate expressed in percentages of registration days varied between 79·5 and 88·8 per cent.[25]

Another indication of the degree of motivation can be found in the fact that at the end of the programme 1982–83, 70 per cent of the SGPs renewed their participation in the new programme 1983–84.

The motivation of the participants was certainly reinforced by various factors such as the voluntary character of the participation, the anonymity of the registration, the regular change of the programmes, the feedback by quarterly reports, and a moderate work-load. The latter represented 12 registrations per 1000 contacts, which equalled an average of 1·57 registrations per week and per GP, which was sufficient to interest the practitioner without overloading him.

Bibliography

1. Bres, P., Les méthodes modernes de surveillance des maladies transmissibles: introduction générale. *Rev. Epidém. et Santé Publ.* **25**, 351–9 (1977).
2. Royal College of General Practitioners, Collective research in general practice. Influenza. *J. R. Coll. gen Pract.* **27**, 544–51 (1977).
3. Collete, B. J. A., The sentinel practices system in The Netherlands. In *Environmental epidemiology* (ed. P. E. Leaverton). Praeger Publishers, New York (1982).
4. Thiers, G., Maes, R., Van Lierde, R., Heyrman, J., Peeters, H., Minne, A., and Pattyn, S., Surveillance van besmettelijke ziekten door een net van peilpraktijken. *Tijdschrift voor Geneeskunde* **12**, 781–94 (1979).
5. Leroy, X., Densité et activité des médecins en Belgique, situation actuelle évolution et perspectives. *Cah. Socio Démo med.*, 157–81 (1984).
6. Anderberg, M. R., *Cluster analysis for applications.* Academic Press, New York (1973).
7. Hartigan, J. A., *Clustering algorithms.* John Wiley, New York (1975).
8. Sheldon, M. G., Rector, A. L., and Barnes, P. A., The accuracy of age–sex registers in general practice. *J. R. Coll. gen. Pract.* **34**, 269–71 (1984).
9. Leroy, X., *L'accès aux soins médicaux III. Données régionales d'offre et de consommation en 1979.* Rapport du Service d'Etudes Socio-économiques de la Santé, réf. D-1983-2735-1, p. 71 (1983).
10. Institut National de Statistique., Recensement de la population et des logements au 1er mars 1981. *Résultats généraux* **1**, 76–95 (1982).
11. Leroy, X., *Fichier socio-démographique des médecins.* Service d'Etudes Socio-économiques de la Santé. Université Catholique de Louvain, 1200 Brussels (1985).
12. Nationaal Instituut voor de Statistiek., *Bevolkingsvooruitzichten, 1981–2025, Deel I, Methodologie en voornaamste resultaten* (1985).
13. Thiers, G., Stroobant, A., Van Lierde, R., Heyrman, J., and Lafontaine, A., Epidémiologie de la rougeole en Belgique. *Arch. B. Méd. Soc., Hyg., Méd. Tr. et Méd. Lég.* **41**, 329–340 (1983).
14. Thiers, G. and Stroobant, A., Enregistrement de données de morbidité par un réseau de médecins généralistes. *Arch. B. Méd. Soc., Hyg., Méd. Tr. et Méd. Lég.* **42**, 3849 (1984).
15. Stroobant, A. and Thiers, G., Surveillance continue de la morbidité par un reseau de médecins "vigies". *Médecine Sociale Préventive* **29**, 276–9 (1984).

16. Stroobant, A., Lamotte, J. M., Van Casteren, V., Cornelis, R., Walckiers, D., and Colyn, Y., Epidemiological surveillance of measles through a network of sentinel general practitioners in Belgium. *Int. J. Epidemiol.* **15,** 386–91 (1986).

17. Stroobant, A., Piot, P., Meheus, A., and Fontaine, J., Les urétrites chez l'homme en Belgique. Résultats de l'enregistrement par un réseau de médecins généralistes. *Rev. Epidém. et Santé Publ.* **33,** 432–6 (1985).

18. Van Casteren, V., Surveillance van de morbiditeit in België door huisartsenpeil-praktijken. Programma 1983–1984 (vervolg). *Huisarts Nu 4, 144 (1985).*

19. Van Casteren, V., Cornelis, R., Stroobant, A., and Walckiers, D., Urinaire infecties in de Belgische huisartsenpraktijk. *Tijdschr. voor Geneeskunde* **42,** 523–9 (1986).

20. WHO, Surveillance des oreillons. Belgique. *Relevé Epidém. hebd.* **32,** 250–1 (1985).

21. Lobet, M. P., Stroobant, A., Mertens, R., Van Casteren, V., Walckiers, D., Masuy-Stroobant, G., and Cornelis, R., Tool of validation of the network of sentinel general practitioners in the Belgian health care system. *Int. J. Epidemiol.* (in press).

22. McWhinney, I. R., Research implications of the Virginia study. In *Content of family practice* (ed. J. P. German), pp. 13–14. Appleton-Century-Crofts, New York (1976).

23. Leroy, X., *Offre et consommation de soins de médecine générale. Analyse régionale. Mécanismes du marché. Indicateurs de besoins.* Rapport pour la Commission Interministérielle de la Politique Scientifique, Bruxelles, 164 pp, réf. XL04 (1978).

24. Crombie, D. L., Research and confidentiality in general practice. *J. R. Coll. gen. Pract.* **23,** 863 (1973).

25. Continue morbiditeits Registratie, Peilstations. *Stichting Nederland Huisarsen-instituut, Ministerie van Welzijn, Volksgezondheid en Cultuur* (ed.). Drukkerij Boeijinga BV, Apeldoorn, 15–18 (1982).

8

Surveillance systems from primary-care data: from a prevalence-oriented to an episode-oriented epidemiology

H. LAMBERTS AND E. SCHADE

The Use and Relevance of the International Classification of Primary Care (ICPC): Introduction

There is ample support for the need for a shift in the orientation of health-information systems and health-services research.[1–5] Whilst the quantity of available information is overwhelming, its quality and structuring, however, often prohibit practical use. It is a paradox that in many countries the cost of health care is generally considered to be too high, while at the same time very little information is available indicating which intervention for which patient at which point during an episode of a defined disease could be considered too expensive, useless, or even dangerous. Without taking into account the patient's original complaint, making diagnoses almost automatically implies medical intervention. The original complaint is then not properly interpreted and coding and classification occurs through the ICD.[6]

White advocates a restucturing of the classification systems used in health care.[3] Depending on where you look and whom you consult, there are anywhere from 17 to about 3000 and even tens of thousands of different 'labels' to assign to the health problems that beset mankind. For our diverse manifestations of ill health and related suffering, there are lay and colloquial terms; there are symptoms, complaints, and problems, there are functional and feeling states, there are chromosomal, molecular, behavioural aberrations, there are impairments, handicaps, and disabilities, there are accidents, injuries, and poisonings, there are fetal deaths and 'voodoo' deaths, and then, there are diseases. The original classification, the International Classification of Diseases, Injuries and Causes of Death the ICD, on the other hand has simply grown in complexity and heterogeneity; in trying to satisfy everybody, it now satisfies nobody. Through nine revisions, at roughly ten-year intervals, the current edition consists of seventeen chapters based on unrelated axes devoted to body systems, clinical manifestations, age-groups, clinical specialities, and known or suspected aetiological 'causes'.

There is no coherent conceptual or organizational theme, to say nothing of theory, and yet this classification and its modifications seek to meet the needs of policy-makers, statisticians, insurance organizations, managers, clinicians, and investigators of all persuasions and preoccupations in a wide range of socio-economic and cultural settings around the world.

One of the first signs of a change in the orientation of health information systems was the implementation of sentinel practices, a strategy which originated in England in 1968. Since 1970 a network of sentinel practices using 45 general practitioners has also functioned in The Netherlands covering about 1 per cent of the population. Apart from this national network, local sentinel systems have been organized by the municipal health services of three big cities: Amsterdam, The Hague, and Rotterdam.[7] The idea of gaining insight into the occurrence of certain diseases and their trends over periods of time with the help of data from general practice has also affected other countries. In the USA and Canada the 'Ambulatory Sentinel Practice Network' has been established, while in Belgium, England, France, Switzerland, Israel, and Australia general practitioners participate in a disease surveillance system.[7-10]

Apart from sentinel systems, especially in England and in the Netherlands, general practitioners collect comprehensive data on all morbidity presented to them over a longer period, such as one year.[10-12] Official notification systems often result in incomplete data, while clinical information from general practice provides far more reliable data on the incidence of common diseases. With direct surveillance in general practice, using multiplier factors, infectious diseases among others can be monitored on a national basis. In various countries multiplier factors have been calculated for diseases such as hepatitis A, measles, gonorrhoea, whooping cough, and infectious gastroenteritis, in order to correct official data. These factors vary in magnitude from 1·5 to over 100. They also can change considerably over a period of time.

General practitioners have thus proved able to provide information quickly on shifts in patterns, as, for example, on the disappearance of measles, the extent of influenza epidemics or on the recurrence of whooping cough. The emphasis on the distribution of infectious diseases has been succeeded by attention to non-infectious diseases, for example 'life-style diseases' and to the potential for prevention of these. In addition the need for information on problems such as contraception, abortion, sports-injuries, diabetes, the use of tranquillizers, depression, and suicidal behaviour is growing. Morbidity data from general practitioners apparently form an essential link in the chain of sources of information necessary for health statistics. This chain, which is available now in several countries, is limited at best to a prevalence-oriented epidemiology based on the structure of the ninth revision of ICD (Fig. 8.1).[6] However, when tested in practice, this chain has proved to be weak.

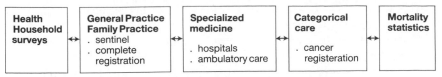

Fig. 8.1. A prevalence-oriented information chain.

The analysis of diagnosis-related information from the primary care setting has drawn two important conclusions:

1. *Numerator problems*—the quality of the classification itself—tend to be underestimated, while *denominator problems*—the exact sex/age composition of the population for which incidences and prevalences are calculated—tend to be overestimated. Lack of definitions for the use of diagnostic rubrics and, even more so, lack of understanding of the relationship between the patient's request for care and the doctor's diagnostic interpretation hamper the interpretation of clinical data. This is especially evident when very reliable data from a well-defined denominator population are available which, then, cannot be readily compared with data collected in another link of the information chain (Fig. 8.1). The high price of a very reliable denominator often does not result in equally reliable clinical interpretation of the findings.

2. *Encounter-based diagnostic information*[13] is insufficient for the interpretation of large variations in prevalence and utilization of health care, both within and between the links in the information chain.

The understanding of the differences in clinical judgement amongst primary-care physicians and specialists when they treat patients with diseases such as diabetes, hypertension, depression, or chronic respiratory disease, is limited because we lack sufficient knowledge of the natural history of disease, systematically collected during complete episodes.[14] This also applies when we want to judge the quality and appropriateness of medical care as it is provided during each phase of an episode, because the relationship between the demands of the patient, the diagnostic interpretation by the physician, and the medical intervention which is the consequence of both, is not clear.[15,16]

WONCA (World Organisation of National Colleges, Academies and Academic Associations of General Practitioners/Family Physicians) provides the forum for general practitioners/family physicians to co-operate and conduct research with regard to the above mentioned problems. As a consequence several Primary Care classifications have been developed and field tested. ICHPPC-1, ICHPPC-2, ICHPPC-2-Defined, and IC-Process-PC, together with the International Glossary of Primary Care, form the basis of ICPC as a comprehensive system to classify simultaneously three of the four elements of the problem oriented SOAP-registration:[17–24]

1. S for *Subjective experience* by the patient of his problem, his demand for care and his reason for encounter.
2. A for *Assessment* or *diagnostic interpretation* of the patient's problem by the provider.
3. P for *Process of care*, representing the diagnostic and therapeutic interventions.

Objective findings—0—cannot be classified with ICPC.

Structure of ICPC

ICPC is a simple, two-axial classification system with mnemonic qualities, facilitating its day-to-day use both by physicians and other primary-care providers (Fig. 8.2). It can be used for decentralized coding with handwritten records as well as for central coding in a computerized system.[21]

Seventeen chapters each with an alpha code, form one axis, while seven components with rubrics bearing a two-digit numeric code form the second axis.

The system was strongly influenced by experiences with other classifications (Fig. 8.3).

1. Component 1, symptoms and complaints, drew upon the experience of the National Ambulatory Medical Care Survey/Reason for Visit Classification (NAMCS/RVC) and on the results of the field trial of the Reason for Encounter Classification, which has now been replaced by ICPC.[15,16,25–27]
2. Components 2–6 contain the main rubrics of the new *International Classification of Process in Primary Care*[20] and are identical throughout the chapters.
3. The classification of psychological and social problems developed by the WHO sponsored Tri-axial Classification Group are virtually duplicated in chapters P and Z.[28]
4. The rubrics of ICHPPC-2-Defined, the ICD-9 compatible diagnostic classification system for primary care, are virtually all distributed over component 7.[19] In ICPC, however, morphology and localization (body systems) take precedence over aetiology so that infectious diseases, neoplasms, injuries, and congenital abnormalities do not form separate chapters as in ICD-9, but are represented in component 7 of each chapter, as is illustrated by vertical lines in Fig. 8.3.

The nomenclature of ICPC forms a bridge between the highly specialized ICD-9 compatible classification systems on the one hand, and lay terminology and common descriptions of symptoms, complaints, and health problems in the community on the other.[29]

	A – General	B – Blood, blood forming	D – Digestive	F – Eye	H – Ear	K – Circulatory	L – Musculoskeletal	N – Neurological	P – Psychological	R – Respiratory	S – Skin	T – Metabolic Endocrine, Nutr.	U – Urinary	W – Pregnancy Childbearing Family planning	X – Female genital	Y – Male genital	Z – Social
1. Symptoms and complaints																	
2. Diagnostic, screening prevention																	
3. Treatment procedures, medication																	
4. Test results																	
5. Administrative																	
6. Other																	
7. Diagnoses disease																	

Fig. 8.2. Biaxial structure of the International Classification of Primary Care.

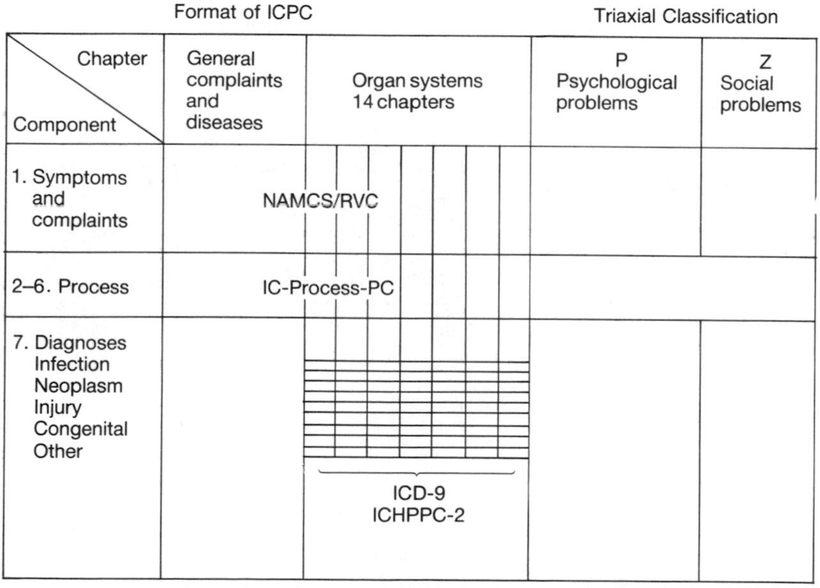

	Format of ICPC			Triaxial Classification	
Chapter / Component	General complaints and diseases	Organ systems 14 chapters		P Psychological problems	Z Social problems
1. Symptoms and complaints	NAMCS/RVC				
2–6. Process	IC-Process-PC				
7. Diagnoses Infection Neoplasm Injury Congenital Other		ICD-9 ICHPPC-2			

Fig. 8.3. Format of ICPC in relation to other classification systems.

Table 8.1 Illustration of the conversion of a main ICPC title and its synonyms to ICHPPC-2, RCGP, and ICD-9

ICPC	ICHPPC-2	RCGP	ICD-9
D73 Other presumed infectious gastrointestinal diseases	002	0015	−008.8
			−009.0
			−009.1
			−009.3
			−009.5
− food poisoning unspec.	002	0015	009−
− food poisoning infectious unspec.	002	0015	009.3
− gastric flu	002	0015	008.8
− infectious gastro-enteritis unspec.	002	0015	009.1
− infectious enteritis unspec.	002	0015	009.1
− infectious colitis unspec.	002	0015	009.0

A conversion of all ICPC rubrics, including approximately 5000 synonyms forming its thesaurus, to the corresponding rubrics of ICHPPC-2, the Classification of Royal College of General Practitioners of the UK and to ICD-9 has recently been completed (Table 8.1).[30] This conversion is available on tape and will be developed in the near future to allow automatic coding with ICPC—and if desired with the three other systems—when a computer system is being used to replace the patient's record.

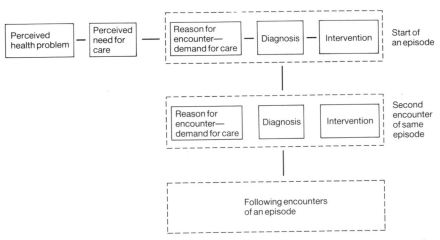

Fig. 8.4. An episode of a health problem—the relation between reason for encounter, diagnosis, and intervention.

Use of ICPC as a 'Reason for Encounter' Classification

The reason for encounter (RFE) is defined as the statement of the reason why a person enters the health-care system with a demand for care. It forms the basic formulation of the patient's subjective need and actual demand for care as it is clarified, understood and classified by the provider and to which he responds with a diagnosis and with a medical intervention (Fig. 8.4 and Table 8.2). Most reasons for encounter are classified in the first component of ICPC (symptoms and complaints) although all components can be used. ICPC has

Table 8.2   The first and the seventh components of chapter D, to be used both as an RFE and as a diagnostic classification

---

D—Digestive

Component 1—Symptoms and Complaints

D01	Generalized abdominal pain/cramps
D02	Stomach ache/stomach pain
D03	Heartburn
D04	Rectal/anal pain
D05	Perianal itching
D06	Other localized abdominal pain
D08	Flatulence, gas pain, belching, wind
D09	Nausea
D10	Vomiting (excl. blood D14/Pregnancy W06)
D11	Diarrhoea
D12	Constipation
D13	Jaundice
D14	Hematemesis/vomit blood
D15	Melaena/black, tarry stools
D16	Rectal bleeding
D17	Incontinence of bowel (faecal)
D18	Change in faeces/bowel movements
D19	Sympt./complt. teeth, gums
D20	Sympt./complt. mouth, tongue, lips
D21	Swallowing problems
D22	Worms/pinworms/other parasites
D24	Abdominal mass (not otherwise specified)
D25	Change in abdominal size/distension
D26	Fear of cancer of digestive system/organ
D27	Fear of other digestive disease
D28	Disability/impairment
D29	Other sympt./complt. digest.

---

continued

Table 8.2   *cont.*

Component 7—Diagnosis/Diseases

D70	Infectious diarrhoea, dysentery
D71	Mumps
D72	Infectious hepatitis
D73	Other presumed infections of digestive system

D74	Malign. neopl. stomach
D75	Malign. neopl. colon, rectum
D76	Malign. neopl. pancreas
D77	Malign. neopl. other and unspecified sites
D78	Benign neoplasms

D79	Foreign body through orifice
D80	Other injuries

D81	Congenital anomalies digestive system

D82	Disease of teeth/gums
D83	Disease of mouth/tongue/lips
D84	Disease of oesophagus
D85	Duodenal ulcer
D86	Other peptic ulcers
D87	Disorders of stomach function/gastritis
D88	Appendicitis
D89	Inguinal hernia
D90	Hiatus (diaphragm) hernia
D91	Other abdominal hernia
D92	Diverticular disease intestines
D93	Irritable bowel syndrome
D94	Chronic enteritis/ulcerative colitis
D95	Anal fissure/perianal abscess (excl. pilonidal cyst S85)
D96	Hepatomegaly
D97	Cirrhosis/other liver disease
D98	Cholecystitis/cholelithiasis
D99	Other disease digestive syst. (excl. hemorrhoids K96)

---

been tested in the RFE mode for approximately 100 000 RFEs, classified by 100 providers in 12 developed and developing countries.[15,16] Additional studies support the feasibility and relevance of classifying the patient's demand for care. The reliability of coding the RFE is not less than that of the diagnosis. Its validity from the patient's point of view however, is not known;

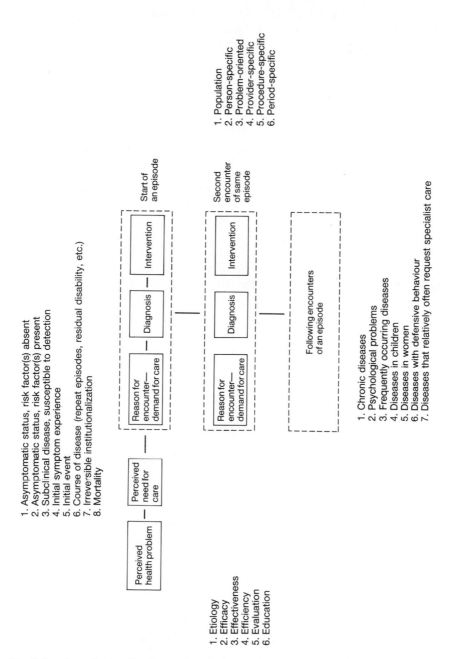

Fig. 8.5. An episode of a disease in relation to four central issues of health services research.

its validity from the provider's point of view is reflected in its relation—or lack of relation—to the diagnosis and the intervention which are the consequence of the patient's demand for care as it is understood by the provider (Fig. 8.5).

ICPC as a Diagnostic Classification

In ICPC, body systems take precedence over aetiology so that chapter A (general) is the last chapter to be considered when coding a disease which because of its aetiology can be found in several chapters. All chapters provide specific rubrics, which include both aetiology and the body system or organ involved in the diseases. The first component can be used in the diagnostic mode if the provider considers this to be convenient. Users are encouraged to record during each encounter the full spectrum of diagnoses in their practice, including organic, psychological, and social health problems. Formulations should be recorded at the highest possible level of diagnostic refinement, but never more specifically than can be defended by the inclusion criteria contained in ICHPPC-2-Defined for that rubric (Table 8.2).

ICPC as a Process Classification

The *International Classification of Process in Primary Health Care* is the latest product of the Classification Committee of WONCA.[20] Its feasibility has been confirmed in an international field test with approximately 80 000 encounters. The structure and the major rubrics of IC-Process-PC are duplicated in the central components 2–6 of ICPC (Table 8.3). Because the process rubrics can also be used to classify the reason for encounter, ICPC allows a broader approach to patient-oriented information.

An Episode-Oriented Health-Information System

Complete episodes of diseases form a very attractive principle to organize patient-oriented health-information systems.[1–5] For this purpose ICPC can be used to collect, to enter, to organize, and to analyse clinical information on episodes of diseases over periods of time.

An episode is defined as a problem or illness in a patient from its onset to its resolution over the entire period of time.[19] Figures 8.4 and 8.5 represent the elements of an episode which can be classified with the help of ICPC: the reasons for encounter, the diagnoses, and the diagnostic and therapeutic interventions. The health problem and the need for care as they are perceived in the population before the start of an episode in the context of health care, is the subject of health-and household-surveys and can be linked if ICPC is consequently used.

Table 8.3 Process components of the ICPC

Standard Process Components of ICPC

The dash (—) shown in the first position must be replaced with the appropriate alpha code for each chapter.

Component 2—Diagnostic and preventive procedures

– 30	Medical examination/health evaluation—complete
– 31	Medical examination/health evaluation—partial
– 32	Sensitivity test
– 33	Microbiological/immunological test
– 34	Blood test
– 35	Urine test
– 36	Faeces test
– 37	Histological/exfoliative cytology
– 38	Other laboratory test NEC
– 39	Physical function test
– 40	Diagnostic endoscopy
– 41	Diagnostic radiology/imaging
– 42	Electrical tracings
– 43	Other diagnostic procedures
– 44	Preventive immunizations/medications
– 45	Observation/health education/advice/diet
– 46	Consultation with primary-care provider
– 47	Consultation with specialist
– 48	Clarification/discussion of patient's RFE/demand
– 49	Other preventive procedures

Component 3—Medication, treatment, therapeutic procedures

– 50	Medication–prescription/request/renewal/injection
– 51	Incision/drainage/flushing/aspiration/removal body fluid (excl. catheterization–53)
– 52	Excision/removal tissue/biopsy/destruction/debridement/cauterisation
– 53	Instrumentation/catheterization/intubation/dilation
– 54	Repair/fixation-suture/cast/prosthetic device (apply/remove)
– 55	Local injection/infiltration
– 56	Dressing/pressure/compression/tamponade
– 57	Physical medicine/rehabilitation
– 58	Therapeutic counselling/listening
– 59	Other therapeutic procedures/minor surgery, NEC

---

continued

Table 8.3   *cont.*

Component 4—Results

– 60	Results tests/procedures
– 61	Results examination/test/record/letter from other provider

---

Component 5—Administrative

– 62	Adminstrative procedure

Component 6—Referrals and other reasons for encounter

– 63	Follow-up encounter unspecified
– 64	Encounter/problem initiated by provider
– 65	Encounter/problem initiated by other than patient/provider
– 66	Referral to other provider/nurse/therapist/social worker/(excl. MD)
– 67	Referral to physician/specialist/clinic/hospital
– 68	Other referrals NEC
– 69	Other reason for encounter NEC

Focusing on episodes as they can be documented in primary health care settings, 4 issues are important:

(a) the several stages of an episode, with its inherent prognosis and with its impact on the functional status of patients;[31]
(b) the epidemiological orientation of the available information: the 6 Es;[32,33]
(c) the orientation of statisitics: the 6 Ps;[32,33]
(d) the major determinants of professional behaviour of general practitioners.[12]

These issues provide the framework for an effective interpretation of data classified with ICPC and also for an efficient selection of episodes—characterized with ICPC—for limited research endeavours as in sentinel practice.

Discussion

The *International Classification of Primary Care* (ICPC) together with its manual and the International Glossary of Primary Care, offers general practitioners as well as epidemiologists, health statisticians and health service researchers, an attractive way of collecting, classifying, organizing, and ana-

Table 8.4

Example

A sixty-year-old male patient presents with vomiting and abdominal pain of two days duration. There is no fever but he also complains of pain in both knees, in his left wrist and some visible swelling, for which he seeks attention.

Reason for encounter	
Abdominal pain	D01
Vomiting	D10
Pain and swelling of wrist	L11
Knee pain	L15

Process	
Partial examination of the digestive tract	D31
Partial examination of the left wrist	L31
X-rays of wrist and knee	L41
Medication prescribed for arthritis	L50

Diagnosis	
Gastro-enteritis	D73
Arthritis	L91

Fig. 8.6. Example of the copying encounter form which allows comprehensive use of ICPC.

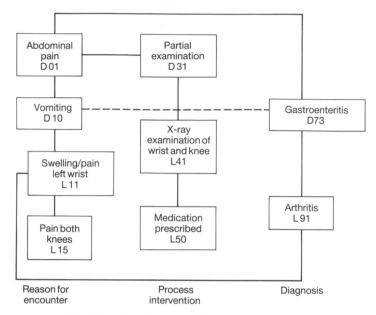

Fig. 8.7   Data linkage within a single encounter.

lysing medical problems. Patient information, which is structured with ICPC, is open to an approach based on four important issues in health services research: data linkage within single encounters and within the string of encounters, forming an episode, becomes easier with ICPC, because the relationship between the patient's demand, the diagnosis and the medical interventions can be dealt with in a logical and straightforward manner and without losing information beforehand, as data storage, analysis, and interpretation become less cumbersome (see Table 8.4 and Figs 8.6 and 8.7).

ICPC is also important for health statistics and health-services research because it makes it easier to aim at episode-oriented data, where important constraints for data collection exist. If one wishes to focus on a limited number of diseases, observed over a limited time as in sentinel practices, the information can still be interpreted in conjunction with data from complete registration projects in general practice and from other sources such as household surveys and clinical information from out-patient and hospital settings.

Bibliography

1. Health Services Research 1984. Planning for the third decade of health services research. *Med. Care* **23,** special issue 377–750 (1985).
2. Variations in Medical Practice, special issue. *Hlth Affairs* **3,** 4–148 (1984).

3. White, K. L., Restructuring the International Classification of Diseases: Need for a new paradigm. *J. Fam. Pract.* **21,** 17–20 (1985).
4. Health Services Research on Primary Care, Program note. National Centre for Health Services Research and Health Care Technology Assessment. US Department of Health and Human Services, Atlanta, Georgia (1985).
5. Feinstein, A. R. *Clinical epidemiology: The architecture of clinical research.* Saunders, Philadelphia (1985).
6. *International Classification of Disease,* Ninth revision. WHO, Geneva (1977).
7. Collette, H. J. A. and Bijkerk, H. Vijftien jaar peilstations Nederland 1970–1984. *Huisarts en Wetenschap* **28,** 207–10 (1985).
8. Green, L. A., Wood, M., Becker, L. *et al.*, The ambulatory sentinel practice network: Purpose methods and policies. *J. Fam. Pract.* **18,** 275–80.
9. Instituut voor Hygiene en Epidemiologie, *Surveillance van de morbiditeit in België door de huisartsenpeilpraktijk: programma 1982–1983.* Ministerie van Volksgezondheid en van het Gezin, Brussels.
10. *Morbidity statistics for general practice,* Office of population censuses and surveys, Royal College of General Practitioners, London (1975).
11. *Continue Morbiditeitsregistratie NUHI 1971–1978 Gewone ziekten; een aantal morbiditeitsgegevens uit een viertal huisartspraktijken,* Nijmeegs Universitair Huisartsen Instituut, Nijmegen (1980).
12. Lamberts, H., *Morbidity in general practice: Diagnosis-related information from the monitoring project.* Huisartsenpers bv, Utrecht (1984).
13. Kilpatrick, S. J. and Boyle, R. M., (eds) *Primary care research: Encounter records and the denominator problem.* Praeger, New York (1984).
14. Brook, H. R. and Lohr, K. N , Efficacy, effectiveness, variations and quality. *Med. Care* **23,** 710–22 (1985).
15. Lamberts, H., Meads, S., and Wood, M., Classification of reasons why persons seek primary care: Pilot study of a new system. *Publ. Hlth Rep.* **99,** 597–605 (1984).
16. Lamberts, H., Meads, S. and Wood, M., Results of the international field trial with the reason for encounter classification. *Méd. Soc. Prév.* **30,** 80–7 (1985).
17. ICHPPC-2 (*International classification of health problems in primary care*). Oxford University Press (1979).
18. ICHPPC-2-Defined (inclusion criteria for the use of the rubrics of the *International Classification of Health Problems in Primary Care*). Oxford University Press (1983).
19. *An International Glossary for Primary Care,* Report of the classification committee of the World Organisation of National Colleges, Academies and Academic Associations of General Practitioners/Family Physicians (WONCA). *J. Fam. Pract.* **13,** 671–81 (1981).
20. *International Classification of Process in Primary Care* (IC-Process-PC). Oxford University Press (1986).
21. *International Classification of Primary Care* (ICPC), Manual for use of ICPC in relevance studies, as prepared by the WHO-working party on ICPC. Department of General Practice, University of Amsterdam (1985).
22. Wood, M., Family medicine classification systems in evolution. *J. Fam. Pract.* **12,** 199–200 (1981).
23. Froom, J., New directions in standard terminology and classifications for primary care. *Publ. Hlth Rep.* **99,** 73–77 (1984).

24. Weed, L., *Medical records. Medical Education and Patient Care. The problem-oriented record as a basic tool.* The Press of Case Western Reserve University,, Cleveland, Ohio (1969).

25. Meads, S., The WHO reason for encounter classification. *WHO Chron* **37,** 159–162 (1983).

26. *A reason for visit classification for ambulatory care,* US Public Health Service, National Center for Health Statistics, DHEW Publication 79, 1352 (1979).

27. *Patient's reasons for visiting physicians: National Ambulatory Medical Care Survey, US, 1977–1978.* Data from the National Health Survey, Hyattsville, Md: Series 13, 56, DHHS Publications 82, 1717 (1981).

28. Lipkin, M. and Kupka, K., (eds) *Psychosocial factors affecting health.* Praeger, New York (1982).

29. Kupka, K., *International Classification of Diseases*: Ninth revision. *WHO Chron.* **32,** 219–25 (1978).

30. Classification of diseases: Problems and procedures. Royal College of General Practitioners, London. Occasional paper 26 (1984).

31. Kasl, S. V., How can epidemiology contribute to the planning of Health Service Research? *Med. Care* **23,** 598–666 (1985).

32. White, K. L., Information for health care: An epidemiological perspective. *Inquiry* **17,** 296–312 (1980).

33. White, K. L., Evaluation of medicine. In *Evaluation of health care* (ed. W. W. Holland). Oxford University Press (1982).

9

Surveillance of perinatal morbidity

H. P. VERBRUGGE AND M. WOHLERT

Introduction

In Western countries perinatal mortality rates have decreased during the last decade.[1] No single factor seems to be responsible for this. Possible explanations have been sought in improved health among pregnant women, in a decrease in the number of births by very young and very old mothers, in the introduction of legal abortion, and in the improvement of preventive services during pregnancy. Changes in the organization and content of obstetrical services and health services concerning the new-born may also, of course, have contributed.[2,3,4,5]

Perinatal mortality yields but a limited picture of the health dynamics associated with pregnancy, birth, and the perinatal period. Thus the decisions to change structures or strategies in this health-service field should also be based on more comprehensive indicators of health including perinatal morbidity and morbidity in childhood.

At the same time, deaths among children born alive will be important end-points in morbidity studies. It is, of course, crucial that agreement is reached about morbidity as well as mortality terminology.

There is no generally accepted definition of the term 'perinatal morbidity'. Some of the subjects for perinatal epidemiological studies have been spontaneous abortion, congenital malformations (see Chapter 10), intrauterine growth retardation, spontaneous pre-term birth, perinatal death, and neonatal illnesses. Aetiological inferences from epidemiological studies require evidence concerning factors in the preconceptional period as well as during pregnancy. In other words, the perinatal period can only be understood as a consequence of a comprehensive, longitudinal process. Paradoxically, however, obstetricians generally consider, for instance, pre-term birth an *end-point*, whereas paediatricians view it as an *initial risk factor*. Perinatal surveillance should encompass both these views, which unfortunately originate from the over-specialized structure of health-care systems.

Perinatal care did not become the object of scientific attention in Western Europe till after the Second World War. Following Butler and Alberman's perinatal cohort study in Great Britain,[6,7] a number of epidemiological studies were carried out in different countries. These studies initially concentrated on perinatal mortality and the organization of health services. Later studies have concentrated on morbidity, along with the decrease in mortality. Improved perinatal care, however, does not always seem to be associated with improved health among the new-born, such as reductions in serious impairments. Close follow-up is thus essential to decide how much morbidity stems from reduced mortality and how much it owes to new or growing aetiological factors and to changes in the perinatal services.

Consequently the collection, analysis, and use of standard perinatal data sets for decisions concerning health care strategies are essential. Standardization across national borders as well as between regions in individual countries seems crucial to facilitate comparisons and to evaluate the outcome of different strategies.

Perinatal Morbidity

Perinatal morbidity stems from conditions and events such as:

(a) Chromosomal abnormalities
(b) Congenital malformations
(c) Pre-term birth
(d) Growth retardation ('small for dates')
(e) Neonatal disease
(f) Other conditions

Congenital malformations are discussed in Chapter 10.

Down's syndrome is the most prevalent condition among *congenital chromosomal abnormalities*, the prevalence being about 1 per 1000 newborn.[8] Important known risk factors are maternal age, a family history, and the existence of certain balanced chromosomal abnormalities in one of the parents. The prognosis of the disorder depends on the presence of malformations, especially cardiac malformations. Surgical treatment of cardiac malformations and antibiotic treatment of infections have reduced the high mortality among children with Down's syndrome. Other autosomal aberrations, for example Patau's syndrome[13] and Edward's syndrome[18] are so rare that their quantitative importance is negligible.

Surveillance of the prevalence of chromosomal abnormalities in newborns is performed in Aarhus County, Denmark.[9] Published evidence has shown among other things, that in spite of an increased screening activity among pregnant women with an anticipated raised risk of giving birth to children with Down's syndrome, the prevalence of the syndrome did not decrease from 1969–79 to 1980–82.[9] Comparisons of findings from amniocentesis and chromosomal examinations among newborns may lead to better management of the prenatal prevention of Down's syndrome.

Pre-term birth is defined by the WHO[10] as birth more than 21 days prior to term. The prevalence of children born pre-term varies according to period and region, from 4 to 6–7 per cent.[11–13] Comparisons are complicated by, for instance, the omission of information about induced deliveries being included or not. Known risk factors are primiparity, bleeding in pregnancy, frequent uterine contractions, maternal underweight, physical work during pregnancy, and previous pre-term delivery.[11,13–17] The importance of urogenital infections is still a matter of debate.[18]

Spontaneous pre-term birth is the most prevalent risk factor for perinatal death and it is, in addition, associated with neonatal morbidity in general as well as persistent handicaps.[12,19] Sick-leave during pregnancy is considered a crucial preventive measure. French studies especially have described specific measures to prevent pre-term birth, data from perinatal surveillance forming part of the information base for the discussion.[20] Further evidence should be gained from the combined use of surveillance data and observations from randomized control trials.

Newborns are defined as *growth-retarded* (*small for dates*) if their weight is below the gestational-week-specific tenth percentile. Some authors use other definitions, which complicates comparisons. Regional demographic and social variations are marked.[21] Generally, boys are heavier than girls, and children born to multiparae heavier than those born to primiparae. It is recommended that the estimation of growth retardation in a child is carried out after correction for gender but not for the parity of the mother.[22]

Important risk factors for growth retardation are low maternal weight prior to pregnancy, reduced weight gain during pregnancy, primiparity, hypertensive illness, and tobacco smoking during pregnancy.[11,22,23] Tobacco smoking has been found to be responsible for 30–40 per cent of all cases of growth retardation in one epidemiological study.[23] Identification of possible cases of growth retardation *in utero* is essential because of the increased risk of perinatal asphyxia, illness, and death.[24,25] Identification of high risk fetuses and relevant measures taken seem substantially to lower the risks mentioned.[11] Perinatal surveillance should lead to the production of national as well as regional gender-specific growth curves, forming the basis for the evaluation of preventive measures during pregnancy. However, as few as 26 per cent of babies with low birthweight for gestational age were identified antenatally in a case record review of randomly selected pregnancies.[26] Priority setting concerning the type of growth retardation—i.e. other anthropometric data such as length and circumference of the head and abdomen, is needed, leading to new ways of classifying types of growth retardation and, consequently, further insight into the bio-mechanisms leading to the conditions. This in turn would be the basis for more specific preventive strategies.

A variety of *illnesses* are prevalent among the newborn including hormonal, respiratory, vascular, and neurological illnesses, disorders, and those affecting other body systems. There are in addition general developmental problems and some related to general well-being. There is little information on which conditions or combinations of conditions are most likely to lead to illness and handicap later in life. Low Apgar score and low pH in umbilical artery blood, for instance, both seem to be predictors, although there is little evidence on the risk of neurological disorders.[27] Further paediatric research is needed to unveil the more specific perinatal indicators of later childhood morbidity, which are suitable for use as part of a perinatal surveillance system.

Surveillance Systems

The following text aims to give a brief overview of attempts to conduct surveillance of children in the perinatal period. The examples are chosen to illustrate different ways of collecting data. Perinatal surveillance systems can be categorized as national or regional, and both are described, as well as the mutual interaction of these systems.

National surveillance systems

The *Nordic countries* have built and organized their health-care systems along similar main lines. The medical notification of the outcome of pregnancy is common to all these countries and is organized in nationwide systems. The amount and type of information notified differs also to a certain extent, as does the technology used for data processing. All births are registered continuously. Fig. 9.1 gives an example of the data content of the surveillance systems in the Nordic countries.

Norway has formulated specific objectives for birth registration, namely:

1. The surveillance of:
    1.1. Morbidity and mortality among women in relation to pregnancy and childbirth.
    1.2. The incidence of congenital deformities, affliction, and injuries of the newborn.
    1.3. The incidence of spontaneous abortion and infant mortality.
2. To study the causal relationships in:
    2.1. Disease and mortality in pregnancy, childbirth, and the post-natal period.
    2.2. Congenital deformities, diseases, and injuries in the newborn
    2.3. Spontaneous abortion and infant mortality.
3. To organize for infants and young children a health service capable of search and follow-up by:
    3.1. Registration of infants with manifest and recognized deformities and injuries at birth.
    3.2. Registration of infants, who because of special circumstances at birth

Infant: Items registered	Denmark	Finland	Iceland	Norway	Sweden
Sex	⊕	⊕	⊕	⊕	⊕
Date and hour of birth	⊕	⊕	⊕	⊕	⊕
Place of birth	○	○	⊕	⊕	⊕
Type of birth institution	⊕	⊕	⊕	⊕	⊕
Single–multiple births	⊕	⊕	⊕	⊕	⊕
Multiple births coded	⊕	⊕	⊕	⊕	⊕
" " total	⊕	⊕	⊕	⊕	⊕
" " number of girls	⊕	⊕	⊕	⊕	⊕
" " number of still births	⊕	⊕	⊕	⊕	⊕
Live birth	⊕	⊕	⊕	⊕	⊕
Still birth:					
Death before/during delivery	⊕	⊕	⊕	⊕	⊕
Presentation of fetus	⊕	−	⊕	−	−
Birthweight	⊕	⊕	⊕	⊕	⊕
Length at birth	⊕	⊕	⊕	⊕	⊕
Birthweight versus duration of pregnancy	○	−	−	−	−
Head circumference	−	⊕	⊕	⊕	⊕
Congenital anomalies	⊕	−	⊕	⊕	⊕
Apgar score	⊕	−	−	⊕	⊕
Other diseases diagnosed in perinatal period	−	−	⊕	⊕	⊕

Items registered	Denmark	Finland	Iceland	Norway	Sweden
ANTENATAL VISITS: Number of examinations:					
by a general practitioner	⊕	−	−	−	⊕
" obstetrician	⊕	−	−	−	⊕
" midwife	⊕	−	−	−	⊕
" surgical department	⊕	−	−	−	⊕
" obstetrical "	⊕	−	−	−	⊕
No antenatal examinations	−	−	−	−	⊕
Total number of examinations	⊕	−	⊕	−	⊕
Number of pregnancies	⊕	⊕	○	⊕	⊕
" of induced abortions	⊕	⊕	⊕	○	⊕
" of spontaneous "	⊕	⊕	⊕	○	⊕
" of live births	⊕	⊕	⊕	⊕	⊕
" of still births	⊕	⊕	⊕	⊕	⊕
" of early neonatal deaths	−	−	−	−	⊕
Date at end of last pregnancy	−	⊕	−	−	⊕
First day of last menstruation	○	⊕	⊕	⊕	⊕
Length of pregnancy estimated correctly	⊕	−	−	−	⊕
Length of pregnancy — weeks	⊕	−	⊕	⊕	⊕
Diagnoses prior to pregnancy	−	−	⊕	⊕	⊕
" during "	−	−	⊕	⊕	⊕
Type of complications	⊕	−	⊕	⊕	⊕
Total number of complications	⊕	−	⊕	⊕	⊕
Intervention prior to delivery	⊕	−	−	⊕	⊕
" during delivery	⊕	−	⊕	⊕	⊕
Type of intervention	⊕	−	⊕	⊕	⊕
Total number of intervention during delivery	⊕	−	⊕	⊕	⊕
Weight of placenta	⊕	−	−	⊕	−
Pathology of placenta	−	−	−	⊕	−
Many white infarctions yes/no	⊕	−	−	−	−
Amniotic fluid	−	−	−	⊕	−
Umbilical cord. length/vessels et al.	○	−	−	⊕	−
Pain relief — type — anaesthesia	○	−	−	○	⊕
The mother related to the father of child	−	−	−	⊕	−

Key:
- − = Not registered
- ○ = Registered
- ⊕ = Registered and computerized

Fig. 9.1. Items registered by the perinatal surveillance systems in the Nordic countries. (Source: Births in the Nordic Countries. Registration of the Outcome of Pregnancy, 1979. NOMESKO, Reykjavik, 1982.)

or during pregnancy may be considered to be especially at risk of developing physical or psychological defects or functional impairments.

The notification systems used in the Nordic countries are described by NOMESKO.[28] Similarities and differences are discussed and also their implications for perinatal care. The inclusion of morbidity data in addition to information on mortality opens up possibilities for rational planning and resource allocation in the health-care sector. Results are published regularly if not quickly, from the surveillance systems.

In *France*, perinatal surveillance is based on representative samples of births in the nation as a whole. Surveys were carried out in 1975, 1976, and

1981, each based on a representative sample of births from public and private maternity units. The data comprised information on the course of pregnancy, living conditions, obstetric history—all observed by doctors and midwives. Information on the delivery and the neonatal period was added. Only 1 per cent of the women and two maternity units in the survey refused to co-operate. Data were obtained on 11 254, 4685, and 5508 births respectively. The official report from the studies[29] dealt with strategies for the development of prevention and care amongst other things.

In *Great Britain*, Butler *et al.*[6] conducted a nationwide survey, as cited earlier. The results of follow-up studies are still being published thirty years later, indicating the impact that the results of perinatal surveillance has had on discussions on health strategy.

In 1978 the National Perinatal Epidemiology Unit was established in Oxford, comprising a team of social scientists and epidemiologically-oriented paediatricians and obstetricians. Two main fields were outlined:

1. 'Perinatal surveillance and research into the context of childbearing'. In addition to the monitoring of trends over a period of time, this research included specific *ad hoc* investigations, some of which focused on child-bearing in a wider social and economic context.
2. 'Evaluation of perinatal practice'. Various facets of perinatal care (social, technological, and pharmaceutical) have been evaluated using a variety of research methods such as reviews, surveys, case-control studies, cohort studies and, (especially) randomized control trials. These have employed a wide range of social, medical, and economic measures of outcome.

In 1985 the unit procured a report summarizing its activities between 1981 and 1984 and listing material that had been published. It also outlined its plans for the future.[30]

The Netherlands have had a notification system for births and deaths since 1840. Until recently there was, however, no centralized system for the surveillance of congenital malformations and pregnancy outcome. In 1983, a cohort consisting of newborns with a gestational age below 32 weeks and/or birthweight below 1500 g was constituted comprising an estimated proportion of 0·5–0·7 per cent of all live births. The objective was to estimate the prevalence of pre-maturity. Antenatal, perinatal, and post-natal data from 109 neonatal wards have been analysed together with data from a 2 year follow-up.[33] Obstetric data have been gathered on a nationwide basis in The Netherlands since 1982.[31] Three years later, about 65 per cent of all obstetricians participated voluntarily. About 60 per cent of all births in The Netherlands are attended not by obstetricians but by midwives and general practitioners in the primary health-care system. In 1985, a nationwide notification system was established, based on information from midwives. The objectives were:

(a) to promote the permanent monitoring of standards used by professional groups as well as individual practitioners;
(b) to encourage continuous mutual evaluation of the services rendered by primary and secondary health care units;
(c) to form a basis for strategy-making;
(d) to form a basis for research as well as professional training.

By the end of 1985 as many as 65 per cent of midwives submitted data to the system. General practitioners have reacted positively but have not yet been engaged. Record linkage, including the previously mentioned specialist system and the midwife system, still poses serious problems.[32,33] Future developments in perinatal surveillance in The Netherlands comprise the notification of neonates (up to 28 days old), including a variety of obstetrical and morbidity data. Preliminary studies have already been conducted.

Finally, as the follow-up of newborns to late childhood is crucial to the development of relevant perinatal predictors of morbidity later in life, it might be mentioned that several Danish nationwide registers contain information on morbidity. Examples are registers concerning cancer, cerebral palsy, chromosomal abnormalities, psychiatric disorders, and visual defects. All citizens in Denmark have an identification number. In spite of this, no register-based studies relating obstetric survey data to later-in-life morbidity data have yet been conducted.

Regional surveillance systems

Since 1965 the Cardiff Births Survey[34] has collected detailed information on all births among residents in a geographical region. For each birth, social, demographic, obstetric data are registered as well as neonatal data up the twenty-eighth day after birth. Since 1980 a regional surveillance system has also been in existence in Aarhus, Denmark. The aims of such systems are to describe the prevalence of congenital malformations, chromosomal abnormalities, pre-term births, and weight-retarded newborns (small for dates), and the incidence of perinatal morbidity and mortality. Further aims are to formulate the bases of more thorough epidemiological investigations as well as the formulation of obstetrical strategies, both preventive and curative. Information sources are obstetrical files chromosomal analyses, and data from standardized interviews concerning social background, work, complications during pregnancy, alcohol and tobacco consumption, and medication.[11] Information about the prevalence of the conditions mentioned above and their development over time has been established, and important risk factors have been identified. Practical consequences are still under consideration, based on suggestions from the surveillance inferences concerning changes in the actual screening procedures before birth and the possibility of prolonged sick-leave during pregnancy.

Forming the Basis for Health Strategies

In the section on benefit and action (in Part 1 of this book) it is stated that the type and amount of information in surveillance systems must balance the need to know with the need to act. One important criticism of the Danish nationwide system might thus be that too much data are registered with too few consequences on health-strategy formulation. Periodic reports are usually several years late, probably due to the amount of data registered. Rational resource allocation and the efficient and relevant use of up-to-date technical equipment should prevent undue delays in publication. In the long run such delays may cause a decrease in data quality because of lack of motivation in those who, through the years, have been collecting data continuously.

The question of how to make a surveillance system a flexible tool for the making and evaluation of health strategies is a difficult one. A combination of nationwide and regional systems seems to be one path to follow. A common general data core should be defined, leaving room for more pene-trating surveillance systems and *ad hoc* epidemiological and clinical studies in selected areas. The regional staff would be close to regional strategy-makers, and experiences from other regions on different health issues might affect the decisions too. The Aarhus perinatal surveillance system is an attempt to com-bine national and regional data and it thus offers far more potential for flexi-bility than might a comprehensive national system. In turn, national strategy makers may learn from the regional experiences, thus generalizing *ad hoc* in-formation from a specific region to the whole nation. Curative and pre-ventive measures should, before they are introduced as routine procedures, be evaluated experimentally—on the basis of survey information as well as *ad hoc* observations—thus ensuring that neither human health, time nor money are risked unnecessarily.

Bibliography

1. Hoffman, H. J., Meirik, O., and Bakketeig, L. S., Methodological considerations to the analysis of perinatal mortality rates. In *Perinatal epidemiology* (ed. M. B. Bracken). Oxford University Press (1984).
2. Baird, D., The interplay of changes in society, reproductive habits, and obstetric practice in Scotland between 1922 and 1972. *Br. J. prevent. social Med.* **29,** 135–46 (1975).
3. Chase, H. C., Perinatal mortality: Overview and current trends. *Clinics in Perina-tology* **1,** 3–17 (1974).
4. Rovinsky, J. J., Impact of a permissive abortion statute on community health care. *Obstetrics Gynecol.* **41,** 781–8.
5. Chamberlain G., Better perinatal health: Background to perinatal health. *Lancet* **ii,** 1061–5. (1979).

6. Butler, N. R., and Bonham, D. G., *Perinatal mortality. The first report of the 1958 British Perinatal Mortality Survey.* Livingstone, Edinburgh (1963).
7. Butler, N. R. and Alberman, E. D., *Perinatal problems. The second report of the 1958 British Perinatal Mortality Survey.* Livingstone, Edinburgh (1969).
8. Hook, E. B., Human chromosome abnormalities. In *Perinatal epidemiology* (ed. M. B. Bracken). Oxford University Press (1984).
9. Nielsen, J., Wohlert, M., Faaborg-Andersen, J. *et al.*, Incidence of chromosome abnormalities in newborn children: Comparison between incidences in 1969–1974 and 1980–1982 in the same area. *Hum. Genet.* **61**, 98–101 (1982).
10. WHO, Recommended definitions, terminology, and format for statistical tables related to the perinatal period, and use of a new certificate for cause of perinatal deaths. *Acta obstet. gynaecol. scand.* **56**, 247–53 (1977).
11. Wohlert, M., *The influence of biological, social, and organisational factors on pregnancy and delivery* [In Danish, with a summary in English]. Department of Obstetrics and Gynaecology. University Hospital of Aarhus, Denmark. Aarhus (1986).
12. Rush, R. W., Davey, D. A., and Segau, M. L., The effect of pre-term delivery on perinatal mortality. *Br. J. Obstet. Gynecol.* **85**, 806–11 (1978).
13. Mamelle, N., Laumon, B., and Lazar, P., Prematurity and occupational activity during pregnancy. *Am. J. Epidemiol.* **119**, 309–22 (1984).
14. Fedrick, J. and Anderson, A. B. M., Factors associated with spontaneous pre-term birth. *Br. J. Obstet. Gynecol.* **83**, 342–50 (1976).
15. Funderburk, S. J., Guthrie, D., and Meldrum, D., Outcome of pregnancies complicated by early vaginal bleeding. *Br. J. Obstet. Gynecol.* **87**, 100–5 (1980).
16. Estryn, M., Kaminski, M., Franc, M. *et al. Revue Française de gynaecologie et d'obstetrique* **73**, 625–31 (1978).
17. Bakketeig, L. S. and Hoffman, H. J., Epidemiology of pre-term birth: Results from a longitudinal study of births in Norway. In *Obstetrics and gynecology 1. Pre-term Labour* (eds M. G. Elder and C. H. Hendricks). Butterworths, London (1981).
18. Minkoff, H., Prematurity: Infection as an aetiologic factor. *Obstet. Gynecol.* **62**, 137 44 (1983).
19. Mayer, P. S. and Wingate, M. B., Obstetric factors in cerebral palsy. *Obstet. Gynecol.* **51**, 399–406 (1978).
20. Papiernik, E., Proposals for a programmed prevention policy of pre-term birth. *Clin. Obstet. Gynecol.* **27**, 614–35 (1984).
21. Keirse, M. J. N. C., Epidemiology and aetiology of the growth retarded baby. *Clin. Obstet. Gynecol.* **11**, 415–36 (1984).
22. Keirse, M. J. N. C., Aetiology of intra-uterine growth retardation. In *Fetal growth retardation* (eds A. von Assche and W. B. Robertson). Livingstone, Edinburgh (1981).
23. Scott, A., Moar, V., and Ounsted, M., The relative contribution of different maternal factors in small-for-gestational-age pregnancies. *Eur. J. Obstet. Gynecol. reprod. Biol.* **12**, 157–65 (1981).
24. Low, J. A., Boston, R. W., and Pancham, S. R., Fetal asphyxia during the intra-partum period in intra-uterine growth retarded infants. *Am. J. Obstet. Gynecol.* **113**, 351–7 (1972).
25. McIlwaine, G. M., Howat, R. C. L., Dunn, F. *et al.*, The Scottish Perinatal Mortality Survey. *Br. med. J.* **12**, 1103–6 (1929).

26. Hepburn, M. and Rosenberg, K., An audit for the detection and management of small-for-gestational-age babies. *Br. J. Obstet. Gynecol.* **93,** 212–16 (1986).

27. Dijxhoorn, M. I., Visser, G. H. A., Fiddler, V. J. *et al.* (1986). Apgar score, meconium, and acidaemia at birth in relation to neonatal neurological morbidity in term infants. *Br. J. Obstet. Gynecol.* **93,** 217–22 (1986).

28. NOMESKO, *Births in the Nordic countries. Registration of the outcome of pregnancy.* Publication No. 17. Reykjavik (1982).

29. Rouquette, C. R., (ed.) *Inserm. Naître en France, 10 ans d'évolution.* Doin, Paris (1984).

30. National Perinatal Epidemiology Unit, *Report on the Unit's Work 1981–1984.* Oxford (1985).

31. Van Hemel, O. J. S., An obstetric data base, human factors, design and reliability. Thesis. Amsterdam (1977).

32. Verloove-Vanhorick, S. P., Review of evaluative studies on intensive care for very low birthweights infants. Medical aspects. In *perinatal care delivery systems: Description and evaluation in EEC countries* (ed. M. Kaminski). Publication of EEC. Oxford University Press (1986).

33. Verloove-Vanhorick, S. P., Verwey, R. A., Brand, R., Bennebroek Gravenhorst, J., Keirse, M. J. N. C., and Ruys, J. H., Neonatal mortality risk in relation to gestational age and birthweight. Results of a national survey of pre-term and very-low-birthweight in the Netherlands. *Lancet* **i,** 55–6 (1986).

34. Chalmers, I., Lawson, J. G., and Turnbull, A. C., Evaluation of different approaches to obstetric care. Part I–II. *Br. J. Obstet. Gynecol.* **83,** 921–33 (1976).

10

Surveillance of congenital malformations and birth defects

JOSEPHINE A. C. WEATHERALL

Introduction—History

Congenital anomalies are not a new phenomenon in the human race. In 1945 when death at birth or during the first year of life accounted for more than 4·5 per cent of infants born, there was little incentive for investigators to look for the cause of human malformations which at that time accounted for less than 10 per cent of the deaths. At such times, it is probable that congenital anomalies, chromosomal anomalies, malformations, and metabolic defects, were present among at least 5 per cent of the births[1,2] but the surviving children were scarcely creating a great problem to paediatricians while infectious diseases were still dominating childhood illness. Many of the malformed children born then, succumbed early in life to infections and did not survive to present some of the problems in living now faced by survivors, such as those with spina bifida or with cardiac defects.

Research into mammalian malformations was in progress in the 1920s and 1930s. Attention was paid most to dietetic factors which were shown for some species to influence the outcome of pregnancy.[3,4] Environmental influences were clearly demonstrated after 1940 for man when Gregg[5] described the relation between infants with specific eye defects and infection of their mothers with rubella during pregnancy. Researchers continued to look at teratogenic substances in animals during the 1940s and 1950s but the toxicologists in the pharmaceutical industry were not then alerted to the possible dangers of drugs used by mothers during pregnancy. When a drug firm produced the very effective sedative drug Thalidomide, in 1958, it was widely used for two years before an epidemic was recognized and another two years before it was firmly established that its consumption was associated, in some cases, with the subsequent birth of infants with gross limb defects.[6,7]

The delays in recognizing the association rested largely on the absence of information on the normal incidence of the conditions in question or, for those parts of Europe where adequate data about infants were being recorded, in arranging suitable and timely analyses of the data. One of the first persons to attempt to ascertain in England the normal level for the gross type of defects which were occurring was Smithells who had recently established a register in Liverpool.[8] Smithells was concerned himself with reviewing defects being collected in Liverpool and therefore was alerted by the frequency of the particular defects which he saw. Many registries are, however, managed by clerical or computer staff who usually have not enough medical knowledge—unless specifically trained—to be alerted by an odd finding. This must have happened with data being processed in the Swedish registry in the late 1950s[9] and in the Birmingham registry in 1959 and 1960.[10] In both registers, the increase in limb defects could have been recognized before 1960.[11]

To detect the cause of malformed babies a record of their occurrence is essential. There are many different types of malformation and metabolic anomalies which altogether occur in only a small proportion (about 5 per cent) of the births. Many types of defects are trivial, some are lethal and in many there is a major handicap. Many combined defects are very rare.

Two main types of recording system are used for surveillance. One method concentrates on early warning. A large number of babies are observed at birth and the defects found at that time or within seven days are reported. Information is centralized and analysed rapidly. Changes in frequency of different types of defect can be assessed, and confirmatory investigations started. Such systems are sensitive to changes, but because data collection is confined to a short period after birth, are vulnerable to artefacts such as newly developed methods for early diagnosis of defects.

A second method concerns recording defects in a defined group of children, no matter at what age the defects are found. Such a system requires a register of affected children to avoid duplication. Geographic definition of the population of parents assists in the search for environmental influences and allows family relationships to be studied. Such a system is usually best carried out in relatively small areas where data collection methods can be standardized and good communication with the doctors making the diagnoses can be maintained.

The Purposes of Surveillance

One of the main and most important objectives in carrying out surveillance of any condition, and particularly surveillance of relatively rare conditions such as congenital anomalies and hereditary diseases, is to establish reliable recording of the events so that increases or decreases in the numbers of cases and other trends are recorded. Such records, once established, may be used for many purposes. Obviously, epidemics—such as the thalidomide epidemic—should be recognized as soon as possible; or if not at first actually noted by the surveillance system, the increase quickly confirmed or denied by using the surveillance data. Some scepticism has been voiced that large national systems will be insensitive to small increases. This is undoubtedly likely, though the notification system established in England and Wales quickly responded to the doubled rate of reporting of congenital hip dislocation following the introduction of screening recommended by the Department of Health in 1966.[12]

Surveillance will also result in some increases which are false alarms. Common sense and sensible statistics will balance the need to maintain a watch which is sensitive enough to detect an increase of a relatively rare defect but not so sensitive that many false alarms are made.[13,14]

The important factor to be borne in mind is to make sure that the data recorded are in a suitable form to be used to investigate problems and thus lead to appropriate action. Some of the areas of health care where information is needed are discussed below.

Genetics

The identification of defects which are determined genetically is important to geneticists and to parents, especially to those seeking advice about reproduction. The presence or absence of a family history will be crucial in establishing a genetic factor and in helping geneticists to establish recurrence risks[15] and to identify the triggering factors in families which show multifactorial genetic predisposition.

Environment and employment

The identification of so called environmental risks may be difficult. For example, claims that fluoridation of water supplies has altered the risks to mothers of producing malformed infants has repeatedly been refuted through the absence of any increases in defects seen in the malformation registers which have recorded defects in an area before and after the introduction of fluoridation. Contamination of water supplies and of foodstuffs does happen,[16-19] as with methyl mercury or chlorobiphenyls. An increase of birth defects, particularly of a new type, in the infants may be one of the first signs of a problem.

Exposure during employment is another source of potential danger to both men and women, and many investigations have been carried out in the last ten years to investigate several suspicions[20,21] such as organic solvents and gases,[22-24] electrical radiations,[25] ancillary medical occupations,[26] herbicides,[27-29] and vinyl chloride.[30]

Reproductive health and medication in pregnancy

There is a persistent fear that the human race will damage itself and its ability to reproduce successfully, by introducing new chemical substances in everyday life or by changing its life-style. Such a fear can be controlled to some extent by maintaining a watch for genetic changes by monitoring the hereditary diseases and by identifying diseases caused by mutations. Possible damage to the fetus caused by alcohol or by smoking have been difficult to establish since abuse of one or other is often associated with many other possibly damaging factors in the life-style of the mother or father. Good record-keeping is clearly important for identifying any association of drugs with birth defects. Most of the recording systems were established as a direct consequence of the Thalidomide epidemic. Surveillance systems are used routinely to investigate associations between drugs and birth defects in England and Wales and in many other countries.[31–33] The main problem, however, in all these investigations, which are usually carried out on a case control basis, is to find adequate data, recorded with equal reliability for case and control mothers, about events which took place at least six months before the time of enquiry, which is usually not started until an abnormal child is born. Similar problems arise in the recording of occupational exposures. To insist on the recording of detailed information about food, drugs, and illness for every pregnant mother in order to be able to investigate reliably any potential causes of malformed infants in less than 5 per cent of them is expensive, labour intensive, and impractical.

Surveillance of outcome of care and prevention

Probably more important is the need to watch the effects of treatment of handicapping conditions and the effects of prevention. Monitoring the effects of life saving operations on infants with spina bifida in the early 1960s showed an evident prolongation of life. However, some of the children were so malformed or mentally retarded that the intervention was of dubious moral value. A change in policy so that children operated on were only those with reasonably intact development of their nervous system resulted in reduced survival rates for some years. This pattern changed again. When antenatal screening for dysraphic anomalies of the CNS was introduced around 1976, survival rates for newborns with spina bifida began to increase again as those children born alive were presumably less severely affected: the severely abnormal babies by then were being detected antenatally and the pregnancies terminated.[34]

Surveillance of preventive procedures is essential to make sure that prevention is being achieved. Immunization of children for rubella should achieve a reduction in children born with hearing, visual, or cardiac defects.[34] The development of valid antenatal screening procedures carried out to identify mothers bearing fetuses with central nervous system defects or with chromosomal defects should lead to a reduction in the births of such infants. However, great care is needed to make sure that all terminations are identified in order that the numbers observed in a birth cohort, at birth and later, can be augmented by those known to have been removed before birth and so give a true estimate of incidence of the condition in the cohort. In those countries where early termination of pregnancy is readily obtainable some mothers who are suspected to be at high risk of bearing an abnormal child, or who

Table 10.1 Early termination of pregnancy on legal ground of expected abnormal fetus. Percent of terminations in parity group. England and Wales, 1982

Length of gestation	Parity					
	0	1	2	3	4	5 or more
Before 12th week gestation	45	47	68	65	67	62
13–19th week	35	32	22	21	22	21
20th week + and NK	20	20	11	13	12	17
All	100	100	100	100	100	100

Source: Derived from *OPCS Abortion Statistics*[55].

have an abnormality in the fetus diagnosed by ultrasound or chorion biopsy before the normal gestation time for AFP screening or amniocentesis (sixteen weeks) may receive a termination. For such an early termination it is unlikely, too, that confirmation of the presence or absence of the abnormality is requested from pathologists. Table 10.1 shows that about two-thirds of mothers, resident in England and Wales, in 1982, having a termination of a third or later child, obtain their termination before the twelfth week of pregnancy. The early removal of abnormal fetuses in high risk mothers needs to be taken into account when a fall is observed in the incidence of defects at birth.[35]

Observation during the gestation period—What data are surveyed?

Most of the congenital anomalies are recognized around birth.[1,2] There is some evidence to suggest that a large proportion of spontaneously aborted fetuses are abnormal, especially with chromosomal anomalies, so that any observation system which includes records for such aborted fetuses may produce apparently high incidence of anomalies.[36] The monitoring of spontaneous abortions is considered by many experts as a means of recognizing early mutational changes in humans. Information about terminated pregnancies with, if possible, pathological confirmation of the diagnosed defects, is essential for the proper interpretation of changes observed in the frequency of defects discovered at birth or later.

At birth surveillance

Many of the recording systems, existing at this time, concentrate on observations of both live and still born infants at birth. Usually the observation period is confined to the period during which the child and the mother are likely to be in hospital or under medical supervision following the delivery of the infant. The gathering of data about the 10 per cent or so of abnormal children is relatively straightforward where there is an existing routine method for recording data about *all infants born*, as may be seen in the Scandinavian countries[37,38] and in the United Kingdom.[37–39] In all these countries the data concerning malformations are a side product of an existing recording system and are more or less checked according to whether a special study exists. The speed with which the data become available, however, will differ according to the methods used for processing them. As the incidence of malformations is relatively low, many births need to be surveyed before differences in incidence can be reliably identified. To increase the numbers observed international collaboration has been developed. In 1974, representatives from many data-collecting systems in Europe, North and South America, and Australia met in Helsinki and agreed to work towards a regular exchange of data. After a study by the epidemiologist, Sylvia Hay, in 1974 and 1975, it became clear that most of the recording systems were able to adopt common practices concerning observation at birth or within a few days after, and to agree the definition of defects observed, so that a regular quarterly exchange of information was started, backed up by annual conferences and, since 1980, by an annual publication.[40,41] By 1983, 22 systems belonged to what has been named the International Clearing House for Birth Defects Monitoring Systems (ICBDMS) (Table 10.2) and together they monitored about 3 000 000 births a year, concentrating on prevalence at birth with a short observation period of not more than nine days after birth.[40]

Longitudinal Observation Registers

In order to find children who are recognized after the perinatal period to have a malformation or congenital anomaly a far more complex system for collecting data is needed. Infants may be referred to many types of clinics, and to obtain accurate information about the diagnosis involves diligent clerical work by medical records clerks, or the enthusiastic co-operation of the various medical persons concerned with child care. It is quite possible for one child to reach several clinics, so careful record linkage in a registry of the abnormal children is essential to ensure that each child is counted as abnormal only once, although it may have several anomalies.

The establishment of registers with observation of the children continuing over a long time period presents considerable difficulties. In Western Europe, the EUROCAT co-ordinated registers, established under one of the Concerted Action Projects of the EEC Medical Research Program between 1978 and 1985[42] are of this type (Table 10.3). All registers aim at an accurate

Table 10.2   Monitoring systems contributing to ICBDMS scheme in 1983

Monitoring system	Coverage	Number of births surveyed (1983)
Australia	Population-based	241 280
Canada: 6 provinces	Population-based	242 223
Czechoslovakia	Population-based	138 132
Denmark	Population-based	51 087
England and Wales	Population-based	632 765
Finland	Population-based	67 160
France: Rhone–Alps–Auvergne	Population-based	86 597
France: Paris*	Population-based	39 457
France: Strasbourg*	Population-based	12 519
Hungary	Population-based	128 160
Israël: 2 hospitals	Hospital-based	8 860
Italy: 140 hospitals	Hospital-based	139 320
Japan: 16 hospitals	Hospital-based	18 903
Mexico: 13 hospitals	Hospital-based	36 641
New Zealand	Population-based	50 521
Northern Ireland*	Population-based	27 459
Norway	Population-based	50 307
South America: 20 hospitals	Hospital-based	45 312
Spain: 32 hospitals	Hospital-based	77 287
Sweden	Population-based	92 026
United States: Atlanta	Population-based	27 937
United States: 1200 hospitals	Hospital-based	760 300

*Also member registers in EUROCAT.
Derived from ICDBMS *Statistics*[40].

ascertainment of all malformations in children born to women living in a geographically defined area. Details of the methods used by each registry differ according to the type of register and area involved.[37] In the UK registers, and in Ireland and Denmark reasonably well organized routine data-collection systems exist about births, hospital admissions, and deaths. Each of these sources can be used as a starting point for further enquiries—usually going back to the hospital notes and sometimes to the doctor having charge of the child. Newly discovered cases coming to hospital can be discovered this way. In Belgium, Italy, Luxemburg, Germany, and France, however, the finding of later cases presents considerable problems. There is usually little difficulty in following up children who attend a given clinic regularly, provided the paediatrician is willing to notify new findings. There is, however, not likely to be any means for identifying cases newly diagnosed later unless some regular health certificate—as used in France at nine and twenty-four

Table 10.3   Registers collaborating in EUROCAT project in 1983

		Approximate annual birth coverage	Proportion of malformed infants discovered more than seven days after birth per cent
Belgium	– West Flanders	7 000	–
	– Hainaut	8 000	5.8
Denmark	– Odense	4 000	12.6
France	– Paris	40 000	2.8
	– Strasbourg	12 500	22.9
West Berlin		17 000	2.6
Italy	– Firenze	9 000	13.2
	– Umbria	7 000	8.2
	– Emilia Romagna	22 000	0.8
Ireland	– Dublin	23 000	23.6
	– Galway	3 500	13.2
Luxemburg		2 000	9.8
Netherlands	– Groningen	7 500	27.3
United Kingdom	– Glasgow	12 500	27.2
	– Liverpool	20 000	13.7
	– Belfast	27 500	9.2
Yugoslavia	– Zagreb	4 000	4.8
Total annual birth coverage		226 500	

Source: Derived from EUROCAT Statistics 1986[43].

months of age—can be exploited. There does not appear to be any single point such as a local general practitioner, to which a given child will be brought for routine or special care, in the health-care systems of these countries. In Groningen[37] special co-operation has been arranged between the Register, the clinicians, the general practitioners and well-baby clinics which appears to be succeeding in finding cases adequately up to one year of age. It will be of interest to see whether the seven obligatory clinical examinations of children in Yugoslavia in well-baby clinics result in successful finding of abnormal children by the recently established EUROCAT registries near Zagreb.[37]

Collection of Data

In conferences organized by the World Health Organization general agreement has been reached about the data needed routinely to be collected about congenitally abnormal infants.[44,45] On the whole as little data as possible, which can be assured of accuracy, should be collected. The same data should, if possible, also be available for all births in the populations under study in order that appropriate denominators are available when differential frequency of malformations in sub-groups of the population is in question. Data about the mothers, their habits, and their social positions are reasonably easily collected during the antenatal period and at birth. Data about events at conception or in early gestation are likely not to be reliable if recorded by recollection at the time of delivery nine months later and particularly likely to be biased if recorded after the birth of an abnormal child. Data about fathers are more difficult to obtain and will remain a problem until routine provision of such information for medical records of human reproduction is established.

The EUROCAT data set has been laid down by agreement between the Registry Leaders during the early stages of the EUROCAT study. The *EUROCAT Guide 1 1984*[46] contains instructions and definitions. There is no reason why more data than are laid down by the EUROCAT instructions should not be collected locally. However, care must be taken to make sure that basic definitions are not interfered with, so that comparability between the registers is maintained. The provision of denominator data—essential for analysis of frequencies—presents a problem for all registries which do not have a total-birth registration system under their control. Most countries have a national-birth registration system: but data processing and publication of analyses are usually delayed, sometimes by years. Some registers based mostly on hospital can rely on the hospital data to provide a denominator; and other registers routinely collect data for a sample of all births in order to expedite the processing and to obtain additional information which is not collected by a national registration system.

Data Processing

Again, the preparation of the recorded data for suitable analyses has been co-ordinated by EUROCAT. As Eurocat relies on transmission of data about each baby from the constituent registries, guide lines for processing have been prepared so that central analyses should be easily checked by the local registries.[46]

With only 5 per cent of all babies born being reported with any defect it will be seen that all these defects are distributed over a very small proportion of the births and many defects are very rare. It is therefore essential either to count particular specific types of defect—as is done for specific infectious diseases among all the possible 'infections'—or to count all the defects in well-defined classes. Malformations can occur in any part of the human body and metabolic disorders can occur in any of the biochemical processes. Therefore the numbers of separate types of defects can be very large. The ninth revision of the *International Classification of Disease*[47] recognizes 168 classes of malformations in chapter 14 which is devoted only to malformations. There are a further nineteen classes of conditions which are reported in children as 'congenital anomalies' but have been listed in other chapters. British paediatricians find that these classes contain too many dissimilar conditions and they have further divided them to a total of about 750 classes.[48] Although EUROCAT stores every malformation recorded to the full BPA code[48] detail in the EUROCAT data files, there are too many classes, many of them rarely used, to allow routine surveillance of every different type. The malformations have therefore been grouped—as described in the EUROCAT guide—into 'Groups' and 'Subgroups' and surveillance is carried out using these. An increase in a particular rare condition may be obscured by watching grouped material and therefore it is desirable in addition to compare detailed tabulations at regular intervals.

A further problem in classifying the babies with defects arises because about 25 per cent of those with malformations are reported with more than one defect. Two defects are reported in about 12 per cent and six or more defects in about 1·5 per cent of babies. The recognition of consistent patterns in these associations, which could amount to more than 5 000 000 000 different combinations is considered to be an important task for anyone monitoring birth defects, since it is clear that the so-far recognized human teratogens do result in babies being born with newly recognized association of particular defects. For example, rubella is associated with eye, ear, and heart defects and Thalidomide with limb and ear defects.

The reporting of any newly discovered 'syndrome' associated with a particular 'cause' can present many difficulties, particularly if the combination of defects is rare and the alleged cause is commonly used. Fetal alcohol syndrome presents such difficulties. Infants are often now reported as having the syndrome without any mention of the particular defects concerned. Often the ascertainment of alcohol consumption in pregnancy has been made retrospectively after the malformations have been discovered or the child has failed to thrive. To establish a causal connection reliably, a study is needed where alcohol consumption is accurately recorded during pregnancy along with other possibly contributing factors. As the major malformation concerned, microcephaly, occurs in only about 14 of every 10 000 births a large number of pregnancies will need to be studied; and the infants followed up, to establish whether the syndrome occurs more commonly in the consumers of alcohol or the non-alcohol consumers. The setting up of such a study to obtain results in a relatively short time is likely to be achieved only by multi-centre co-operation, and could very well be a research task undertaken by co-operating registers.

Conclusion

As interest in congenital anomalies has increased during the 1960s and 1970s so have the questions about causes of malformations. What good has surveillance achieved either in identifying new teratogenic substances or in discovering how malformations are caused? Which monitoring systems have had alarms that have resulted in the identification of new teratogenic substances? Increases have occurred and been investigated—for example, gastroschisis in Sweden,[40] hypospadias in Latin America[49] and in Hungary,[50] and an increase in reduction deformities of the thigh in Rhone–Alps Region of France.[51] In none of these cases has a specific teratogen been identified, but usually the increase can be explained by some demographic factor or change in procedure of data collection. The Rhone Alps registry has, however, pointed to an association between sodium valproate medication for epilepsy and subsequent birth of infants with spina bifida which on further investigations has led to an awareness that sodium valproate is not such a safe drug for use in pregnancy for the epileptic mother as had been supposed by some doctors. The recognition of Isotretinoin used for treatment of acne as a danger to the fetus has also been assisted by the use of registries.[52]

Good evidence about the likelihood of occurrence of malformations has also assisted the defence in legal cases where a fetus has allegedly been damaged by its mother's exposure to a specific drug during her pregnancy, which after the Thalidomide disaster has become a very emotive issue. Cases concerning alleged damage by Debendox are still being contested in the courts. When a large number of women consume a successful anti-nauseant drug, such as Debendox, during pregnancy it is probable that around 5 per cent of them will, by chance, give birth to an infant which has a congenital anomaly of some kind.[53–55]

In the present climate of concern about health of the environment and of legal actions for alleged damage to the unborn fetus, not to mention possible long-term effects of radiation accidents, it is likely that surveillance of birth defects will become a regular part of the public health in developed countries.

Bibliography

1. Myrianthopoulos, N. C., *Malformations in children from one to seven years—a report from the Collaborative Perinatal Project.* Alan R. Liss, New York (1985).
2. Vowles, M., Methybridge, R. J., and Brimblecombe, F. S. W., Congenital malformations in Devon, their incidnece, age and primary source of detection. In *Bridging in health—reports on studies for health services in children*, Oxford, Nuffield Provincial Hospitals Trust, 201–15 (1975).
3. Nelson, M. N., Production of congenital anomalies in mammals by maternal dietary deficiencies. *Paediatrics* **19**, 764–76 (1957).
4. Wilson, J. G., Is there specificity of action in experimental teratogenesis? *Paediatrics* **19**, 755–63 (1957).

5. Gregg, N. McA., Congenital cataract following German measles in the mother. *Trans. Ophthalmol. Soc. Aust.* **3**, 35–45 (1941).
6. McBride, W. G., Thalidomide and congenital abnormalities. *Lancet* **ii**, 1358 (1961).
7. Lenz, W., Kindliche Missbildungen nach Medikament—Einnahme Währen der Gravidität. *Dtsch Med. Wochenschr.* **86**, 2555 (1961).
8. Smithells, R. W., The Liverpool congenital abnormalities registry. *Dev. Med. Child Neurol.* **4**, 320–4 (1962).
9. Winberg, J., Investigation of the possible relation between congenital malformations and drugs ... in Sweden among 435,000 children born 1955–1962. *Sven Laekartidn* **61**, 722–41 (1964).
10. Leck, I. M., and Millar, E. L. M., Incidence of malformations since the introduction of Thalidomide. *Br. med. J.* **ii**, 16–20 (1962).
11. Källén, B., and Winberg, J., Multiple malformations studied with a national register of malformations. *Paediatrics* **44**, 410–7 (1969).
12. Weatherall, J. A. C., De Wals, P., and Lechat, M. F., Evaluation of information systems for the surveillance of congenital malformations. *Int. J. Epidemiol.* **13**, 193–6 (1984).
13. Chen, R., McDowall, M., Terzian, E., and Weatherall, J. A. C., Eurocat Guide to monitoring methods for malformation registers. *EUROCAT Epidem.* 3034 UCL, 1200 Brussels (1983).
14. Weatherall, J. A. C., and Haskey, J. C., Surveillance of malformations. *Br. med. Bull.* **32**, 39–44 (1976).
15. Owens, J. R., Simkin, J. M., and Harris, F., Recurrence rates for neural tube defects. *Lancet* **i**, 1282 (1985).
16. Ashton, J., Pollution of the water supply in Mersey and Clwyd—a cause of concern. *Community Med.* **7**, 299–303 (1985).
17. Moriyama, H., A study on the congenital Minimata disease. *J. Kumamoto Med. Soc.* **41**, 506–32 (1967).
18. Amin Zaki, L., Elhassani, S., Majeed, M. A. *et al.*, Intra-uterine methyl mercury poisoning in Iraq. *Paediatrics* **54**, 587–95 (1974).
19. Funatsu, I., A chlorobiphenyl induced fetopathy. *Fukuoka Acta Med.* **62**, 139–49 (1971).
20. Ericson, A., Källén, B., Meirik, O., and Westerholm, P., Gastro-intestinal atresia and maternal occupation during pregnancy. *J. occup. Med.* **24**, 515–18 (1982).
21. Bjerkedal, T., Occupation and outcome of pregnancy (in Norwegian). Rapporter 80–9 Statistisk Central Byra, Oslo (1980).
22. Ericson, A., and Källén, B., Survey of infants born in 1973–1975 to Swedish mothers working in operating rooms during their pregnancies. *Anesth. Analg.* **58**, 302–5 (1979).
23. Holmberg, P., Central-nervous-system defects in children born to mothers exposed to organic solvents during pregnancy. *Lancet* **ii**, 177–9 (1979).
24. Hanson, J. W., and Oakley, G. P., Spray adhesives and birth defects. *J. Am. Med. Ass.* **236**, 1010 (1976).
25. Källén, B., Malmquist, G., and Moritz, U., Delivery outcome among physiotherapists in Sweden: Is non-ionising radiation a fetal hazard? *Arch environ. Hlth* **37**, 81–84 (1982).
26. Baltzar, B., Ericson, A., and Källén, B., Delivery outcome in women employed in medical occupations in Sweden. *J. occup. Med.* **21**, 543–8 (1979).

27. Donovan, J. W., Case control study of congenital anomalies and Vietnam service. Sydney Australia Commonwealth Institute of Health, University of Sydney (1983).

28. Erickson, J. D., Mulinare, J., McClain, P. W. *et al.*, Vietnam veterans' risks for fathering babies with birth defects. *J. Am. Med. Ass.* **252**, 903–12 (1984).

29. Smith, A. H., Fisher, D. O., Pearce, N., and Chapman, C. J., Congenital defects and miscarriages among New Zealand 2,4,5-T sprayers. *Arch. environ. Hlth* **37**, 197–200 (1982).

30. Infante, P. F., Wagoner, J. K., McMichael, A. J., Waxweiler, R. J., and Falk, H., Genetic risks of vinyl chloride. *Lancet* **i**, 734–5 (1976).

31. Greenberg, G., Inman, W. H. W., Weatherall, J. A. C., Adelstein, A. M., and Haskey, J. C., Maternal drug histories and congenital abnormalities. *Br. med. J.* **ii**, 853–6 (1977).

32. Ericson, A., Källén, B. and Lindsten, J., Lack of correlation between contraceptive pills and Down's syndrome. *Acta obstet. gynaecol. scand.* **62**, 511–14 (1983).

33. Jick, H., Holmes, L. B., Hunter, J. R., Madsen, S., and Stergachis, A., First trimester drug use and congenital disorders. *J. Am. Med. Ass.* **246**(4), 343–6 (1981).

34. Weatherall, J. A. C., A review of some effects of recent medical practices in reducing the numbers of children born with congenital abnormalities. *Hlth Trends* **14**, 85–8. HMSO, London (1982).

35. Owens, J. R., Harris, F., McAllister, E., and West, L., 19 year incidence of neural tube defects in an area under constant surveillance. *Lancet* **ii**, 1032–5 (1981).

36. Yamamoto, M. and Watanabe, G., Epidemiology of gross chromosomal anomalies at the early embryonic stage of pregnancy. *Contr. Epidem. Biostatist.* **1**, 101–6. Karger, Basel (1979).

37. De Wals, P., Weatherall, J. A. C., and Lechat, M. F., *Registration of congenital anomalies in Eurocat centres 1979–1983*. Cabay, Brussels and Louvain-la-Neuve (1985).

38. Ericson, A., Källén, B., and Winberg, J., Surveillance of malformations at birth: a comparison of two record systems run in parallel. *Int. J. Epidemiol.* **6**, 35–41 (1977).

39. Cole, S. K., Evaluation of neonatal discharge record as a monitor of congenital malformations. *Community Med.* **5**, 21–30 (1983).

40. *Annual Reports of International Clearinghouse for Birth Defects Monitoring Systems*. 1980–1983 available from E. Knudsen, National Board of Health, 1 St. Kongensgade DK 1264 Copenhagen K, Denmark.

41. Källén, B., Hay, S., and Klingberg, M., Birth defects monitoring systems. *Issues and Reviews in Teratology* **2**, 1–22. Plenum Press, New York (1984).

42. Weatherall, J. A. C., *The beginnings of Eurocat*. Cabay, Brussels and Louvain-La-Neuve (1985).

43. De Wals, P., and Lechat, M. F., *Surveillance of congenital anomalies*. EUROCAT report 1, Epid 3034, UCL, Brussels (1986).

44. WHO, *Report on consultation on World Health Organization Program of Congenital Malformations, 24–28 July 1972*. WHO Report DSI/72:7, WHO, Geneva (1972).

45. Report on World Health Organization Consultation HMG/Cons 85.6., *The methodology for birth defects monitoring*. WHO, Geneva (1986).

46. De Wals, P., Mastroiacovo, P., Weatherall, J. A. C., and Lechat, M. F.,

EUROCAT Guide 1 for the registration of congenital anomalies. Cabay, Brussels and Louvain-La-Neuve (1984).

47. I.C.D., *International Statistical Classification of Diseases, Injuries and Causes of Death*, ninth revision 1975. WHO, Geneva (1978).
48. British Paediatric Association Classification of Diseases., B.P.A., London (1979).
49. Montelone, N. R., Castilla, E. E., and Paz, J. E., Hypospadius: An epidemiological study in Latin America. *Am. J. med. Genet.* **10**, 5–19 (1981).
50. Czeizel, A., Tóth, J., and Erödi, E., Aetiological studies of hypospadius in Hungary. *Hum. Hered.* **29**, 166–71 (1979).
51. Robert, J. M., Guibaud, P., and Robert, E., A local outbreak of femoral hypoplasia or aplasia and femur-fibula-ulnar complex. *J. Genet. Hum.* **29**, 379–94 (1981).
52. CDC Atlanta USA, *Isotretinoin—a newly recognised teratogen*. Morbidity and Mortality Weekly Reports 33/13, 171–3 (1984).
53. Smithells, R. W., and Sheppard, S., Teratogenicity testing in humans—a method demonstrating safety of Bendectine. *Teratology* **17**, 31–5 (1978).
54. *The Pharmaceutical Journal*, Debendox—Mr Ashley writes to the Minister. *Pharmaceut. J.* **236**, 549 (1986).
55. *OPCS Abortion Statistics Series AB, 1982*. HMSO, London (1984).

11

Cardiovascular disease surveillance

G. DE BACKER, U. LAASER, AND H. WENZEL

Cardiovascular disease (CVD) is a leading cause of death and disability all over the world. This includes a large variety of CV disorders:

1. Defects of the cardiovascular system are believed to represent a high proportion of all congenital anomalies.
2. Rheumatic heart disease is still a burden in most developing countries.
3. Cerebrovascular disorders cause functional disability and death in a large proportion of the elderly population.
4. Coronary heart disease (CHD) is still present in epidemic proportions in most industrialized societies.

These statements are based on analyses of statistics which in turn are derived from 'passive' surveillance of populations, usually national vital statistics. These sources of information are usually reliable enough to support such general statements as those made above.

Limitations of Vital Statistics

However, if one wants to study these problems in more detail, major limitations of vital statistics become apparent. The information collected for producing vital statistics is generally restricted to routine data about deaths or disabling disorders and even then its validity is uncertain.

If one wants to study geographical or temporal changes in the incidence of CVD either as a 'natural experiment' or within the framework of experimental epidemiological research, one needs precise and accurate data; for that purpose vital statistics may not be sufficient; studies on the validity of death certificate diagnoses have found them to be incomplete or even erroneous for 20–40 per cent of cases.[1-6] This causes serious limitations in the use of vital statistics, particularly in studies with a relatively small number of events.

Moreover, the validity of vital statistics may change over time in a given community and may also differ between populations at any given time. This can create biases in mortality rates as well as conceal real differences. This is particularly true if one considers a specific disease entity, for instance ischaemic heart disease (IHD), and may be less so for the comparison of mortality rates for larger disease groups, such as cardiovascular diseases.

Although vital statistics are helpful for studying the distribution of CVD between and within communities, standardized and 'active' surveillance of CVD by direct measurement in defined communities will be needed if reliable and precise data are required.

A Plea for Heart Attack Registers

The potential usefulness of community surveillance of CVD was already emphasized by a working group of WHO in 1968[7] when the CHD mortality rate was at a peak level in most industrialized countries. This working group discussed the feasibility of, and the need for, ischaemic heart-disease registers in defined communities. They concluded that:

Registers would
. . . facilitate the study of aetiology, pathogenesis and it was hoped, prevention of attacks. They would provide information on the occurrence of coronary disease in the community and its human, social and economic costs.
. . . provide measures of how existing services matched needs.
. . . provide a basis for the evaluation of new and old methods of management by comparing the experience of groups in the population managed in different ways.
. . . highlight areas where treatment was inadequate.
. . . and would be invaluable in research by providing representative cases for study and a sample framework for clinical trials.

In a few centres, the plea for the implementation of ischaemic heart-disease registers was acknowledged and registers were introduced.

The interest in community surveillance of CVD received a second boost some years later, when it became evident that CVD mortality was changing at a different rate between populations.

In Fig. 11.1 an international ranking of the percentage change in age standardized death rates from ischaemic heart disease from 1970 to 1983 is presented for men aged 40–69. This figure is derived from data published by WHO.[8] Large improvements were observed in countries such as Belgium, Australia, and the USA, whereas in several Eastern European countries sharp increases were seen in the same time period. The understanding of these heterogeneous trends could be of great importance for public health policy, but even now, 20 years after the start of the decline of CHD mortality in the USA it is not possible to state the precise causes of these changes. We do not even know whether these changes in CHD mortality rates are accompanied by comparable changes in non-fatal CHD incidence and/or by changes in case-fatality rates. Hypotheses abound and come from medical and surgical experts as well as from public health and preventive cardiology researchers. At an expert meeting in 1978 in Bethesda, USA, it was concluded that no precise answers to these hypotheses could be given and several

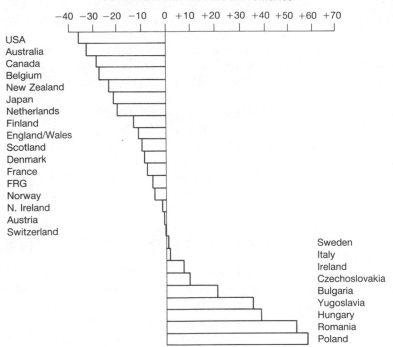

Fig. 11.1. Percentage change in age-standardized death rates from ischaemic heart disease for males aged 40–69 years in 1970–83.

recommendations were made for studying the determinants of CVD mortality trends in detail.[9]

The methods suggested include more detailed surveillance and analysis of mortality data as well as surveillance of morbidity. This can be achieved by establishing registers for CVD in well-defined communities over a sufficient time period. Besides the surveillance of the incidence of the disease one should also monitor the changes in medical care as well as changes in the major CVD risk factors.

However, numerous problems can be anticipated with community surveillance of CVD.

Problems Related to Surveillance of Cardiovascular Mortality and Morbidity

In retrospect it is surprising to realize that in the 1950s and 1960s when CHD-mortality was on the increase in most western societies, no attempts were made to obtain precise and accurate data at a national level. The magnitude and severity of the epidemic should have made national surveillance programmes a health priority.

This does not mean that no research on the matter was conducted. Gillum[10] reviewed most of the short- and long-term surveillance studies from which it became clear that major differences existed in the definition of the disease entity, in sources from which data were collected, in the retro- or prospective character of the studies or in the main targets the investigators were trying to achieve.

It was only in the early 1970s that a major collaborative attempt was made to standardize community surveillance of CHD through heart-attack registers.[11] This study, co-ordinated by WHO, ended in 1973 and received insufficient attention in the years that followed. It involved 19 communities in which, during 1971, myocardial infarction was registered in the total population below the age of 65 years. The population studied comprised 3.6 million people aged 20–64. Altogether 14 000 acute heart attacks were observed in one year. Important information was collected on the evolution of the attack, the availability of medical assistance, the case fatality, the natural history over a one-year period, etc.

Several problems that could be anticipated with community surveillance were discussed, including the completeness of case ascertainment, diagnostic criteria, timing of events, etc. These registers have provided a clear picture of CHD as it affects the community; the implications for public-health policy were numerous but have been inadequately translated into practice. These registers provide exactly the information needed to develop and test community control programmes.

After 1973 some of the centres decided to continue registration in a similar or simplified form. From these efforts temporal changes in CHD incidence during the 1970s have become available in some communities.

In Table 11.1 results from some of these studies[12-15] are summarized and compared with the national ischaemic heart-disease mortality trends. In Stockholm the incidence of myocardial infarction increased with no change in case fatality rate (CFR) while the national IHD mortality trends were favourable for women and stable for men. In Auckland the incidence and CFR of myocardial infarction did not change from 1974 to 1981 while the national IHD mortality rates declined in New Zealand by 25 per cent and 17 per cent in men and women respectively. In Auckland a significant decline in the rate of sudden death was observed. The findings in Finland were more consistent while in the USA the experience in the Kaiser Permanente Study favoured the effect of prevention of the disease. These and other experiences have posed questions to the unexplained time trends in CHD mortality. It became clear that a sustained collaborative effort was needed in different communities to learn more about the precise reasons for the phenomenon. It should be re-emphasized that the acute myocardial infarction community register programme of WHO has been of the greatest help in the further development of community surveillance of CVD. The WHO initiative has also

Table 11.1   National mortality trends and CHD incidence studies

National IHD mortality (8)			Incidence studies			
Country	Period	Trend %	Population	Period	Incidence AMI	CFR
SWEDEN			STOCKHOLM[12]			
Men	1972–82	+ 0.7	Men	1974–80	+2.9%/yr	No change
Women	1972–82	− 19.4	Women	1974–80	+2.2%/yr	No change
NEW ZEALAND			AUCKLAND[13]	1974–81	No change	No change
Men	1971–81	− 23				
Women	1971–81	− 17				
FINLAND			FINLAND[14]			
Men	1970–80	− 13	Men	1972–81	− 14%	− 7%
Women	1970–80	− 23	Women	1972–81	− 19%	− 10%
USA			KAISER			
Men	1970–80	− 36	PERMANENTE[15]	1971–77	− 27%	No change
Women	1970–80	− 39				

been of value in establishing clear-cut diagnostic criteria for CVD such as sudden death, ischaemic heart disease, congenital disorders, stroke, and arterial hypertension.

In the absence of standardized and simple diagnostic criteria the comparability of study materials becomes impossible and this has been the case for too many years regarding CVD surveillance. However, despite these improvements in methodology we still do not have sufficient proof that the present criteria result in valid and comparable event rates at an international or national level.

If it is considered possible to develop a valid and complete CVD register in the community, other problems can be anticipated especially if these registers have to function over a prolonged time period.

Diagnostic methods may change or new therapeautic techniques may obscure the results from previous data. Such problems are not theoretical but happen as for example after the introduction of thrombolysis and coronary artery balloon dilatation.

Another problem area relates to the observation in different cohort studies that myocardial infarction can occur without typical symptoms in a fairly high proportion of the population. One can easily imagine that in a certain community the patients' or doctors' attitudes towards certain symptoms can change, resulting in an increased detection of atypical or asymptomatic infarcts. Thus, one has to be cautious about sources of bias that can affect the outcome of collaborative community surveillance programmes. Despite its limitations the method as developed in the early 1970s from the heart-attack registers is still the basis from which new programmes start; improvements in diagnostic criteria and updates in classification make them more specific and quantitative. A more extensive and prolonged application of it will disclose other problems but in the meantime it will provide a rich data base and a useful tool for evaluating various CVD community programmes. If such systems can be stable over time they could serve as a model for health surveillance systems in general, relying as much as possible on existing structures of information and improving their quality.

Surveillance of Determinants of CVD

The community surveillance of CVD as it has been developed over the last decades has focused primarily on sickness and mortality. Few attempts have been made to monitor the health-care system or changes in CV risk factors at the community level.

The attempts made to study changes in health-care delivery and effectiveness were based on hospital experiences or clinical trials. It is almost impossible to apply these results to the community.

In the last decades preventive and curative cardiology have changed dramatically with the introduction of coronary care units and of specialized units for acute care delivery outside the hospital, the development of programmes of comprehensive cardiac rehabilitation and tertiary prevention, the nationwide programmes of arterial hypertension detection and treatment, the newer techniques for limiting or preventing acute myocardial infarction, and the new surgical techniques to prevent recurrence or other complications, etc. It is, however, impossible to know if these developments have anything to do with the temporal changes in CVD mortality rates.

No attempts were made to study the effects of the developments in a systematic way in defined communities or to examine their efficiency at the population level.

The surveillance programmes that have been designed for the eighties include monitoring of changes in medical treatment and provide a valid methodology. They include community indices of drug use, coronary artery disease surgery rates, monitoring the development of new approaches to CHD, such as thrombolysis and dilatation techniques as well as changes in the acute coronary care delivery systems outside hospitals.

Besides the possible effects of developments in medical care on CVD mortality rates, changes in coronary risk factors could influence incidence and case-fatality rates. There are indeed several arguments to suggest that the temporal changes in CVD mortality have to do with alterations in life-styles and risk indicators. However, reliable and precise data to support these hypotheses are again lacking, either because the changes have been observed in cohort studies in selected population groups or because the temporal changes have been from different population studies.

Monitoring of risk-factor trends and of life-style behaviour in total communities has started only in recent years either by examination of repeated cross-sectional samples of defined communities or by repeated examinations of a sample cohort. Such surveillance programmes face numerous problems, such as assuring an acceptable survey response-rate or keeping the survey methods sufficiently stable over time. Standardized methods for surveilling the major coronary risk factors, such as arterial blood-pressure, smoking habits, and blood cholesterol are available and have been successfully applied in collaborative epidemiological studies. The methodologies for monitoring life-styles, such as nutrition, physical activity, and psychosocial variables are much less developed and present great difficulties for international application. Major advances have been made in recent years particularly with the help of the EEC.[16]

Ongoing Research into Community Surveillance of CVD

As it has been explained before, the interest in community surveillance of CVD has been on the increase in recent years and several large scale and long-term programmes have been developed. Four examples are given, illustrating different approaches. A complete list of all ongoing or planned programmes is beyond the scope of this paper.

The Stanford Five-City Project

The Stanford Five-City Project is a trial of the effort of community health education on cardiovascular risk factors, morbidity, and mortality.[17] In the three reference communities the surveillance programme will provide information on secular trends in CHD incidence, risk factors, and medical treatment over a long-term period. This project is a good example of how community surveillance can function as an operational system for evaluating intervention programmes; this could be applied either in the field of primary, secondary, or tertiary prevention.

The Minnesota morbidity and mortality surveillance programme (MMMP)

In the MMMP[18] changes in CHD incidence, case-fatality, hospital care, and risk factors are examined in a major effort to find explanations for the temporal changes in CHD death rates observed in the US since the 1960s. The population of Minneapolis-St Paul (approximately 2 million) is studied using the following hypotheses:

1. The observed decline in IHD mortality is due to a decline in incidence of myocardial infarction and to a decline in the case-fatality rate of hospitalized cases.

2. The decline in IHD mortality is associated with downward trends in population levels of the standard risk-factors.
3. Trends in IHD case-fatality are associated with trends in pre-hospital and in-hospital care of myocardial infarction.
4. Changes in levels of the standard risk-factors are associated with changes in specific health behaviour patterns.

This surveillance programme is also linked to a quasi-experimental epidemiological study to test the hypothesis that modification of standard risk-factors in the population is associated with a decline in ischaemic heart disease.

Multinational monitoring of trends and determinants of cardiovascular diseases

Another approach, involving particularly the heterogeneity in CHD mortality trends, was developed by WHO's cardiovascular unit in Geneva. After a series of meetings a protocol and a manual of operation were drafted for a 'Multinational monitoring of trends and determinants of cardiovasular disease' summarized as the MONICA-project.[19] It involves community surveillance of coronary heart disease (acute myocardial infarction) and cerebro-vascular disease (stroke).

The two main hypotheses regarding coronary heart disease are:

1. There is no relationship between ten-year trends in a measure of coronary risk obtained from community levels of total serum cholesterol, diastolic blood-pressure and cigarette consumption and ten-year trends in CHD incidence rates.
2. There is no relationship between ten-year trends in case-fatality rates and ten-year trends in medical care after the attack.

In order to test these and other hypotheses four main groups of variables are monitored:

1. Incidence rates of coronary heart disease defined as the sum of fatal and non-fatal acute myocardial infarction.
2. Case-fatality rates: percentage of fatal attacks within twenty-eight days of the onset of symptoms.
3. Risk-factor levels in the community: by repeated surveys of independent random samples of the community.
4. Several aspects related to the treatment of acute heart attacks.

The project is now fully implemented in 27 countries: 41 centres representing 118 reporting units and covering more than 12 million subjects and is expected to continue for 10 years. Additional studies have been derived from the main project on the international level and include more detailed surveillance of drug use, surveillance of nutritional habits, studies on psychological variables, and on physical activity patterns.

It is clear that in the majority of the MONICA participating centres several secondary objectives are set using the community surveillance programme as an excellent tool for evaluating research projects. In many centres the surveillance programme provides essential information on the effect of cardiovascular preventive programmes.

Registration and follow-up of congenital heart diseases

EUROCAT is a result of concerted action of the EEC for the epidemiological surveillance of congenital anomalies.[20] As a sub-project of EUROCAT, a registration of congenital heart disease at present is done in different centres in Western Europe. The general objective is to measure the prevalence and distribution of congenital heart disease in different geographically defined populations in Europe and to assess the survival and outcome of affected children. Specific and additional objectives are described elsewhere.[21]

In conclusion, although community surveillance of CVD has always been of prime importance for public health, insufficient attention has been paid to it for too many years. More recently surveillance systems have been developed and encouraging progress is being made. Hopefully this development will continue and will be extended to other major health problems.

Bibliography

1. Engel, L. W., Strauchen, J. A., and Chiazze, L., Accuracy of death certification in an autopsied population with specific attention to malignant neoplasms and vascular diseases. *Am. J. Epidemiol.* **111,** 99–112 (1980).
2. Cozurin, L. I., Wolf, P. A., and Kannel, W. B., Accuracy of death certification of stroke: The Framingham Study. *Stroke* **13,** 818–21 (1982).
3. Gittelsohn, A. and Senning, J., Studies on the reliability of vital and health records. I. Comparison of cause of deaths and hospital record diagnoses. *Am. J. publ. Hlth* **69,** 680–9 (1979).
4. Gillum, R. F., Feinleib, M., Margolis, J. R., Fabsitz, R. R., and Brasch, R. C., Community surveillance of cardiovascular disease: The Framingham cardiovascular disease survey. *J. chron. Dis.* **29,** 289–99 (1976).
5. Kuller, L. H., Lilienfeld, A., and Fisher R., Sudden and unexpected deaths due to natural causes in adults: A comparison of deaths certified and not certified by the medical examiner. *Arch. environ. Hlth* **13,** 236–42 (1966).
6. Scherde, E., Over de beperkingen van de officiële sterftestatistieken. *Huisarts en Wetenschap* **26,** 286–8 (1983).
7. WHO, Ischaemic Heart Disease Registers. Regional Office for Europe, Copenhagen (1968).
8. Uemura, K. and Pisa, Z., Recent trends in cardiovascular disease mortality in 27 industrialised countries. *World Hlth Stat. Quart.* **38** (1985).
9. *Proc. Conf. on Decline in Coronary Heart Disease Mortality*, US Government Printing Office, Washington, DC. USPHEW 79, 1610 (1979).
10. Gillum, R. F., Community surveillance for cardiovascular disease. Methods, problems, applications—a review. *J. chron. Dis.* **31,** 87–94 (1978).

11. WHO, Myocardial infarction community registers. Public Health in Europe, No. 5. Regional Office for Europe, Copenhagen (1976).
12. Alfredsson, L. and Ahlbom, A., Increasing incidence and mortality from myocardial infarction in Stockholm County. *Br. med. J.* **286,** 1931–3 (1983).
13. Beaglehole, R., Bonita, R., Jackson, R., Stewart, A., Sharpe, N., and Fraser, G. E., Trends in coronary heart disease event rates in New Zealand. *Am. J. Epidemiol.* **120,** 225–35 (1984).
14. Koskenvuo, M., Kaprio, J., Langindinio, H., Romo, M., and Pulkkinen, P., Changes in incidence and prognosis of ischaemic heart disease in Finland: A record linkage study of data on death certificates and hospital records for 1972 and 1981. *Br. med. J.* **290,** 1771–5 (1985).
15. Friedman, G. D. Decline in hospitalizations for coronary heart disease and stroke: The Kaiser Permanente experience in Northern California: 1971–1977. In ref. 9, 109–14 (1979).
16. De Backer, G., Tunstall-Pedoe, H., and Ducimetière, P., Surveillance of the dietary habits of the population with regard to cardiovascular diseases. EURONUT Report 2 (1983).
17. Fortman, S. P., Haskell, W. L., Williams, P. T., Varady, A. N., Hulley, S. B., and Farquhar, J. W., Community surveillance of cardiovascular diseases in the Stanford Five-City Project. *Am. J. Epidemiol.* **123,** 656–69 (1986).
18. Gillum, R. F., Blackburn, H., and Feinleib, M., Current strategies for explaining the decline in ischaemic heart disease mortality. *J. chron. Dis.* **35,** 467–74 (1982).
19. Tunstall-Pedoe, H., Monitoring trends in cardiovascular disease and risk factors: the WHO 'MONICA' project. *WHO Chron.* **39**(2), 3–5 (1985).
20. De Wals, P., Weatherall, J. A. C., and Lechat, M. F., *Registration of congenital anomalies in EUROCAT-centres, 1979–1983.* Cabay, Louvain-la-Neuve, (1985).
21. EUROCAT guide 2 for the registration and follow-up of congenital heart disease. EUROCAT working group on CHD. *Louvain-la-Neuve News*, pp. 1–21 (1986).

12

Nutritional surveillance in Europe: an operational approach

A. KELLY

Introduction

Accurate, reliable, and timely information is required for the detection, control, and prevention of nutrition-related public health problems. Nutritional surveillance systems have been developed during the last decade to meet this requirement. Surveillance is accomplished by observing, analysing, and reporting regularly on a wide range of variables indicative of food consumption patterns, nutritional status, and health impact. Such information then provides an empirical basis for decision-making and policy-planning. In a sentence, nutritional surveillance means 'to watch over nutrition in order to make decisions which will lead to improvements in nutrition in populations'.[1]

The term 'Nutritional Surveillance' (NS), was adopted during the World Food Conference in Rome in 1974, arising from which a joint FAO/ UNICEF/WHO Expert Committee was convened to set out a general methodology suitable for global application.[2] Since then, more than two dozen countries, almost entirely in the developing world, have implemented, in one form or another, a NS system. A wealth of experience has accumulated, although many practical difficulties, both technical and institutional, remain to be overcome.[1,3,4]

Clearly, from the perspective of the developed economies of the West, the need for NS (or indeed, for explicit food and nutrition policies, as distinct from purely agricultural policies) has been less obvious. As the problems of food scarcity and unequal distribution were largely overcome, diseases and health problems associated with dietary deficiency have, for the most part, disappeared. Ironically, it is now apparent that the existence of a surplus food supply has actually given rise to a series of new health problems. In a recent report from EURO-NUT[5] it was affirmed that one of the major public health problems facing EEC countries is the high prevalence of the so-called 'diseases of affluence', i.e. coronary heart disease, atherosclerosis, hypertensive disease, diabetes mellitus, colo/rectal cancer, breast cancer, etc. These represent a primary cause of premature death and hospitalization in our society, the cost of which in both economic and social terms is immense. But, in tandem with those conditions arising from dietary excess or imbalance, some residual problems of undernutrition persist in the traditionally vulnerable groups within our society; for example, the very young, the elderly, and now, due to continuing large-scale unemployment, the economically stressed. In addition, the existence of food additives raises new scientific questions concerning a wide range of health problems.

While the precise role of diet in the aetiology of certain diseases is, as yet, unclear, there is broad agreement that diet represents a significant contributory factor. In recognition of this, a large number of expert committees, both national and international[6,7] have deliberated and produced, as prerequisites for nutrition planning and health promotion, dietary guidelines which are remarkably similar.[8] A further prerequisite is a decision-support system to aid the planning process by correcting deficiencies in knowledge, and by presenting a coherent picture of the environment as it changes; such is the *raison d'être* of nutritional surveillance.

In the following pages nutritional surveillance will be introduced from an operational perspective, by considering, in outline, basic information needs, a minimal model for an NS system, followed by a description of the major components of the system. In the main, these features are illustrated by reference to the Irish experience which may be taken as generally applicable to any European country.[9] Indeed, considerable interest is now being expressed in the development, and possible co-ordination, of NS systems in Europe, both within the EEC, and in a wider context, by the Regional Office of the World Health Organisation in Copenhagen. In May 1986, a EURO-NUT sponsored workshop took place in Athens and was attended by delegates from the 12 EEC member states as well as representatives from Scandinavia. It was clear from this meeting that most, if not all, of the elements required to establish NS programmes (discussed below) are currently present in these countries. All that is lacking is the establishment of national units with responsibility for the co-ordination and integration of existing information sources. A report, based on this meeting, is to be published by EURO-NUT during 1987[10] and a book dealing with the methodology of NS and directed primarily at planners and decision-makers will be produced by WHO-EURO, also in 1987.

Clearly, parallels exist with nutritional surveillance systems already operational in Asia, Africa, and South America. However, these have been designed to cope with radically different problems, structures and facilities from those obtaining in the West, and it will be necessary to evolve new methodologies to facilitate medium- to long-term nutrition planning to cater for our future needs in Europe.

The Surveillance System

Information needs

Designing an optimal, yet economic, information system to meet particular needs is by no means a simple exercise. No system can anticipate all contingencies, but rather must contain sufficient flexibility to be responsive to changing perceptions and demands over time-scales of decades. Therefore, a critical question, though hardly a trivial one, is: "What basic information is required for effective nutrition planning?" A general response might very well include the following (see, for example, Pines[11]):

(a) who is malnourished;
(b) in what ways;
(c) in what circumstances;
(d) why;
(e) how are conditions changing with time?

Before one can attempt to answer these questions, some form of conceptual model reflecting our present understanding of the interrelationships between three interacting systems, namely:

FOOD SUPPLY→FOOD CONSUMPTION→HEALTH IMPACT

must be constructed to provide a framework from which to proceed. Such a model is referred to as a 'food chain', a simplified version of which is shown in Fig. 12.1. This flow diagram depicts the essential macro-level elements which must be monitored. The model is plausible, and encourages revision with experience and as further understanding is gained through medical and epidemiological research.

Surveillance data base

Having indicated the initial data requirements, then ideally these would be met by recourse to extensive field surveys. However, such large-scale surveys are prohibitively expensive, and are unlikely to be repeated on a sufficiently regular basis to meet planning needs in a changing environment. Instead, data already available through routine sources (for example in Agriculture and Health), or readily obtainable, are fully utilized to furnish a feasible and adaptable assessment tool. The core data sets (indicated in Fig. 12.2) are typically derived from statistics on national food production/supply, household surveys, food prices (collectively referred to as 'Dietary surveillance'), morbidity and mortality rates, fertility, data on infant feeding practice and birthweight, and height and weight measurements for schoolchildren and adults (referred to as 'Health impact surveillance'). These are continually updated as, and when, new sources become available. Of course, data do not constitute information, and therefore extensive statistical analyses are

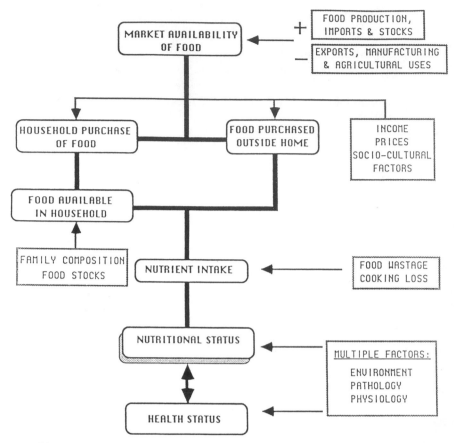

Fig. 12.1. Simplified model of the food chain and associated determinants.

required to understand and suitably summarize such diverse material. Irrespective of the form of analysis, results should be:

(a) *relevant*—that is, findings must be characterized in functional terms i.e. by age, sex, region, income, etc. to enable problem definition and possible targeting of intervention;

(b) *reliable*—reasonably so, as high degrees of precision are rarely essential to the decision-making process; unlike basic research, no attempt is being made to investigate causal mechanisms;

(c) *valid*—accurate or unbiased estimates for a properly identified group;

(d) *timely*—the regular updating of information to retain its utility;

(e) *appropriately formulated*—clearly presented in a form that is both concise and useful to planners.

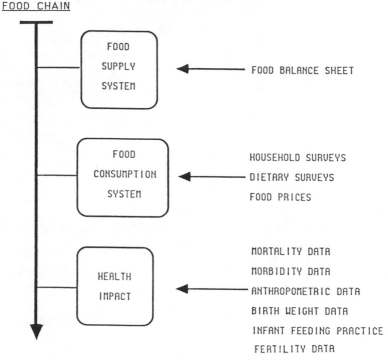

Fig. 12.2. Primary sources of information for surveillance data base.

To answer certain detailed questions, particularly regarding consumption patterns and attitudes, core data are necessarily supplemented by periodic, possibly small-scale surveys of targeted groups. In addition, use is made of a wide range of research undertaken by nutrition scientists and epidemiologists operating outside the NS programme. Consultation and information exchange with sectoral interests, data suppliers, scientists, and experts are fundamental to the successful operation of NS. Figure 12.3 illustrates this information cycle as it is developing in Ireland. The Expert Committee referred to in this figure has been appointed by the Minister for Health and consists of representatives drawn from all sectors having an interest in food, nutrition, health, and education. This committee's role is to strengthen the inputs to the NS system as well as to provide for an informed and critical appraisal of the findings, and, based on the latter, to identify various problem areas and then to propose a set of policy options for consideration by the Ministry of Health.

Note that the focus is entirely on information requirements for planning, and not primarily for scientific purposes. In effect, surveillance measures what is needed for policy guidance, even if it can only be measured poorly! As decisions affecting matters of policy are rarely made on the strength of the

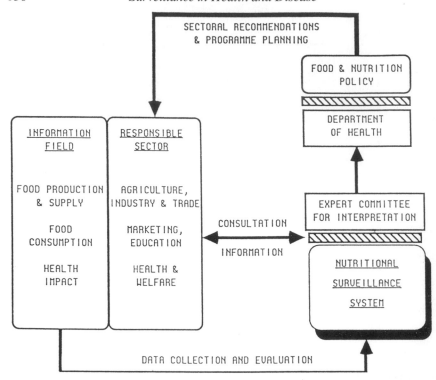

Fig. 12.3.   Information cycle in the Irish nutritional surveillance programme.

data alone, frequently it is the case that such decisions are robust to poor quality data. Härö discusses a number of misconceptions regarding data quality which can arise in the interactions of data producers, data analysts, scientists, and decision-makers.[12]

Costs

In Ireland, we have found that financing a NS programme is reasonably inexpensive. Assuming that the operation is based in a research environment of a Ministry, which provides office accommodation, etc. then there are three major items of expenditure in relation to the running of a NS system namely: (i) data acquisition, (ii) computing, and (iii) manpower. We can examine each of these in turn.

Data acquistion   Broadly speaking, there are three sources of data available to the system:

1. *Official statistics*—food balance sheets, households surveys, vital statistics, and (possibly) morbidity data, etc. These are collected regularly

for routine purposes by the state or state agencies, e.g. the Ministry of Health, the regional health authorities, the Central Statistics Office, and medical and/or social research institutes. Such data are invariably free or available at a nominal charge to 'official' users.

2. *Survey data*—specific surveys conducted by the NS unit to provide detailed information on a sample of the population or a sub-group of interest. Depending both on the purpose of the study and the available resources, such surveys need not entail a large expenditure. Indeed, the ongoing nature of a surveillance system encourages the planning of a series of small-scale (either complementary or overlapping) surveys over a period of several years, thus ensuring a modest outlay in any given year—an important consideration when seeking annual funding.

3. *Ad hoc sources*—consumer purchasing patterns are studied by food producers, retailers, and marketing boards and such information can, in certain circumstances, be made available to the surveillance system. In addition, a substantial amount of relevant work is usually being undertaken by researchers within a country and may be integrated into the NS system. Costs associated with gathering data from either of these sources are likely to be minimal.

Computing It is our experience that, during the course of a year, several hundreds of hours of computing may be required for purposes of data processing. This includes:

(a) data editing/preparation;
(b) statistical analyses;
(c) generation of graphics for the presentation of findings; and
(d) report production.

Items (c) and (d) are performed on sophisticated personal computers, as is much of (a) and (b). However, access to a mainframe is certainly required for manipulating very large data files and consequently some few tens of hours of CPU (Central Processing Unit) time on a large time-sharing system are budgeted for annually.

Manpower Again, our experience indicates that the minimal requirement is for a programme manager, a research assistant, and a number of researchers and advisors available for temporary assignment for periods ranging from one to six months for specific projects.

Some additional costs

Two further costs are worth mentioning. The first relates to the production of an annual report which is intended not only for the Ministry of Health, but is also distributed on request to: nutritionists, dietitians, clinicians, teachers, public health nurses, the media, marketing boards, and commercial firms. The second concerns the holding of an annual workshop to which representatives of all sectors having an interest in diet and public health are invited. This workshop serves several purposes, namely, to disseminate the latest findings of the surveillance system, to obtain feedback from our data providers and other experts, and, not least, as a public relations exercise in support of the NS programme. The latter is crucial, given our dependence on national agencies and other bodies for data provision.

It was stated above that nutritional surveilance can conveniently be separated into two distinct sub-systems, viz. dietary surveillance and health impact survellance. In the remainder of this paper, both of these sub-systems are examined in brief, with greater emphasis on dietary surveillance in view of the coverage of mortality and morbidity data provided elsewhere in this book.

Dietary Surveillance

The overall objective of dietary surveillance is to assess dietary habits, but at what level and with what effectiveness? What data are available or must be acquired? Dietary information may be identified at three separate levels:

1. Dietary patterns at *national level* in terms of structure—the relative importance of the major food components, i.e. cereals, meat, vegetables, etc., in the national diet; quality—calories, protein, fat, dietary fibre, etc.; evolution—the changing dietary profile with time.
2. Dietary patterns at the level of *subgroups of households*, again in terms of structure—choice of foodstuffs, i.e. family purchasing/consumption patterns; quality—mean group consumption of macro- and micronutrients; and evolution—pattern of group consumption with time.
3. Dietary patterns at the level of *sub-groups of individuals*, this is similar to level 2. In addition to dietary practice, information on knowledge and attitudes can also be sought at this level.

Data relating to levels 1 and 2 may be obtained from Food Balance Sheets and Households Surveys, respectively—both available in the European region, while level 3 requires periodic sample surveys. These relationships are shown in Fig. 12.4. The capabilities of each are described below. The definitions used are those provided by Klaver *et al.*,[13] with slight modifications.

National level—Food Balance Sheets (FBS)

Definition A national Food Balance Sheet is an account of the annual production of food, changes in food stocks, imports and exports, and distribution of food over various uses within the country. Daily per capita food availability is expressed in grams of food, energy and some additional nutrients.

FBS data are likely to be available from two sources: (i) from the annual

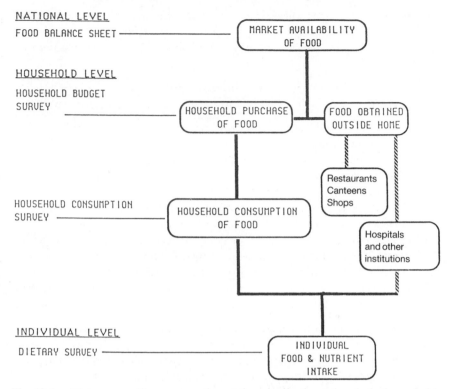

Fig. 12.4. Dietary surveillance operating at three levels: the national, the household, and the individual level.

published statistics of the FAO[14] or OECD,[15] or (ii) nationally, from the agency responsible for their compilation. Significant differences may exist between these two sources. Such differences arise because the FAO imposes a standard format on all contributors (useful for inter-country studies); this format may be considered deficient or limiting for within-country studies, and national statistics should be sought.

Utility These data give information on the current and evolving structure of a national diet in terms of the major food commodities and selected macro-nutrients which are disappearing into consumption. Time dependence on economic and demographic factors can be investigated, and short-term forecasts can be produced with a view to anticipating change resulting from market developments, and/or intervention activities. Also, relationships between trends in nutrient consumption and chronic disease patterns can be sought in an initial attempt to elucidate the role of diet in the latter. Inter-country comparisons, using both cross-sectional and time series data, can be informative. The latter must be interpreted with due caution because of residual uncertainties arising from differing food accounting practices by individual countries (see below), even after the standardization required by FAO.

Limitations   The following comments may apply in part or in whole when making comparisons within a given country over time or between countries:

1. Border trade and home production can significantly affect the availability of certain foods.
2. Recording accuracy differs substantially for different foodstuffs, as certain items are produced centrally (for example, sugar), while others are not (for example, vegetables).
3. Recording accuracy may improve or deteriorate with time for different products, and is likely to differ between countries.
4. For certain items, product weight may be recorded (for example, whole carcass for livestock) which includes inedible portions.
5. Certain items may be omitted (for example, alcohol, offal, fish).
6. Conversion of available foodstuffs into nutrient equivalents must be treated with caution, if not scepticism.

One factor tends to minimize or offset the above limitations, that is the accumulated expertise of the government agency (and FAO) responsible for compiling national figures. Repeating the exercise on an annual basis for several decades will result in a large degree of consistency and a corresponding measure of reliability. Therefore, we conclude that the reported absolute levels of per capita availability are not particularly meaningful for our purposes; only relative comparisons, year by year, are reasonable. Figures 12.5

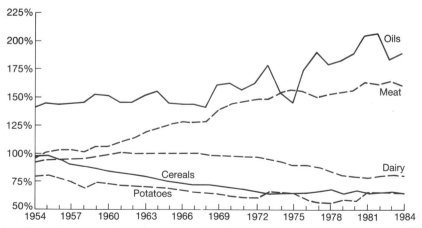

Fig. 12.5.   Relative change in selected major foodstuffs. Base year 1936. (FBS, Ireland.)

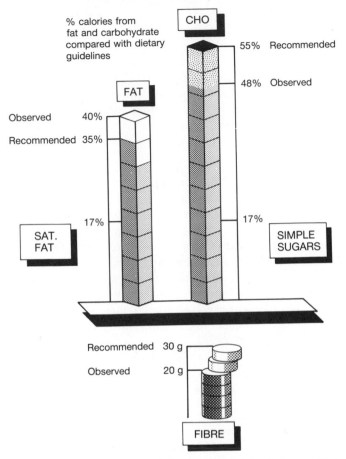

Fig. 12.6. National dietary pattern (1986) compared to dietary guidelines (FBS, Ireland.)

and 12.6 show a sample of the output from these data illustrating the change in the national dietary pattern.[9]

Household level—household budget and consumption surveys

Definition   Two forms of national household food surveys may be identified:

1. Household food consumption in an economic sense is the sum of the food commodities *purchased*, or obtained by other means, by the household. (Price data are then necessary to convert to food quantities.)
2. Household food consumption in a nutritional sense is the food and beverages *consumed* by the household.

These provide either indirect (1) or direct (2) estimates of the food entering the household during a specified period. Most European countries conduct household surveys on a periodic basis, primarily to update the national consumer price index; both expenditure on, and quantities of foodstuffs purchased are usually recorded. Within the EEC, the Statistical Office is now compiling harmonized cross-country information, including expenditure on selected foodstuffs, from national household budget surveys.[16] The United Kingdom appears to be the only European country performing a dedicated annual household food survey.[17]

Utility   These surveys investigate dietary habits in *subgroups of households* in the population. Thus, the influence of a number of social, demographic, and economic factors (for example, social class, household composition, region, income, etc.) on the household purchase or consumption of foodstuffs can be modelled. Relative expenditure on different food groups cross-classified by the above variables will prove informative, especially in relation to policy issues on pricing, food subsidies, fortification, and marketing. Also, household expenditure on food relative to total expenditure may help to identify potentially at-risk groups (of households). Specific household types can be identified and examined; for example, households with a particularly low or high consumption of specific foods, or households with person(s) over 65 years of age living alone. Availability of data from previous surveys would enable consumer eating-patterns to be studied longitudinally. Foodstuffs may be converted to equivalent nutrients and similarly analysed.

Limitations   Unlike the Food Balance Sheet, household surveys in Europe come in a variety of forms with a greater or lesser emphasis on food. The points which follow are necessarily general in nature and, as in the case of FBS data, are indicative of the factors which must be considered when analysing these data:

1. Details on foods consumed outside the home, for example in canteens or restaurants, may not be available.
2. Alcohol consumed outside the home may not be included.
3. Household food stocks may not be accounted for.
4. Waste from a variety of sources may need to be estimated, and households of differing composition are likely to differ significantly in this.
5. Aggregation of individual food items into broader food categories is inevitable and results in loss of information. New products may be subsumed into existing categories.
6. If expenditure is recorded rather than quantities, then reliable price-per-item information must also be obtained.

7. The conversion of foods into nutrient equivalents depends on the availability of suitable national food tables.
8. As data are only available at household level no information is provided on consumption patterns of household members.

Due to cost factors, household surveys are normally only conducted on a five- to seven-yearly basis, although, because of the short-term conservative nature of nutrient intake (though not of individual food items), developing patterns are subject to timely detection.

Individual level—dietary surveys

Definition A dietary survey is designed to obtain quantitative and/or qualitative information on food consumption by groups of individuals.

Utility As neither the Food Balance Sheet nor the Household Survey are intended to provide information on the actual consumption of food by individuals, dietary surveys have a role to play in problem definition. That role is to establish the adequacy or otherwise of dietary consumption (of all or particular nutrients) in specific and clearly identified subgroups of individuals within the population, such as: elderly persons living alone, young unmarried mothers, middle aged males, or other at-risk groups. The purpose of these surveys is not the nutritional screening of the individual, but rather the characterization of the dietary profile (or attitudes, or knowledge) of sections of society with the intention, if necessary, of designing an appropriate form of intervention. For this purpose, small scale, or so-called 'micro' surveys, may be particularly efficient, and these can also be used in regular follow-up studies. For example, a major difficulty encountered with the national household surveys is that they fail to provide information on food consumed outside the home by family members (as only expenditure is recorded). Moreoever, the increasing interest and concern being expressed in relation to exposure to food contaminants, pesticides, growth stimulants, and artificial agents, requires a detailed knowledge of the dietary habits of those groups under investigation—this is unlikely to be fully met by most national household budget surveys (as presently constituted).

Limitations Each form of dietary survey has its own limitations. There will be no attempt here to consider these as they have been adequately dealt with in the literature. Callmer *et al.* consider the criteria for selecting a dietary survey method appropriate to the level at which inferences are to be made.[18] Additional references are to be found in the EURO-NUT Report No. 1.[5]

Surveillance of Health Impact

Unbalanced nutrition contributes to the incidence of certain diseases. Conversely, selected morbidity and mortality rates as well as fertility rates may be interpreted as indicators of nutritional status. Their collective impact on public health throughout Europe, in terms of premature death, hospitalization, and disability give cause for grave concern. Effective intervention to tackle this unnecessary burden calls for an improved understanding of the development of chronic disease in populations and associated behaviour patterns, and this in turn requires that relevant morbidity and mortality patterns be monitored, as well as other measures of health status and environmental conditions. Some health indicators are discussed now in the specific context of nutritional surveillance (and more generally elsewhere in this book).

Mortality rates

Primarily by virtue of their availability, completeness, and comparability (but see below), standardized mortality statistics have been used traditionally to indicate the level of community health and the change in health status over time, forecast future demand for services, and provide inter-country comparisons.[19,20] In addition to reports on vital statistics, information on heart disease and certain cancers may be obtainable from incidence registers. Unacceptably high rates for ischaemic heart disease have prompted political action to initiate wide-ranging primary prevention programmes, e.g. the North Karelia Project[21] and a number of similar projects in other European countries, and the United States, in addition to long-term monitoring programmes, such as WHO's MONICA project.

Utility   Trends in age/sex standardized mortality statistics for selected diseases are examined to estimate their incidence and prevalence by region and social class. Period and cohort models are available to describe such trends. Relationships between trends in national dietary patterns and chronic diseases can be sought using multivariate analysis techniques in an initial attempt to explore the association and to derive testable hypotheses. Economic and social effects may be studied using techniques such as potential years of life lost,[22] or through cost–benefit analysis as shown for smoking by Oster *et al.*[23]

Limitations   The limitations of mortality data have been discussed often in the context of epidemiological research.[20,24,25] However, from the NS perspective, the major drawback of these data is that they tell us nothing of the condition of the survivors.

Morbidity rates (Hospital based)

Hospital In-Patient Enquiry (HIPE) schemes based on admissions or discharges, provide information on conditions of interest requiring hospitalization, but not necessarily resulting in death. In some countries (for example UK) a Hospital Activity Analysis may also be available.

Utility   These data may be analysed in a manner similar to mortality data, although information is available additionally on duration of stay in hospital, which allows for an economic component to the analysis.

Limitations   HIPE data are rarely complete or fully reliable. They are also subject to a number of the problems experienced in using mortality data—for example, variation in diagnostic criteria, especially where multiple conditions are present, and errors in the denominator in calculating standardized rates. A severe difficulty in calculating rates is caused by the recording of events, i.e. admissions or discharges, and double counting is inevitable if patients are admitted more than once during a year. Again, prevalence and incidence estimates of rates of disease (for certain conditions more so than others) based on hospital data alone, will be underestimated. Further information on the prevalence of conditions not serious enough to require hospitalization, may be extracted from a variety of sources: morbidity surveys on population samples, General Practitioner's files (discussed in detail elsewhere in this book), certificates issued for school or industrial absenteeism, and prescription rates for drugs.

Additional sources of data

A variety of data are available which can be interpreted in a manner useful to the surveillance system.

Anthropometry   Growth and development in children are easily observed and readily measured, and such measurements are often routinely available from national programmes of pre-school and school-health examinations. Anthropometric indices are internationally used as nutrition status indicators, both in nutritional screening of individual children and in subgroup assessment. General population studies of adults are less routine (except in the narrower context of health insurance, or where national conscription applies), but provide crucial information on the prevalence of obesity—an important risk indicator for certain chronic diseases and now regarded as a major public health hazard in many Western nations. One adult group for whom height and weight data are normally available through pre-natal clinical records are pregnant women.

Birthweight   Birthweight statistics are available from maternity hospitals or from a central register. Infant mortality and morbidity are closely linked to birthweight, and the association between birthweight and maternal nutrition is well documented. Low-birthweight can be used to identify at-risk groups in terms of age marital status, social class, and location. The birthweight curve for a hospital (or region) may be modelled to establish the proportion and characteristics of the three components, i.e. low, optimal, and high, and the results may be compared by area and over time.

Fertility   Fertility may be a sensitive indicator of the consequences of the consumption of a variety of food additives; for example, pesticides in grain and cereals. For surveillance purposes, national statistics on birth are available. Birth rates do, however, only reflect part of the fertility picture. Abortion rates would also need to be taken into account, as would chromosomal changes in sperm and human tissues. Such information is, however, not readily to hand for population health surveillance. Surveillance on congenital malformations in relation to intake of food additives might produce some information of value in this field (see Chapter 10).

Infant feeding practice   Human milk is the most nutritious diet for the infant during the early months of rapid growth and offers added protection against infection. It is important to determine the extent of breast feeding regionally, and to identify those characteristics—both maternal and socio-demographic, which influence maternal choice. An understanding of these factors enables advisory and support services to be effectively targeted. This information should be obtainable from maternity records, but coverage and reliability can be poor.

Conclusion

In recent years the importance of nutrition for health has been increasingly recognized from a scientific standpoint, while the spiralling cost and severely limited capacity of curative medicine to control the diseases of affluence have added a strong economic impetus to further research in this field, given its considerable disease prevention potential. The available evidence has prompted international agencies, national governments, and professional bodies to produce recommendations for modifying the diet of populations or subgroups with the purpose of preventing nutrition-related diseases.

Dietary guidelines may be viewed as but one aspect of a comprehensive food and nutrition policy, which must be developed through the collaboration of the health sector with the food and agriculture industries, and which must take into account social and economic considerations as well as health needs. At the very minimum, such a policy must consider the medium- to long-term implications of decisions by other sectors (within a country and equally importantly, at EEC level) which may directly or indirectly affect nutrition conditions. Instruments available for implementation of policy include economic, technological, and educational measures, which can be applied at various points in the food chain from production through industrial processing to marketing and consumption. For the purposes of such policy-making, a requirement exists for reasonably accurate and timely information identifying trends occurring in food supply, food consumption and health effects. This is the function of nutritional surveillance.

Bibliography

1. Mason, J., Habicht, J. P., Tabatabai, H., and Valverde, V., *Nutritional surveillance*. WHO, Geneva (1984).
2. WHO, *Methodology of nutritional surveillance*. Technical Report No. 593. WHO, Geneva (1976).
3. UNICEF, *Background papers for workshop on social and nutritional surveillance in eastern and southern Africa*. UNICEF/EARO. Nairobi, Kenya (1982).
4. UNICEF, *Report on the Botswana workshop on clini-based nutritional surveillance systems and integrated data bases*. UNICEF/EARO. Nairobi, Kenya (1984).
5. Hautvast, J. and Klaver, W. (eds), *The diet factor in epidemiological research*. EURO-NUT Report 1. Agricultural University, Wageningen, The Netherlands (1982).
6. COMA, *Diet and cardiovascular disease*. Department of Health and Social Security, HMSO, London (1984).
7. WHO, *Prevention of coronary heart disease*. Technical Report No. 678. WHO, Geneva (1982).
8. WHO, *Guidelines for health nutrition, and for the prevention of diseases of major public health importance in Europe* (in preparation). WHO/EURO, Copenhagen (1986).
9. Kelly, A., *Nutritional surveillance in Ireland: Report for 1985*. Medico-Social Research Board, Dublin (1986).
10. Kelly, A., *Nutritional surveillance in Europe: A critical appraisal* (in preparation), EURO-NUT. Agricultural University, Wageningen, The Netherlands (1987).
11. Pines, J., The community nutrition planning process. In *Nutrition in the community* (ed. D. S. McLaren). John Wiley, New York (1983).
12. Hard, A. S., Information systems for health services at the national health level. In *Systems for health services* (cd. G. McLachlan). WHO, Copenhagen (1986).
13. Klaver, W., Knuiman, J., and van Staveren, W., Proposed definitions for use in the methodology of food consumption studies. In *The diet factor in epidemiological research*. EURO-NUT Report 1, Agricultural University, Wageningen, The Netherlands (1982).
14. FAO, *Food production yearbook* **37**. FAO, Rome (1984).
15. OECD. *Food consumption statistics, 1973–1982*. OECD, paris (1985).
16. EUROSTAT, *Family budgets: Comparative tables* **1**. EUROSTAT, Luxembourg (1984).
17. Derry, B. J. and Buss, D. H., The British national food survey as a major epidemiological resource. *Br. med. J.* **288**, 765–7 (1984).
18. Callmer, E., Haraldsdottir, J., Loken, J., Seppanen, R., and Solvoll, K., Selecting a method for a dietary survey. *Narings-Forskning* **29**, No. 2. Sweden (1985).
19. Black, D., Report of the working group on inequalities in health. Department of Health and Social Security. HMSO, London (1980).

20. Brzezinski, Z., *Mortality in the European region.* WHO, Copenhagen (1985).
21. Puska, P., Nissinen, A., and Tuomilehto, J., The community-based strategy to prevent coronary heart disease: Conclusions from the ten years of North Karelia Project. *Ann. Rev. publ. Hlth,* **6,** 147–93 (1985).
22. Romeder, J. and McWhinnie, J., Potential years of life lost between ages 1 and 70: An indicator of premature mortality for health planning. *Int. J. Epidemiol.* **6**(2) (1977).
23. Oster, G., Colditz, G., and Kelly, N., *The economic costs of smoking and benefits of quitting.* Lexington Books, Toronto (1984).
24. Alderson, M., *International mortality statistics.* Macmillan, London (1981).
25. Doll, R. and Peto, R., *The causes of cancer.* Oxford University Press (1983).

13

Surveillance of cancer

D. PARKIN

Introduction

Surveillance systems of cancer have been mainly used for the development of aetiological hypotheses by the study of the occurrence of disease in different areas, subgroups of the population and over time.

The planning of health services requires information on the size and distribution of the cancer problem and also on the effectiveness of preventive or therapeutic services. Because for most cancers there is a long and variable interval between exposure to carcinogens and clinical onset of disease, surveillance systems have only limited usefulness in the identification of discrete environmental hazards.

In this chapter we review the different types of data on cancer morbidity and mortality, and their availability in the countries of the European Economic Community (EEC). The uses to which such data have been put are also discussed.

Measurement: Cancer Data

Statistics on cancer occurrence

The single most useful measure for cancer surveillance is the incidence rate, which is an indicator of the risk of disease, and can be used to estimate service need. Incidence defines the load of new cases arising per unit time, and hence priorities and requirements for treatment facilities. Measurement of incidence requires the identification of all new cases of disease in a defined population, and hence some kind of case-finding mechanism, and record-linkage to ensure that persons are not confused with events. The cancer registry is the usual method of collecting such data. However, cancer registration is a relatively recent development, the oldest functioning registries having been in existence for at most fifty years.[1] For surveillance purposes mortality rates have been more widely used, since these have been available for a much longer period, and usually for larger populations. In these circumstances, the mortality rate is usually being used as a proxy measure of incidence. Death rates will be very similar to incidence for cancers with poor survival (for example, oesophagus, stomach, liver, lung). For cancers with a more favourable prognosis such as colon and breast, the incidence rate will be considerably higher than mortality and any inferences which are made from the latter about variation in incidence of disease assume that survival rates are reasonably constant. However, when survival rates are changing substantially as a result of improved methods of treatment (for example, Hodgkin's disease, childhood leukaemia), then mortality rates will be a poor guide to incidence. Mortality, rather than incidence, is the appropriate measure in certain circumstances, however, particularly when the objective of surveillance is to estimate the effectiveness of treatment or early detection programmes.

Mortality statistics   Death rates are widely available as a result of the introduction of legislation requiring that the fact and cause of death in a community be certified, usually by a medical practitioner. The International Classification of Diseases (ICD) provides a uniform system of nomenclature and coding, and a recommended format for the death certificate. When mortality statistics are presented it is the underlying cause of death which forms the axis of classification; this may not equate with the presence of a particular tumour. Although the ICD contains a carefully defined set of rules and guidelines which allow underlying cause to be selected in a uniform manner, interpretation of the concept probably varies considerably; for example, when death occurs from pneumonia in a person previously diagnosed as having cancer. Comprehensive mortality statistics thus require that good diagnostic data are available on decedents, which are transferred in a logical, standardized fashion to death certificates which are then accurately and consistently coded, compiled, and analysed.

There have been many studies of the validity of cause of death statements in vital statistics data. The methods used involved the comparison of the cause of death entered on the death certificate, with a reference diagnosis derived from autopsy reports,[2] detailed clinical records,[3,4] or cancer registry data.[5] Such studies reveal that the degree of accuracy of the stated cause of death declines as the degree of precision in the diagnosis increases. Thus, although the total number of deaths from cancer of all types may be only slightly underestimated, the distribution by site of cancer may be incorrect. There is a tendency to over-record non-specific diagnoses instead of the correct location (for example, large intestine instead of rectum), and accuracy is sometimes lower in those dying at older ages, or at home.

The study of Puffer and Wynne-Griffith[3] in twelve separate cities (ten in Latin America plus Bristol and San Francisco) showed that much of the apparent difference in mortality rates between them could be explained by variation in certification practices. This study took no account of differences which would have been introduced if the certificates had also been coded in each centre. Percy and Dolman[6] studied this by sending 1246 death certificates from the Third National Cancer Survey in the United States for coding of 'cause of death' in seven countries in Europe and North America. Comparisons at the three-digit level of the ICD showed that all seven centres coded the same underlying cause of death for only 53 per cent of certificates. Large variations existed for individual sites and it was concluded that differences in the application of rules for selecting underlying cause of death seriously affect cancer mortality statistics.

There are further potential sources of bias in the study of time trends in mortality. A wider availability of diagnostic resources (biochemical, radiological, and endoscopic) or an increase in hospitalization of elderly patients will mean that fewer diagnoses of cancer are missed, and that the sites of origin of the tumours are determined more accurately. This will apply particularly to cancers which are difficult to diagnose on clinical grounds alone (e.g. pancreatic cancer, lung cancer). In addition, for certain sites of cancer, time trend studies are complicated by changes in the classification system with successive revisions of the International Classification of Diseases. Table 13.1 shows the result of changes introduced with the ninth revision in 1978 on the number of cancers certified as 'bone' (ICD 170)—the new revision specified rules to ensure that 'metastatic bone cancer' was not included in this category.

The great advantage of mortality statistics is their comprehensive coverage, and their availability. All national vital statistics departments produce analyses of mortality rates by cause; in addition, the data are sent to WHO in Geneva on computer tape or by questionnaire. They relate only to entire national populations, however, and if detail on subdivisions of the population are required, national sources must be consulted. These mortality data are presented in tabular form in the World Health Statistics Annual. In addi-

Table 13.1 Mortality from bone cancer: effect of ICD revision (ICD-8 vs. ICD-9)

Year		No. of deaths certified to ICD-170	
		USA	England & Wales
ICD-8	1977	1721	417
	1978	1737	465
ICD-9	1979	1190	316
	1980		293
% Change 1978–1979		− 32%	− 32%

Source: Percy—Unpublished data.
5

| | 3-digit | 1955–1982 |

*Short list: 'A' list of ICD 6, 7, 8, Basic Tabulation List of ICD-9 3-digit: ICD 7–9.
†na = not applicable.

tion, in recent years WHO has set up a system of standardized computer tapes which allow extraction of the data in more detail or in different formats. There are three files relevant to cancer: a general mortality file (deaths by age, sex, and cause), a special cancer mortality file (deaths by age, sex, and detailed site), and a denominator file on population by sex and age. The availability (mid-1985) of data from the countries of the EEC is shown in Table 13.2. For the majority, there is information by three-digit ICD categories since 1955, the seventh revision being in use until 1968 (1971 in Luxemburg and Portugal), and since 1979 the 9th revision has become standard. The table also shows two indicators which are often used to judge quality of data. It is known, for example, that about one-fifth of the deaths coded to 'Senility and ill defined conditions' in Europe are likely to be due to cancer.[7] Unfortunately, it is not possible to adjust the cancer deaths by reassigning deaths from the senility category, since it is known that many countries already perform routine, mechanical 'corrections' to reduce the numbers in this group. Similarly, the number of cancer deaths without specification of site of primary, or where it is given in only vague terms, is shown. In general, as far as can be judged from such figures, quality of data is fairly good.

Morbidity statistics   A direct estimate of cancer incidence must be obtained by collecting data on cases of cancer in the population. Statistics based on utilization of health services (for example, clinic attendances or hospital discharges) are often available but since these are event-based it is usually not possible to relate them to incidence rates. Incidence rates of cancer are derived from population-based cancer registration[8] which involves the collection of information on all new cases of cancer in a defined population. The first such registry in Europe which is still functioning, the Danish Cancer Registry, was founded in 1942 and there has been a steady growth in the number of cancer registries, and in the population covered, since that time.

A registry must collect information on cancer cases from diverse sources, and link together the documents pertaining to a single individual (or more correctly a single tumour), so that as far as possible no new case of cancer is missed, and no case is recorded twice. Sources of information may be special notification forms completed by physicians and sent to the registry—in some countries there is a legal basis for this provided by compulsory notification. However, most registries rely in addition, or as an alternative, upon the use of documents completed for other purposes. Hospital discharge abstracts, treatment records (especially from oncology or radiotherapy units), and pathology reports referring to cancer are the most common source documents. Most registries also make arrangements to obtain from vital statistics offices copies of death certificates which mention cancer as a causative or contributory factor. Registries will usually attempt to elicit further information on cases of cancer which first come to their attention in this way, but in

Table 13.2

Country	Detail*	Years available	% deaths attributed to senility ill-defined conditions (A136 & A137)		Quality indicators % malignant neoplasm deaths assigned to ill-defined or unknown sites (195–199)	
			M	F	M	F
Belgium	Short list	1954, 1980–1982	8	10	6	10
	3-digit	1955–1979				
Denmark	Short list	1951–1954	4	4	4	6
	3-digit	1955–1982				
France	Short list	1950–1954	6	9	10	12
	3-digit	1955–1981				
FRG	Short list	1952–1954	3	4	7	9
	3-digit	1955–1983				
Greece	Short list	1961–1965	8	11	17	19
	3-digit	1966–1982				
Ireland	Short list	1950–1954	1	1	5	5
	3-digit	1955–1981				
Italy	Short list	1951–1954	2	4	6	9
	3-digit	1955–1980				
Luxembourg	Short list	1967–1978	5	6	?	?
	3-digit	1979–1982				
Netherlands	Short list	1950–1954	5	5	4	6
	3-digit	1955–1983				
Portugal	Short list	1955–1982	12	18	na†	na†
	3-digit	—				
Spain	Short list	1950–1954	4	6	6	9
	3-digit	1955–1979				
UK	Short list	1950–1954	<1	1	4	5
	3-digit	1955–1982				

*Short list: 'A' list of ICD 6, 7, 8, Basic Tabulation List of ICD-9
3-digit: ICD 7–9.
†na = not applicable.

147

its absence practice varies as to whether to reject such cases, or record them as 'Death Certificate Only' (DCO) cases. The proportion of cases of cancer first coming to the attention of the registry in this way is a useful indicator of completeness of registration.[9] If it is high, this implies that recorded incidence rates are likely to be too low. If a proportion of fatal cancers come to light only as a result of death certificates, then presumably a corresponding percentage of non-fatal cases is also being missed. Estimates of completeness of registration among non-fatal cases can be produced using information on time of diagnosis and reporting of cases first notified to the registry by death certificate.[10] In some countries (for example, France and Belgium) the medical part of the death certificate (which includes the diagnostic information) is anonymous, so that it is impossible to systematically link death certificates with registered cancers.

A further index of completeness of registration is a comparison of registrations with deaths in the same period and population, and for the same cause. Unless incidence is declining at a very rapid rate, then incidence should exceed mortality, the ratio being determined by the survival rate. Some care is needed in interpretation, however, since the registry diagnosis is likely to be more precise than that recorded at death certification (see above). Caution is also necessary when interpreting time trends in cancer incidence from a registry in which the completeness of registration is changing, since better ascertainment will give rise to apparent increases in the absence of any true change.

The quality of information recorded at cancer registration is likely to be superior to that at death registration and considerably more information about the patient and his/her tumour (including histological type and extent) can be recorded. A crude index of 'quality' of registry data is the calculation, for each site, of the percentage of diagnoses based upon histological examination—a high figure being taken to imply that precise information was available to allow correct identification of tumour site and histology. However, it should be noted that a high percentage of histologically verified neoplasms might equally imply that case ascertainment by other than pathology reports was defective.

A few studies have attempted to assess accuracy of information recorded in a registry. West[11] found, for example, that according to his interpretation of the clinical records, 6·3 per cent of registrations in Wales had been allocated an incorrect three-digit ICD code. A review of lung cancer registration in the Swedish Cancer Registry[12] found that 1·7 per cent of registrations were incorrect. However, for histological diagnoses there is usually a much larger discrepancy between registered diagnosis and that of the independent reviewer, depending upon the precision of histological type specified.[11-13]

Cancer registries record all newly diagnosed cases as 'incident', thus avoiding a problem of death certification—namely the decision as to whether a cancer has 'caused' a particular death. Some problems of comparisons between countries or due to revisions of ICD are thus much less evident. However, a new difficulty arises in deciding what constitutes an incident case. Prostate cancer, for example, is extremely common in subclinical form in the elderly—in the USA 25 per cent of males autopsied at age 70 have a prostate cancer.[14] If registries record autopsy-detected cancers as incident, then rates will vary according to the autopsy rate. When screening programmes which aim to detect early cancers (for example, breast or colon cancer) are introduced, the total number of new invasive cancers should not, in theory, change. There is some doubt whether this is true; in the lung cancer screening programme in the Mayo Clinic, screened groups continue to show an excess number of cancers over the unscreened,[15] and it has been suggested that screening brings to light cases of disease which would never have become clinically apparent. In addition, screening permits the diagnosis of *in situ* cases which should always be reported separately from invasive cancers. In the USA, incidence rates for breast cancer show a rise, whereas mortality is more or less constant.[16] Since there is no evidence of improving results of treatment, this may well represent the diagnosis and registration of previously inapparent lesions.

Incidence rates derived from cancer registries are also considerably more restricted in availability than mortality. The establishment of cancer registration in Europe has been a very haphazard process, in some countries there has been a (more or less) official policy to support and fund registries, elsewhere individual initiative of research orientated clinicians and pathologists has often been a major factor. The current status of cancer registration in the EEC countries is summarized in Table 13.3.

As an alternative to cancer registration, data on incidence of cancer can be obtained from morbidity surveys. These may be *ad hoc* studies limited to identifying specific tumours, which are essentially the same as cancer registration, except that the time-scale is limited, and the survey purely retrospective. General morbidity surveys record all cases of disease appearing in a sample of the community, for example, the surveys of morbidity at primary care level undertaken in The Netherlands and Great Britain (see chapters on Surveillance in primary care). The problem with such community level surveys is that for comparatively rare causes of morbidity, such as cancer, there are relatively few cases among the large number of contacts recorded by primary care workers, so that the populations studied are too small to yield very useful information.

Other statistics

Mortality data may be used to evaluate effectiveness of early detection programmes, and decrease in mortality is also the goal of treatment services. In fact, treatment is usually evaluated in terms of survival rates. Computation

Table 13.3 Population-based cancer registries in EEC countries, 1985

REGISTRY*	Data collection started	Approx. population covered	Data in cancer incidence in five continents	Notes
BELGIUM	—	—		A National Cancer Registry was established in 1983. This is a continuation and extension of the annual reports on cancer produced by the Ministry of Health/Oeuvre Belge du Cancer since 1947, which are based on claims made to the Unions Nationales de Mutualités (five large confederations of sickness funds).
DENMARK Danish Cancer Registry	1942	5.1 million	Vols I–IV since 1953	
FRANCE Bas-Rhin (Strasbourg)	1975	883 000	Vol. IV (1975–77)	Registries have also been started in Tarn (Albi), Hérault (Montpellier), Vaucluse (Avignon) and North Ardèche (Annonay). There is a digestive tract cancer registry in Côte d'Or (Dijon) and registries of childhood cancer in Lorraine (Nancy) and Alpes-Côte d'Azur (Marseille). The Enquête Permanente Cancer collects data on cases treated in the 22 Cancer Centres in France, and publishes regular statistics, notably on survival. These centres cover about 25% of all cancer cases; recruitment patterns vary by institution and by cancer site.
Doubs (Besançon)	1976	472 000	Vol. IV (1977)	
Isère (Grenoble)	1979	950 000	—	
Calvados (Caen)	1981	560 000 (all sites)	—	
FEDERAL REPUBLIC OF GERMANY Hamburg	1954	1.7 million	Vols. I–IV (since 1960)	There is a specialised registry for childhood cancer in Mainz, and for bone tumours in Heidelberg. Legal restrictions preserving confidentiality of medical records have greatly hindered extension of cancer registration.
Saarland	1966	1.1 million	Vols. III, IV (1968–77)	
GREECE	—	—	—	No population based registry. An Annual Statistical Survey of Cancer has been performed since 1967, organized by the Statistical Service of the Ministry of Social Services, which relies upon notification of cancer cases treated in hospitals. Coverage variable by region.
IRELAND Southern Tumor Registry (Cork)	1977	500 000	—	

Table 13.3 *cont.*

ITALY				In recent years, population-based registries have been founded in Latina, Toscana (Firenze), Genova, Bologna and Trieste. In total, around 6 million (11% of the population) are covered. A childhood cancer registry is present in Torino.
Piemonte (Torino)	1965	1 100 000	—	
Lombardy (Varese)	1974	778 000	Vol. IV 1976–77	
Parma	1976	400 000	—	
Sicily (Ragusa)	1980	270 000	—	
LUXEMBOURG	—	—	—	
NETHERLANDS				A registry was established in Rotterdam in 1982, and 5 further registries started data collection in 1985 in Leiden, Nijmegen, Utrecht, Leiderdorp, and Tilburg with the aim of providing national coverage.
SOOZ, Eindhoven	1955	1 million	—	
PORTUGAL				No published report available.
Viana do Castelo	1975	200 000	—	
SPAIN				New registries have been started in Murcia and Guipuzcoa (San Sebastian) and for digestive cancers only in Mallorca (Palma).
Zaragoza	1960	802 000	Vol. III, IV 1967–77	
Navarra (Pamplona)	1970	484 000	Vol. IV 1973–77	
Tarragona	1980	513 000	—	
UNITED KINGDOM				There is a national network of population based registries in each region which submit abstracts to a central bureau responsible for national cancer incidence statistics. In England and Wales the Office of Population Censuses Surveys collects data from 11 regional registries, and in Scotland the Information Services Division of the Health Department receives data from five regions. The quality of data varies somewhat between these regional registries (ref. 65).
England & Wales	National coverage 1962	49.2 million	Certain regional registers e.g. in Vol. IV:	
Scotland	National coverage 1958	5.1 million	Scotland 1973–77 England: N. Western 1973–77 W. Midlands 1973–76 Mersey 1975–77 S. Metropolitan 1973–77 Oxford 1974–77 Trent 1974–76	
N. Ireland		1.5 million		

*Only registries which began data collection prior to 1982 are listed here.

151

of survival depends upon the follow-up of a group of cancer patients, and the calculation of the numbers surviving after different intervals of time. The usual method is the actuarial or life table method, and there are different ways of allowing for 'normal' or non-cancer mortality in the followed-up patients. The most familiar is the 'Relative Survival' which computes the observed mortality rate in the cancer patients as a ratio of that expected in the population from which they come.[17]

Prevalence of cancer is often advanced as a useful measure in cancer surveillance,[18] indicating the number of patients alive who require medical care. However, there is no standard definition of a prevalent case of cancer. In theory, it should refer to someone once diagnosed as having cancer who is still alive, but then long survivors who are 'cured' are included, and it is not a useful measure of need for service. A compromise might be to regard only patients alive between 0 and 5 (say) years after diagnosis as 'prevalent' cancers, but the estimation of this figure would require good data on incidence and survival. The use of prevalence to denote cases still receiving treatment, or undergoing follow-up clearly has no value as an indicator of service need, since it will be largely dependent upon the availability of facilities and personnel.

Uses of cancer statistics

Exposure to aetiological factors
One of the goals of continuous measurement of cancer occurrence, or risk, is to assess the importance of differences in environment and individual behaviour in cancer causation. In theory, surveillance may reveal new or unexpected hazards, but in practice this has rarely happened. Variation in incidence rates over time, identification of regions of high or low incidence, and abnormal rates of disease in occupational or other groups provoke a search for corresponding differences in exposure to possible aetiological agents. Proof of a causative link, however, requires *ad hoc* individual-based studies.

Time trends The continuous evaluation of time trends in incidence and mortality has been advanced as a means of identifying the emergence of new environmental hazards. The problems involved in such surveillance have been well reviewed.[19] The first is that, since most individual cancer types are relatively rare (especially if they are defined in terms of histology as well as site), then large populations, long time-periods, or very big changes in risk are needed if the change in incidence is to be statistically significant. As noted above, apparent changes in incidence, especially over long time-periods, can be due to changing diagnostic ability, or coding rules. Conversely, for common cancers, the introduction of a new carcinogenic factor which affects only limited subgroups of the population will lead to only a small increase in the overall incidence in the entire population. Yet if surveillance is extended to the frequent examination of changes in incidence or mortality by geographic area, sex, age-group, etc, then many statistically 'significant' changes will emerge by chance.

Although passive surveillance is most likely to be successful when changes involve rare cancers, in fact most such 'epidemics' have been identified by astute clinicians, and the reality and magnitude of the increase later validated by cancer registration. Examples are the occurrence of angiosarcoma of the liver in vinyl-chloride workers,[20] and mesothelioma in persons exposed to asbestos.[21] The clinical suspicion of the role of post-menopausal oestrogens in the aetiology of endometrial cancer was strongly supported by concurrent observations of a very rapid increase in incidence in white females aged over fifty in the early years of the 1970s.[22]

For the epidemiologist, time-trend data more usually present hypotheses concerning aetiology which require testing by other means. Examples are the apparent rapid increases in certain tumours which may be confined to specific age-groups such as testicular cancer,[23,24] or represent a generalized increase in successive birth cohorts, as in malignant melanoma.[25] Sometimes there is no evident explanation even for quite marked time changes, such as the progressive decline in stomach cancer, observed everywhere (see Fig. 13.1).

Time-trend data may also help to substantiate aetiology. Recent trends in lung cancer mortality show declines amongst males in early middle age in UK and Finland which can only be explained by changes in cigarette design and tar yields in addition to consumption patterns. In these two countries cigarette smoking by young adults became established so long ago that their lung cancer rates had stabilized by the late 1950s, i.e. before reductions in tar levels began.[26] These studies show how important it is to study time trend data in different birth cohorts; however, this requires that data be available over long time-periods—as a minimum for fifteen years.

Geographic comparisons The study of geographic differences in incidence and mortality from cancer have been very important in the generation of aetiological leads. Although international comparisons are of enormous value in this respect, cancer surveillance is usually thought of in terms of variation in disease frequency within the same country. It has become standard practice to examine variations in mortality by administrative areas in order to uncover the existence of particular environmental factors important in aetiology, for example, dietary items, pollutants, radiation.

A particularly effective way of presenting data on cancer occurrence in administrative subunits of the population is the Cancer Atlas. Atlases show-

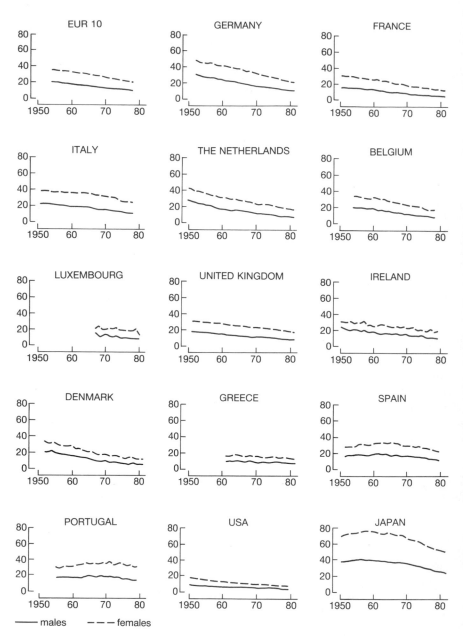

——— males   - - - females

Fig. 13.1. Stomach cancer death rates over time. *X*-axis = calendar year; *Y*-axis = age-adjusted (world standard) mortality per 10^5.

ing variation in mortality rates from different cancers have been produced for Belgium,[27] Federal Republic of Germany,[28] Italy[29] The Netherlands,[30] Spain,[31] and England and Wales.[32] If data are available, similar maps can be prepared using incidence rates, as has been done for Scotland.[33] Cancer maps inevitably produce a large number of apparently significant associations, many of which are due to chance. Other associations shown are those which might have been anticipated from known distribution of risk factors (for example, higher incidence of smoking related cancers in urban areas). Nevertheless, there are often sufficient interesting leads to prompt further study at a local level. In Belgium, the differences in mortality rates of digestive tract cancers[34] were later confirmed by differences in frequency of occurrence[35] which could in part be related to different dietary patterns. The publication of cancer atlases also generates a great deal of public interest, especially from those living in areas of apparently increased risk!

Refining the unit of analysis to very small local areas shows that very marked variations in incidence and mortality can exist, as between adjacent communes for carcinoma of the oesophagus in Brittany (Fig. 13.2) and this suggests the presence of important environmental factors. A widely used technique is to correlate disease rates and various socio-economic, demographic, or environmental variables, using for analysis small geographic units or aggregates with similar characteristics. The limitation of such studies is usually the non-availability of data on exposure of interest for the geographic units concerned. Often, as in the ecological analysis in Finland,[36] only generalized associations with cancer risk such as urbanization and standard of living emerge, and it is not possible to define the precise aetiological factors. This is not surprising in the absence of an exposure which is closely associated with location. Even for industrial exposures, unless a large percentage of the population of the areas is involved with the industry concerned, quite large relative risks will be missed.[37] Nevertheless, the study of cancer mortality at county level in the USA has lead to clear correlations with various industries,[38,39], and in Italy suspicion of excess cancer mortality or incidence in some small but highly industrialized cities led to the investigation of possible chemical exposures.[40] Although several studies have suggested a link between gastric cancer and environmental nitrate, specifically in drinking water, the evidence that such an association is real is unconvincing.[41] Chilvers and Conway[42] showed that there was no association between cancer risk and the concentration of fluoride in drinking water in England and Wales.

The evaluation of cancer occurrence by small areas frequently reveals localities with excess risk, and investigation may uncover an apparent clustering of cases in space and time, suggestive particularly of an infectious aetiology. Most interest has been in the leukaemias and lymphomas, and a variety of statistical methods proposed to identify statistically significant

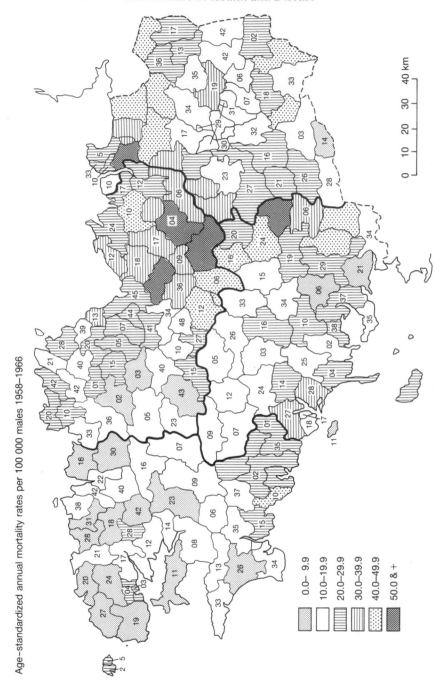

Fig. 13.2.   Cancer of oesophagus in Brittany. (From Tuyns and Massé[66].)

aggregates;[43] however, only for Burkitt's lymphoma is there sufficiently convincing evidence of such clustering.[44]

Personal variables   Several personal variables are recorded sufficiently frequently in routine statistical sources as to permit examination of their association with the occurrence of cancer.

Occupation has commanded most attention, since it presumably relates to a set of relatively clearly defined environmental exposures. The recording of information concerning occupation on death certificates, and on census schedules, allow the calculation of mortality rate (or proportional mortality ratios) for different occupations and cancer sites. The most extensive analyses of this kind have been in England and Wales; Logan[45] reviewed the decennial occupational analyses between 1851 and 1971 for cancer mortality, and at the some time presented comparable international data. There are several problems involved in these analyses, particularly in relation to the accuracy with which the statement of occupation given by the next of kin after death accurately reflects the major occupation during the lifetime of the deceased (who will often have retired, or changed jobs, prior to death); nevertheless, such studies provide a relatively simple method of monitoring potential occupational hazards. The possibility for cancer registries to perform such routine surveillance has been suggested, but quality of information on occupation and the statistical problem of multiple comparisons present difficulties.[46] On the other hand, the possibility of identifying all incident cancers, in the absence of selection bias, allows estimation of the aetiologic fraction of given exposures, such as occupation for the general population.[47]

A different approach is to use routine surveillance systems (cancer registration, death registration) as the case-finding mechanism for prospective cohort studies. If the exposure variable is also available from some routine statistical source, then the exercise of follow-up is essentially one of record linkage. An example of this is the follow-up of 1 per cent sample of workers identified at the 1971 census in England and Wales, using the national cancer registry to study cancer incidence in relation to occupation.[48] However, data on exposure may have to be derived from different sources—sometimes the cohort members provide the necessary information, but other records may be available allowing the exposure groups to be defined on the basis of past experience (for example, the studies of exposure to radiation for ankylosing spondylitis),[49] or the potential carcinogenicity of previous drug therapy.[50-52] A particular example which uses the cancer registry to both define the cohort and outcome was the study of the effects of radiation in the treatment of cancer of the cervix.[53] In special circumstances, the need for long-term surveillance of populations exposed to high levels of potential carcinogens has led to the establishment of registers, for example for the 220 000 residents of Seveso, exposed to dioxin in 1976.[54]

Place of birth is frequently recorded on death certificates and at cancer registration and can be exploited to investigate incidence and mortality rates in relation to migration. Studies of migrants, between or within countries, are of particular interest to epidemiologists in that they provide clues as to the relative importance of genetic factors and environment, and the latent period of environmental 'exposures', in cancer aetiology. Studies of other subgroups which differ in terms of life-style and/or genetic makeup, for example ethnic or religious groups, have been immensely important in the generation of aetiological hypotheses, but such studies are of little potential in Europe where surveillance systems rarely collect the relevant data.

Evaluation of cancer control

Although statistics on disease occurrence have been widely exploited by epidemiologists to elucidate causes of cancer, most surveillance systems would justify their existence in terms of their role in the planning and evaluation of health care.

Preventive programmes are frequently monitored in terms of reductions in exposure in the target population (for example, the reduction in the prevalence of cigarette smoking). However, surveillance systems should be able to identify whether the objective of such programmes, i.e. reductions in the incidence of cancer, have been achieved. There have been relatively few controlled trials of preventive strategies, and those reported have not been designed to detect effects on cancer incidence. Thus most evaluation will require before—after comparisons within the population into which the intervention has been introduced. There will usually be a long interval between the institution of preventive measures, and the results in terms of changed incidence. Figure 13.3 shows the results to be expected, based on a computer simulation, from the introduction of a programme to reduce smoking uptake by young people.[55] Nevertheless, as described above, the results of reduced prevalence of smoking and toxicity of cigarettes are now evident as a lower risk of lung cancer in young males in Finland and UK.

Evaluation of the efficacy of cancer control measures in the occupational setting is more difficult due to the small size of the exposed populations. Similarly, slight modifications in the general environment (drinking water, air pollution, background radioactivity), even if they have an impact on cancer occurrence, cannot be detected by routine epidemiological surveillance.

Most screening programmes for cancer aim for early diagnosis, and subsequent reduction of mortality; an exception, however, is screening for cervix cancer where discovery and treatment of a precursor condition can also prevent the onset (incidence) of clinical disease. Although there have never been any controlled trials of cervix-cancer screening programmes, their effectiveness is now reasonably certain, thanks to a large number of descriptive, cohort, and case control studies (for review see ref. 56). In theory, then, the

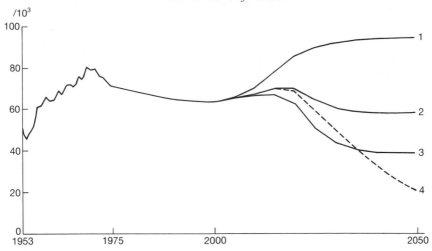

Fig. 13.3. Age-adjusted incidence rates ($/10^5$ person–years) for lung cancer in males in Finland 1953–75, and forecasts for the rates in 1980–2050 derived by means of a simulation model with the following assumptions. In each consecutive 5-year period in 1976–2050, 10 per cent of the smokers in each smoking category will stop, and one of the following alternatives holds true: (1) α% of non-smokers aged 10–14 years, β% of those aged 15–19, and γ% of those aged 20–24 years will start smoking. $\alpha = 60$, $\beta = 30$, $\gamma = 10$; (2) Same as (1) but $\alpha = 30$, $\beta = 15$, $\gamma = 5$; (3) Same as (1) but $\alpha = 15$, $\beta = 7.5$, $\gamma = 2.5$; (4) Same as (1) but the values of α for consecutive 5-year periods starting from 1976–80 are: 30, 24, 18, 12, 6, and 0 (remaining intervals), those for β are: 15, 12, 9, 6, 3, and 0 (remaining intervals), and those for γ are: 5, 4, 3, 2, 1, and 0 (remaining intervals). (From Hakulinen and Pukkula[55].)

effectiveness of cervical cytology screening could be easily evaluated by following trends in incidence (or mortality) in the community. In practice, this is rather more difficult than apparent since there are quite marked underlying trends in incidence which may complicate interpretation—for example, the apparent lack of effect of screening in England and Wales[57] is misleading— the programme has had a moderate success, but in the face of a strong underlying increase in risk of disease in young women.[58]

Breast-cancer screening by mammography also appears to be effective in reducing mortality.[56] The coming years will probably see increased implementation of such programmes, which will require monitoring by mortality rates in the screened areas. The mortality rate from breast cancer in most European countries shows a progressive increase (Fig. 13.4), any apparent change must be judged against this underlying trend; the problem of interpreting incidence data in the face of active screening programmes has been mentioned.

The evaluation of the effectiveness of treatment programmes has traditionally relied upon the measurement of survival. Survival rates are the normal

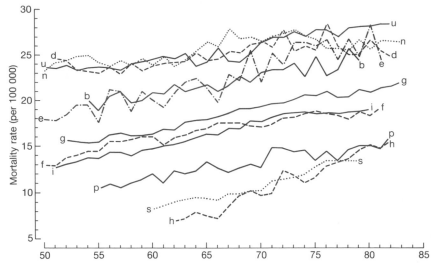

Fig. 13.4. Breast cancer mortality: Europe 1950–85. *Key*: b = Belgium; d = Denmark; e = Ireland; f = France; g = Fed. Republic of Germany; h = Greece; i = Italy; n = The Netherlands; p = Portugal; s = Spain; u = England and Wales.

endpoints in clinical trials of cancer therapy, and it seems natural to use population survival to evaluate the results of therapy on a population basis— that is for all cancers of a particular type. Thus it is possible to examine time trends in survival, as well as differences within various subgroups of the population.[59] However, great care is needed in interpreting the survival rate; it is a composite index which reflects several tumour factors (stage at diagnosis, histologic type) and patient factors (age, race, socio-economic circumstances) as well as treatment efficacy. Enstrom and Austin[60] question whether, given these problems and the difficulties involved in estimating population-based survival rates (see above), evaluation might not be more easily performed by a simple comparison of incidence and mortality rates. The most impressive improvements in survival have been in a rather limited number of cancers—Wilm's tumour, childhood leukaemia and Hodgkin's disease—whilst for the major solid tumours of adults (lung cancer, stomach cancer, breast cancer) there appears to have been practically no change.[61]

   Although the treatment and aftercare of cancer patients aim for more than a simple improvement in survival, and various measures have been devised to quantify health, or quality of life,[62] it has to be admitted that none is capable of application on a wide enough basis to qualify as surveillance techniques.

Planning of services

Provision of health-care services should logically depend upon an indication of need, which can be regarded as a measure of the amount or burden of particular conditions, and their amenability to interventive measures. Although various ways in which information on incidence of cancer have been used in service planning have been discussed by Wrighton[63] it is not known how often provision is in fact based upon objective criteria. Because of the long latent interval between exposure and clinical disease, trends in cancer incidence tend to be relatively stable, with regular increases (or decreases) in risk between successive cohorts. This means that projections of past cancer incidence (or mortality) trends to provide estimates of future rates of disease are relatively accurate.[64] The use of routine cancer data to predict future need for services should, in theory at least, be a useful planning tool.

Conclusions

Once the organization for delivery of health care passes a rudimentary level, information for planning and evaluation purposes becomes essential. The sources are usually vital statistics systems, or activity analysis (utilization statistics) from the health care system itself. Both sources have been widely exploited by epidemiologists interested in disease causation, as well as by health-care planners. Statistics on cancer are also available from cancer registries, the existence of which is due in part to the fact that for cancer, in contrast to many chronic diseases, the definition of onset and existence of the disease state is relatively clear. With the mounting pressure for cost containment in health services, information systems have come under scrutiny, and will increasingly need to justify their role. Surveillance systems form a vital component of all cancer control programmes. At the simplest level they provide data on cases, deaths, life years lost, etc. which together with future projections are important in establishing priority areas for prevention, treatment, and rehabilitation. Surveillance systems are a useful resource in epidemiological research, and a knowledge of aetiology is obviously essential in the planning of prevention strategies. Evaluation of health care interventions is ideally carried out by controlled trial designed to answer specific questions. This is rarely feasible, however, and usually routine data-collection systems have to be adapted for this purpose. Their general overall suitability for this must be kept constantly under review, and those which are sufficiently flexible to respond to changing demands, for example the cancer registry, should be prepared to adapt their data collection and presentation accordingly. These needs must be set against the frequent requirement for data covering relatively long time-periods (effectiveness of cancer control measures will rarely be evident in a short interval), so that major changes to existing systems should not be undertaken lightly.

Bibliography

1. Wagner G., Cancer registration: Historical aspects. In Parkin, D. M., Wagner, G.

and Muir, C. S. *The role of the registry in cancer control.* IARC Scientific Publications 66, Lyon (1985).

2. Heasman, M. A. and Lipworth, L., *Accuracy of certification of cause of death.* Studies in Medical and Population Subjects 20. HMSO, London (1966).

3. Puffer, R. R. and Wynne-Griffith, G., *Patterns of urban mortality.* Scientific Publication 151, Pan American Health Organization, Washington (1967).

4. Bosch, F. X., Garcia, A., Orta, J., Juvanet, J., Camproden, A., and Pumarola, A., The accuracy of medical certifications of cancer deaths and of cancer diagnosis in the municipal area of Barcelona in 1979. *Rev. Esp. Oncologia* **30**, 17–24 (1983).

5. Percy, C., Stanek, E., and Gloeckner, L., Accuracy of cancer death certificates and its effect on cancer mortality statistics. *Amer. J. publ. Hlth* **71**, 242–50 (1981).

6. Percy, C. and Dolman, A., Comparison of the coding of death certificates related to cancer in seven countries. *Publ. Hlth Rep.* **93**, 335–50 (1978).

7. Hansluwka, H., Cancer mortality in Europe, 1970–74. *World Hlth Stat. Quart.* **31**, 159–94 (1978).

8. McLennan, R., Muir, C. S., Steinitz, R., and Winker, A., *Cancer registration and its techniques.* IARC Scientific Publications 21. Lyon (1978).

9. Waterhouse, J. A. H., Muir, C. S., Shanmugaratnam, K., and Powell, J., *Cancer incidence in five continents*, Vol. 4. IARC Scientific Publications 42. Lyon (1982).

10. Benn, R. T., Leck, I., and Nwene, U. P., Estimation of completeness of cancer registration. *Int. J. Epidemiol.* **103**, 362–7 (1982).

11. West, R. R., Accuracy of cancer registration. *Br. J. prevent. social. Med.* **30**, 187–92 (1976).

12. Larsson, S., Completeness and reliability of lung cancer registration in the Swedish Cancer Registry. *Acta path. microbiol. scand.* **79A**, 389–98 (1971).

13. Stalsberg, H., Lymphoreticular tumours in Norway and in other European countries. *J. Natl. Cancer Inst.* **50**, 1685–702 (1973).

14. Breslow, N., Chan, C. W., Dhom, G. *et al.*, Latent carcinoma of prostate at autopsy in seven areas. *Int. J. Cancer* **20**, 680–8 (1977).

15. Fontana, R. S., Early detection of lung cancer: The Mayo lung project. In *Screening for cancer* (eds P. C. Prorok and A. B. Miller). UICC Technical Report Services, Vol. 78, Geneva (1984).

16. Doll, R. and Peto, R., *The causes of cancer.* Oxford University Press (1981).

17. American joint committee on cancer staging and end results reporting. *Reporting of cancer survival and end results 1982.* American Cancer Society, Chicago (1982).

18. Hakama, M., Hakulinen, T., Teppo, L., and Saxen, E., Incidence, mortality and prevalence as indicators of the cancer problem. *Cancer* **36**, 2227–31 (1975).

19. Muir, C. S., McLennan, R., Waterhouse, J. A. H., and Magnus, K., Feasibility of monitoring populations to detect environmental carcinogens. In *Environmental pollution and carcinogenic risks.* IARC Scientific Publications 13, INSERM Symposia Series 52 (1976).

20. Creech, J. L. and Johnson, M. N., Angiosarcoma in the manufacture of polyvinyl chloride. *J. occup. Med.* **16**, 150–1 (1974).

21. Wagner, J. C., Sleggs, C. A., and Marchand, P., Diffuse pleural mesothelioma and asbestos exposure in the north western Cape province. *Br. J. indust. Med.* **17**, 260–71 (1960).

22. Austin, D. F. and Roe, K. M., Increase in cancer of the corpus uteri in the San Francisco—Oakland standard metropolitan statistical area, 1960–1975. *J. Natl. Cancer Inst.* **62**, 13–16 (1979).

23. Clemmensen, J., Trends and risks Denmark 1943–1972. *Acta path. microbiol. scand.*, Suppl. 261, 1–286 (1977).
24. Davies, J. M., Testicular cancer in England and Wales: Some epidemiological aspects. *Lancet* **i**, 928–31 (1981).
25. Muir, C. S. and Nectoux, J., Time trends in malignant melanoma of the skin. In *Trends in cancer incidence* (ed. K. Magnus). Hemisphere, Washington (1982).
26. International Agency for Research on Cancer, *Tobacco smoking.* IARC monographs, Vol. 38. Lyon (1986).
27. Rijckeboer, R., Janssens, G., and Thiers, G., *Atlas of cancer mortality in Belgium,* 1969–1976. Ministry of Public Health and the Family, Brussels (1983).
28. Becker, N., Frentzel-Beyme, R., and Wagner, G., *Krebsatlas der Bundesrepublik Deutschland.* Springer-Verlag, Berlin (1984).
29. Cislaghi, C., Decarli, A., Morosini, P. L., and Puntoni, R., *Atlante della mortalità per tumori in Italia 1970–1972.* Lega Italiana per la Lotta contro i Tumori, Milano (1978).
30. Netherlands Central Bureau of Statistics, *Atlas of cancer mortality in the Netherlands 1969–1978.* Dept. of Health Statistics, The Hague (1980).
31. Lopez-Abente, G., Escolar, A., and Errezda, M. (eds), *Atlas del cancer en Espana.* Victoria-Gasteiz (1984).
32. Gardner, M. J., Winter, P. D., Taylor, C. P., and Acheson, E. D., *Atlas of cancer mortality in England and Wales 1968–1978.* John Wiley, Chichester (1983).
33. Kemp, I., Boyle, P., Smans, M., and Muir, C. S., *Atlas of cancer in Scotland 1975–1980. Incidence and epidemiological perspectives.* IARC Scientific Publications 72 (1985).
34. Ramioul, L. and Tuyns, A. J., La distribution géographique des cancers du tube digestif en Belgique. Inégale répartition de la mortalité par cancer de l'estomac et par cancer du rectum. *Acta gastro-ent. belg.* **40**, 129–49 (1977).
35. Tuyns, A. J., Reginster, G. and Ravet, L., Une étude épidémiologique sur les cancers du tube digestif en Belgique. Etude interuniversitaire: Alimentation et santé. *Rev. Med. Liège* **40**, X, 1–7 (1985).
36. Teppo, L., Pukkala, E., Hakama, M., Hakulinen, T., Herva, A., and Saxen, E., Way of life and cancer incidence in Finland. *Scand. J. Soc. Med.*, Suppl. 19, 5–84 (1980).
37. Goldsmith, J. R., Geographical pathology as a method for detecting occupational cancer. *J. occup. Med.* **19**, 533–9 (1977).
38. Hoover, R. and Fraumeni, J. F. Cancer mortality in US counties with chemical industries. *Environ. Res.* **9**, 196–207 (1975).
39. Blot, W. J. and Fraumeni, J. F. Geographic patterns of lung cancer: Industrial correlations. *Am. J. Epidemiol.* **103**, 539–50 (1976).
40. Riboli, E., Bai, E., Berrino, F., and Merisi, A. Mortality from lung cancer in an acetylene and phthalic anhydride plant: A case reference study. *Scand. J. Work Environ. Hth* **9**, 455–62 (1983).
41. Fraser, P. Nitrates: Epidemiological evidence. In *Interpretation of negative epidemiological evidence for carcinogenicity* (eds N. J. Wald and R. Doll). IARC pp. 183–94. Scientific Publications 65, Lyon (1985).
42. Chilvers, C., and Conway, D. Cancer mortality in England in relation to levels of naturally occuring fluoride in water supplies. *J. Epidemiol. Community Hth* **39**, 44–47 (1985).

43. Smith, P. G. Spatial and temporal clustering. In *Cancer epidemiology and prevention* (eds L. D. Schottenfeld and J. F. Fraumeni). Saunders, Philadelphia (1985).
44. Day, N. E., Smith, P. G., and Lachet, B. The latent period of Burkitt's lymphoma: The evidence from epidemiological clustering. In *Burkitt's lymphoma. A human cancer model* (eds G. Lenoir *et al.*). IARC Scientific Publications 60, Lyon (1985).
45. Logan, W. P. D. *Cancer mortality by occupation and social class 1851–1971.* IARC Scientific Publications 36. Studies on Med. and Pop. Subjects 44. Lyon and HMSO, London (1982).
46. Jensen, O. M. The cancer registry was a tool for detecting industrial cancer risks. In *The role of the registry in cancer control* (eds D. M. Parkin, G. Wagner, and C. S. Muir). IARC Scientific Publications 66. Lyon (1985).
47. Pastorino, U., Berrino, F., Gervasio, A., Pesenti, V., Riboli, E., and Crosignani, P. Proportion of lung cancers due to occupational exposure. *Int. J. Cancer* **33,** 231–7 (1984).
48. Fox, A. J. The role of OPCS in occupational epidemiology: some examples. *Ann. occup. Hyg.* **21,** 393–403 (1979).
49. Court-Brown, W. M. and Doll, R. Mortality from cancer and other causes after radiotherapy for ankylosing spondylitis. *Br. med. J.* **ii,** 1327–32 (1965).
50. Clemmensen, J. and Hjalgrim-Jensen, S. Does phenobarbital cause intracranial tumours? A follow-up through 35 years. *Ecotoxicol. Environ. Quality* **1,** 255–60 (1981).
51. Reimer, R. R., Hoover, R., Fraumeni, J. F., and Young, R. C. Acute leukaemia after alkylating-agent therapy of ovarian cancer. *New Engl. J. Med.* **297,** 177–81 (1977).
52. Howe, G. R., Lindsay, J., Coppock, E., and Miller, A. B. Izoniazid exposure in relation to cancer incidence and mortality in a cohort of tuberculosis patients. *Int. J. Epidemiol.* **8,** 305–12 (1979).
53. Day, N. E. and Boice, J. R. (eds). *Second cancer in relation to radiation treatment for cervical cancer.* IARC Scientific Publications 52, Lyon (1983).
54. Fini, A., Puntoni, R., Gennaro, V., Rosa, A. M., and Vercelli, M. L'enregistrement du cancer dans la zone de Seveso. Proc. VIII réunion du groupe pour l'Epidémiologie et l'enregistrement du cancer dans les pays de langue latine, Raguse, Italy, 12–13 May. Int. Agency for Research on Cancer, Lyon (1983).
55. Hakulinen, T. and Pukkala, E. Future incidence of lung cancer: Forecasts based on hypothetical changes in smoking habits of males. *Int. J. Epidemiol.* **10,** 233–40 (1981).
56. Parkin, D. M. and Day, N. E. Evaluating and planning screening programmes. In *The role of the registry in cancer control* (eds D. M. Parkin, G. Wagner, and C. S. Muir). IARC Scientific Publications 66, Lyon (1985).
57. Editorial. Cancer of the cervix: death by incompetence. *Lancet* **ii,** 363–64 (1985).
58. Parkin, D. M., Nguyen-Dinh, X., and Day, N. E. The impact of screening on the incidence of cervix cancer in England and Wales. *Br. J. Obstet. Gynaecol.* **92,** 150–7 (1985).
59. Hanai, A. and Fujimoto, I. Survival rate as an index in cancer control. In *The role of the registry in cancer control* (eds D. M. Parkin, G. Wagner, and C. S. Muir). IARC Scientific Publications 66, Lyon (1985).
60. Enstrom, J. E. and Austin, D. F. Interpreting cancer survival rates. *Science* **195,** 847–51 (1977).

61. Page, H. S. and Asire, A. J. *Cancer rates and risks*, 3rd ed. NIH Publication 85-691. US Department of Health and Human Services (1985).
62. Spitzer, W. O., Dobson, A. J., Hall, J. *et al.* Measuring the quality of life of cancer patients. *J. chron. Dis.* **34,** 585–97 (1981).
63. Wrighton, R. J. Planning services for the cancer patient. In *The role of the registry in cancer control* (eds D. M. Parkin, G. Wagner, and C. S. Muir). IARC Scientific Publications 66, Lyon (1985).
64. Hakama, M. Projection of cancer incidence: experience and some results in Finland. *World Hlth Stat. Quart.* **33,** 228–40 (1980).
65. OPCS. *A report of the advisory committee on cancer registration*. Series MB1 6. London, HMSO (1981).
66. Tuyns, A. J. and Massé, L. M. F. Mortality from cancer of the oesophagus in Britanny. *Int. J. Epidemiol.* **2,** 241–5 (1973).

14

Surveillance for communicable disease

M. L. MORO AND A. McCORMICK

A. Italy: Introduction

The Italian health system underwent major changes in 1978. A New Act (Law n. 833) established a National Health Service by which the State took over the finance and planning of health care from various sources. Until then this had been provided by a network of health insurance companies. Major and far-reaching transformations in the system subsequently began, involving the structure of the different health services and emphasizing new aims and functions. Moreover, the stress on preventive activities to reduce the occurrence of disease in the population has promoted a new approach to surveillance of disease, including communicable disease. In particular, the Istituto Superiore di Sanità (ISS) has been granted new tasks of collecting, collating, and analysing data for epidemiological purposes. Thus the opportunity occurred for a centre at national level to co-ordinate the surveillance of communicable diseases in man.

A comprehensive and complex Act such as the National Health Service Act could not be expected to switch from an old health-care system to a new one in a few years without problems, which are still being experienced, but many interesting experiences have been gained.

Historical Background

Case reports of infectious diseases were first used in Italy to implement Public Health measures in 1348. The Republic of Venice during an outbreak of pneumonic plague, (the 'Black Death'), appointed three guardians of public health to exclude ships with affected people aboard from reaching the piers. This is probably the first public health measure taken by an official government in Europe. Fifty years later the Republic of Venice again constrained ships coming from plague stricken areas to stay outside the harbours for forty days. For the first time quarantine was introduced as a means to control the spread of infectious diseases.[1]

Only five centuries later a nationwide reporting system was set up to provide data on morbidity and mortality of infectious diseases. Since 1881 a death certificate has been completed at the time of death by the doctors, initially on a voluntary basis, but it became officially required by law in 1888. In the same year an act requiring mandatory reporting of communicable diseases was passed.[2] The first list included eleven notifiable diseases which had been amended and modified in subsequent years.

Major changes in the national notification system were introduced in 1934 by the Unified Text of Health Acts:[3] sixty-four diseases were included in the list, all to be notified by a common form on an individual basis. A six months' sentence was the penalty for doctors convicted for failure to report cases with serious consequences. At that time, preventing the spread of the disease was a matter of identifying cases in order to isolate them from the community—individual surveillance, rather than establishing preventive measures. Mortality data and notification were collated and published at national level by the Home Office until 1958 and after this date by the Istituto Centrale di Statistica (ISTAT).

The 1934 Unified Text is still in force; amendments have been formulated but they have not been yet approved.

Data on sexually transmitted diseases and tuberculosis have also been routinely collected during the last century: dermovenereal clinics have been run by the State since 1923 and chest clinics since 1927. However, data collected at national level by the Health Minister have not been published until very recently.

Hence most current data sources on infectious diseases in Italy are the legacy of a system geared to the isolation and treatment of individual cases of disease rather than to prevent their occurrence in the community.

The National Health Act issued in 1978[4] greatly modified the health-service organization. The National Health Service represents a comprehensive system organized at three administrative levels: national, regional (21 regions) and local (693 'Unità Sanitarie Locali' (USL)), each with a population ranging between 50 000 and 200 000 people. The USL represents the most fundamental change in the newly organized NHS: it is responsible for integrated delivery of health care. Public hospitals and community services are directly run by the USL, while GP's and most clinical laboratories are private, but enter into a special arrangement with the NHS.

Thus opportunity occurred for improvements in surveillance activities and prevention. However, at this stage difficulties are still being experienced throughout the country due to an uneven transition from the old to the new system, with certain changes not implemented uniformly.

Current Data Sources in Italy

For more than a hundred years mortality certifications and notifications have been the two main sources of routine data on infectious diseases.

1. Mortality data

Advantages   Mortality data have been collected and published in Italy since 1880. Secular trends for specific diseases can be analysed and improvements due to control measures evaluated; for example, the dramatic decrease in poliomyelitis and diphtheria deaths after vaccinations were made compulsory in the 1950s. As in other countries (see p. 000) mortality data are of limited value in monitoring trends in infectious diseases because of improvements in prophylaxis and treatment. They are still useful for surveillance of some diseases, such as tetanus, which has a high case fatality and uneven vaccine coverage in adults.

Disadvantages   Cause-specific mortality data are published after a long delay: although a monthly publication is provided by ISTAT, only tuberculosis deaths are mentioned separately. Cause-specific death rates with sufficient detail for infectious diseases are published with a 3–4 year delay. Therefore they are less useful for detecting variations in mortality from certain infectious diseases; for example, influenza in winter.

Published data refer to primary cause of death only. Occasionally (i.e. once in the last ten years) special publications are available, reporting concurrent causes of death on a national basis only.

2. Notifications of infectious diseases

The reporting of infectious diseases has been in recent years the arena for suggestions and proposals in order to achieve a better system in Italy. At present there are two separate methods of collecting infectious diseases notifications. In 1981 appreciation of delay in data transmission in the official system of reporting run by ISTAT led the ISS to establish experimentally a new system, called Rapid Surveillance System for Infectious Disease (Sistema Informativo Rapido delle Malattie Infettive—SIRMI).

Notification system (ISTAT)

Sixty-six diseases are notified by law in Italy: to the sixty-four included by the 1934 Act, Legionellosis was added in 1983, and AIDS in November 1986.

GPs are required to report to the USL all notifiable diseases both suspected and diagnosed, which come to their attention. For each notified case the Public Health Department of the USL completes a form, which enlists data on name, age, sex, date of onset, residence, and whether the case is suspected or confirmed. The forms are forwarded by mail to the region and from there, every month, to the ISTAT.

Advantages   Notifications represent the only ready source of information on the number of cases of infectious diseases by time, age and sex, and geographical area. Overall and specific incidence rates are obtained. As notification data have been published since the beginning of the century, secular trends can be identified.

Disadvantages As with the mortality statistics, notifications also are burdened by a considerable time-lag before publication. The most rapid publication of notified cases, the monthly newsletter for infectious diseases, appears after a four-month delay. This makes these data useless for rapid identification of an increase in the frequency of a disease. Thus the system lacks the necessary feedback.

Moreover, the large number of notifiable diseases (not all worth notifying) overload GPs and USL. Amendments have been proposed to revise and reduce the list, for example, by limiting reports of some infections (for example Scabies and Pediculosis) to outbreaks in communities, to selected endemic areas of others (for example, Hydatidosis, Leishmaniasis, and Amebiasis), or to confirmed cases only (for example Mumps, Tuberculosis, Gonorrhoea, Brucellosis).

Lack of feedback and work overload is believed to cause a diffuse under-reporting, although no studies have been carried out to assess its extent, except one on a single disease: Santoro *et al.*[5] estimated the proportion of measles notification to be only 10 per cent of the actual number of illnesses occurring in the community, ranging from 2·5 per cent in the south of Italy to 25 per cent in the north. A survey carried out in 1979 to determine the reasons for under-reporting of several notifiable diseases showed that those most often mentioned were apathy, fears of breaching confidentiality, and excess work-load.[6]

Rapid surveillance system for infectious diseases (SIRMI)

In 1981 the ISS set up an experimental system of rapid reporting of infectious diseases to overcome the deficiencies highlighted above.[7] The aims of the new system were:

(a) to allow a swift reporting and analysis of infectious diseases by reducing the number of those notifiable and allowing transmission of data by telephone;
(b) to establish an information feedback by means of a weekly epidemiological bulletin sent to the USL and health workers.

The SIRMI started collecting information from only three out of twenty-one regions, but now all of them have agreed to collaborate. The number of notifiable diseases included in the SIRMI is nineteen. Notifications are sent on a voluntary basis. Reports are transmitted by telephone from the USL to the regions and then to the ISS. A weekly epidemiological bulletin (Bolletino Epidemiologico Nazionale—BEN), issued by the ISS, publishes the total number of cases by region reported during the previous week. From January 1985, rates by region for twelve diseases were also provided.

Advantages   Rapid data analysis allows detection of large outbreaks. For example in 1984 a marked increase in cases of viral hepatitis and typhoid fever in southern Italy was recognized through the SIRMI.[8] Information feedback allows preventive measures to be implemented and strengthens the links within the public health network, as exemplified by increasing requests of collaboration from the USL (for example, for outbreak investigations). Moreover, flexibility of this system has recently allowed the introduction of the aetiological differentiation of viral hepatitis, although it has not yet been requested by law.

Disadvantages   Since only the total number of cases by disease is reported, pattern of diseases in specific population groups cannot be described. Moreover, SIRMI improves the means of data transmission and feedback only; therefore the problems of underreporting and of diagnostic differences among geographical areas remain.

Other Sources of Data

1. Laboratory reports

There is still no network of Public Health Laboratories reporting centrally in Italy, although several laboratories join specific programmes, such as the surveillance of legionellosis, salmonellosis, and influenza.

2. Hospital discharge data

The ISTAT collects data on all in-patients discharged from public hospitals in the first seven days of each month. One record in four is processed. Hospital discharge data cannot be analysed and used at national level because of the small sample, the poor disaggregation and the considerable time lag before publication. Some regions have now started to collect data on all patients discharged from public and private hospitals, so more comprehensive information on hospital patients may be available shortly.

3. Vaccination uptake

In Italy vaccination against the following diseases are mandatory: poliomyelitis, diphtheria, tetanus. Rubella, pertussis, and measles vaccinations are strongly recommended. Vaccination against TB, typhoid fever, and rabies are compulsory only for certain groups at risk. Doses of vaccine for compulsory vaccinations administered by each USL are periodically notified to the regional authorities. Thus at national level the proportion of fully immunized children is unknown even for compulsory vaccinations, because only doses of vaccine are registered and not the number of children vaccinated.

Special Surveillance Programmes

Following a large outbreak of Legionellosis in 1980,[9] halted by case reporting and appropriate control measures, surveillance of legionellosis at national level was started in 1983. 41 public laboratories, scattered over Italy, were supplied by ISS with *Legionella pneumophila* serogroup 1 antigen. This network of laboratories reports to the ISS all new cases with a serologically confirmed diagnosis.

In 1984 a surveillance programme for viral hepatitis, a serious cause of morbidity in Italy, was started.[11] The official notification (ISTAT) does not differentiate between the various types of acute viral hepatitis. USL have been asked to notify reported cases by including the serological diagnosis. Clusters of cases or outbreaks are investigated through case-control studies, carried out to assess the most likely sources and mode of transmission of acute viral hepatitis.

Since January 1985 regional authorities have been requested to report for every case of meningococcal meningitis, demographic data, serogroup, and antibiotic resistance of the isolates.[12]

In January 1983 a voluntary reporting system for Acquired Immune Deficiency Syndrome (AIDS) was set up.[13] Cases are reported on a standard questionnaire, following a standard case definition. Most reports come from hospital doctors. Since September 1984, the generalized lymphadenopathy syndrome has also been under surveillance, and surveillance of HIV-antibody positive subjects will follow as soon as screening of blood donors has been implemented.

Hospital-acquired infections are not routinely reported in Italy. A prevalence survey in 130 hospitals was held in 1983 in order to describe the pattern.[14] After that, continuing surveillance programmes in high-risk areas as Intensive Care Units and Surgical Departments have been implemented.

B. United Kingdom: Introduction

The United Kingdom (UK) comprises England, Wales, Scotland, and Northern Ireland. Whilst rapid communication of information ensures that each country is aware of what is happening in the remainder of the UK, surveillance is carried out separately by England and Wales, Scotland, and Northern Ireland. The collection, analysis, and distribution of information are similar in all four countries, but there are some differences. National surveillance is co-ordinated in England and Wales by the Communicable Disease Surveillance Centre (CDSC) at Colindale in London, in Scotland by the Communicable Diseases (Scotland) Unit (CD(S)U) at Ruchill Hospital in Glasgow, and in Northern Ireland by the Department of Health and Social Services (DHSS(NI)) in Belfast.

Historical Background

Surveillance in the UK dates from the sixteenth century when the clergy were required to keep a register of those who were christened, married, or died within each parish. At about the same time Bills of Mortality were published during epidemics of the plague and in 1662 Graunt used these statistics to compare 'one year, season, parish or other division of the city, with another'.[15] General Register Offices were established in London and Dublin in 1836[16] and in Edinburgh in 1855, leading to a national system of death registration, although it was not until 1874 in England, Wales and Ireland that the doctor was required by law to provide a written statement of the cause of death.[17] The Public Health Act of 1899 enforced notification of specified infectious diseases in every district in the UK.[18]

The present Public Health Laboratory Service of England and Wales was founded in 1946 from the Emergency PHLS of 1939;[19] epidemiological surveillance of laboratory diagnosed infection began soon after by the Epidemiological Research Laboratory, and in 1977 the Communicable Disease Surveillance Centre was established within the PHLS to co-ordinate national surveillance.[20] The Communicable Diseases (Scotland) Unit (CD(S)U) was set up in Glasgow in 1967.[21]

Data on hospital discharges have been available in England and Wales since 1953,[22] in Scotland since 1961 and in Northern Ireland since the 1970s. By 1987, data on diagnosis of all discharges will be processed centrally (replacing the 10 per cent sample until that date in England and Wales), except in Northern Ireland where only about 80 per cent of hospitals include diagnosis among the data they report.

The number of children vaccinated is available and this system has developed as new immunisation procedures have been introduced.

Since 1980 doctors belonging to the Medical Officers of Schools Association have reported weekly to CDSC episodes of illness among children in a sample of boarding schools.

In 1985 the British Paediatric Surveillance Unit was established to co-ordinate work by CDSC and the British Paediatric Association on several diseases of mutual interest.

Since 1801 information derived from the decennial censuses has provided the denominator for the notification of infectious diseases and for deaths. At the time of the 1981 census, the population of England and Wales was estimated to be just over 49 million, that of Scotland to be just over 5 million, and that of Northern Ireland to be about 1 million.

Current Sources of Data

1. Death certification and registration

In the UK each condition mentioned on the death certificate is now coded. Mortality data are published weekly, monthly, quarterly, and annually in varying degrees of detail. However, entries with a mention of certain communicable and other diseases (AIDS, Reye's syndrome, whooping cough, poliomyelitis, tetanus, salmonellosis, malaria, typhoid, and other less common notifiable diseases) are copied each week for inclusion in special surveillance programmes.

Advantages The information is available quickly. For instance, the total number of deaths, and deaths due to respiratory infections and influenza are published weekly, and used to assess the impact of influenza each winter.[23] Statistics for mortality from individual infections are available for many deaths, so that seasonal and other trends can be studied.

Disadvantages Many communicable diseases do not cause death or do so on rare occasions. Revisions of the International Classification of Diseases (ICD), or changes in interpretation of the coding rules cause problems in interpreting trends: a change in the application of rule 3 in England and Wales at the beginning of 1984 roughly halved the number of deaths assigned to pneumonia. Identification of a disease depends upon the correct diagnosis being entered on the certificate.[24] Any member of the public may obtain a copy of any entry and this may deter the doctor from entering the correct diagnosis (for example, AIDS) on the death certificate; however, it is possible for the doctor to send further information for statistical purposes about a death, which will not be entered on the public record.

2. Notification of infectious diseases

The list of diseases which are statutorily notifiable nationally varies slightly in the different countries of the UK. Notifications by disease are reported each week to the Office of Population Censuses and Surveys (OPCS) in England and Wales, to the Common Services Agency (CSA) of the National Health Service (NHS) in Scotland, and to the Department of Health and Social Services (DHSS(NI)) in Northern Ireland. The Public Health Acts provide certain legal powers relating to the investigation of persons thought to be suffering from an infectious disease, and permitting action to be taken to prevent the spread of infection.[25]

Advantages   Data on the numbers of notifications are published quickly, so that the progress of epidemics can be monitored, and preventive local or national action taken if appropriate. Notifications are reported by districts for which the population estimates are known, so that rates can be calculated and local and national comparisons made. Many diseases notified are not routinely confirmed in the laboratory, and notifications provide the only available estimate of incidence. For some infections, national records have been published since near the beginning of the century, so that trends can be studied over many years.

Disadvantages   Not every communicable disease is notifiable, although districts have the power to make other diseases notifiable locally such as has been done with rubella. Some infections are never confirmed, so that it is possible for the clinical diagnosis to be wrong. In addition, it is well known that the national reports are an underestimate of incidence,[26–28], but useful for trends. There are no accepted case definitions.

3. Reports of laboratory identifications

Nearly all microbiology laboratories in England, Wales, and Northern Ireland voluntarily report positive identifications of specified infections each week to the PHLS Communicable Disease Surveillance Centre. A similar reporting system exists in Scotland. Public Health Laboratories also report the results of investigation of environmental specimens such as water, food, and milk.

Advantages   These reporting systems provide precise data on proven infections, with personal, clinical, and epidemiological details, some in free text. Data are analysed and the results distributed to laboratories and health-care workers by the end of the week following that to which the data refer. The system is flexible, so that new infections can be reported, and additional items of information requested. Statistics on some laboratory reported infections—for example, psittacosis—are not readily available through any other source.

Disadvantages   Except in the case of foodborne outbreaks, the number of specimens tested in each laboratory is not reported, and so the denominator is not known. Selection of patients from which samples are taken may give rise to a false impression of the pattern of incidence; for instance, the rate of identifications of rubella is higher among women aged 15–44 years than in any other group. For some infections there is no suitable laboratory test and many patients with the commoner clinically obvious infections do not have samples taken. Reporting from individual laboratories is not always consistent or complete, due to heavy work-loads, but it is hoped that as laboratories acquire computers the burden of reporting will be eased.

4. *Reports from Medical Officers for environmental health*

In England and Wales Medical Officers for environmental health are asked to inform CDSC of any outbreaks occurring within their district. They are also required by law to report to CDSC serious outbreaks of any disease irrespective of whether or not the disease is notifiable.

Advantages Most of the outbreaks reported are of foodborne disease, and the reports include the number of people affected, the number at risk, the number from whom samples have been taken, and the number from whom an organism has been isolated. This provides denominators for each reported outbreak. Some outbreaks which would not otherwise be reported become known to CDSC by this method.

Disadvantages Some outbreaks may not be reported. There is some confusion about what constitutes a 'serious' outbreak which must by law be reported.

5. *Reports from general practice*

The Research Unit of the Royal College of General Practitioners in Birmingham set up in 1966 a national system for reporting new episodes of illness, including the common communicable diseases, presenting to a sample of practices each week.[29] This scheme currently covers a population of about 200 000, a 0·4 per cent sample of the population of England and Wales. The list of diseases to be reported includes many which are not notifiable under the Public Health Act such as chickenpox, herpes zoster, rubella, mumps, infectious mononucleosis, influenza, and other respiratory diseases (see Chapter 7).

Advantages This reporting system is of particular value because it provides incidence data on infections which present in general practice but are not usually referred for secondary care, which are not notifiable and for which no appropriate laboratory test is routinely available. It is therefore complementary to the laboratory and notification systems. General practitioners taking part in this scheme report notifiable diseases at about twice the rate of statutory notifications received from all general practitioners. The data are available within ten days. Each contributing practice keeps an age/sex register which provides a fairly accurate denominator for the calculation of age-specific rates.

Disadvantages The number of practices is small, and are not geographically, and may not be demographically, representative. The population sample is small so that results may be difficult to interpret on a weekly basis. Large areas of the country are not represented and others perhaps over-represented. It is only feasible to collect data on common infections. It is hoped to double the number of practices contributing over the next three years, which, with careful selection, will help to overcome some of these problems.

6. In-patient data

Acute hospitals in the UK record data for management purposes on every patient who dies in or is discharged from hospital; these data include the diagnoses made during the admission and operations performed.

Advantages   Hospital data are useful for those infections, such as meningitis and tetanus, which usually require admission to hospital.

Disadvantages   There is a long interval before the data are published. Before 1987 in England and Wales these provided a national estimate from a 10 per cent sample, giving a wide margin of error for infections which are rarely the cause for admission to hospital. In England and Wales, only the number of discharges is currently readily available, so that patients who are readmitted or are admitted to more than one hospital are counted more than once. These problems will not arise when a new national recording system is implemented in 1987; all deaths in and discharges from hospital will be reported by regions to the national centre and it will be possible to enumerate individuals rather than occurrences.

7. Out-patient data

Although no diagnostic information is routinely available for all out-patient or accident and emergency department attenders, chest clinics and departments for the investigation and treatment of genito-urinary diseases regularly report the diagnosis of all cases seen.

Advantages   This system which includes data by diagnosis, sex, age-group, and country of source of infection provides the only data available on sexually transmitted diseases; for tuberculosis more details of cases are provided.

Disadvantages   Patients who are treated in clinics other than those for sexually transmitted diseases or chest clinics, or who are treated by their general practitioner are not included. Because episodes not patients are reported, an individual may be reported many times. Some clinics report contacts given treatment as cases.

8. Boarding-school data

Episodes of illness requiring confinement to bed on medical advice are reported weekly to CDSC by about fifty-five boarding schools in England and Wales.

Advantages   Information about illness in an age group which is infrequently seen by the general practitioner is available.

Disadvantages   Boarding schools are relatively closed institutions so that incidence and spread of infections may follow a different pattern to that seen in an open community.

9. Immunization data

Childhood immunization against diphtheria, pertussis, tetanus, poliomyelitis, and tuberculosis is offered routinely to all children throughout the UK, and rubella to girls and to women of childbearing age. Immunization uptake rates are calculated using the population in the relevant age group as the denominator.

Advantages   These data are used to monitor the acceptance of immunization at a local level and also nationally.

Disadvantages   High migration rates make it difficult to keep accurate records of children immunized, and to calculate reliable denominators. General practitioners do not always report those they immunize. The national child-health computer record system is now used in the majority of health districts, which has made record keeping easier.

10. Special surveillance programmes

Each winter influenza is surveilled by CDSC using various indices including laboratory reports, reports from general practice, and mortality data. From the sources used the earliest indicators of an impending epidemic have been found to be reports from general practice and total death registrations.[23]

Certain rare syndromes are also reported. Paediatricians provide data on a number of diseases such as Reye's syndrome,[30] haemolytic uraemic syndrome, haemorrhagic shock encephalopathy syndrome, and Kawasaki disease. These reports are supplemented by cases identified from laboratory reports and death registrations.

In September 1982 a programme for the surveillance of AIDS was set up by CDSC in England and Wales. Clinicians report cases under their care, laboratories report opportunist infections in patients who come within the Centres for Disease Control definition of AIDS, and the OPCS sends copies of all death registrations with a mention of Kaposi's sarcoma or AIDS.[31]

Routine Feedback of Information

Weekly reports are issued by CDSC (laboratory reports and selected notifications), OPCS (notifications, births, total deaths and deaths from selected causes, reports from general practice and meteorological data), CD(S)U (laboratory reports and notifications), and DHSS(NI) (laboratory reports and notifications).

Similar reports are issued monthly by DHSS(NI) and quarterly by CDSC and OPCS, and comprehensive reports are produced annually.

Examples of Successful Surveillance

Long-term surveillance based on routinely collected data shows how the incidence of some infectious diseases, for example, diphtheria, measles, and whooping-cough, has changed both in the total number of cases, cyclical distribution, age distribution, and in association with immunization rates. Surveillance of malaria, for example, on the other hand indicates an increase, probably due to an increase in malaria in many parts of the world, and to increased travel abroad, particularly by immigrants returning for holidays without prophylaxis to their country of origin. Reports of travellers infected by malaria and the enteric fevers in different parts of the world provide the basis on which advice on appropriate immunization and prophylaxis is given to those intending to travel.

National surveillance of routinely collected laboratory reports may indicate trends or the appearance of rare infections originating from a common source which could not be identified by a single laboratory. In 1981 and 1982 thirty-three reports of *Salmonella ealing* from 13 laboratories over an area in the north of England were found to be associated with the slaughter and processing of halal poultry for Muslim consumption by one individual who carried chickens in his van to different towns and killed them when demand required. An outbreak of Legionnaires' disease associated with the use of a whirlpool in a Brighton hotel was identified after investigation of the first two cases which were diagnosed in laboratories 200 miles apart. In 1982 three reports of *Salmonella napoli*, a species rarely reported in England, from three laboratories initiated an investigation which soon identified imported chocolate as the source; it was estimated that rapid action prevented 200 hospital admissions and many thousands of cases by early withdrawal of the product.[32] Fifteen cases of *Salmonella goldcoast* were reported in 1984 from ten laboratories; the common source was identified as the aspic glaze on imported pâté, which was withdrawn. In 1985 *Salmonella ealing* infections predominantly among children under one year of age were found to be associated with infected milk feed, which was subsequently withdrawn from the market.

Surveillance of infections acquired abroad among holiday-makers who subsequently present with illness in different parts of the country may indicate a common source. In 1983 an outbreak of *Salmonella typhi* infection occurred among guests in a hotel on a Mediterranean island, and a kitchen worker in the hotel was identified as the source.[33]

Discussion

Systems for communicable disease surveillance in Italy and the UK differ because of the differing characteristics of their peoples, administrative arrangements for the health-care provision, and the rate at which development has been possible.

Routine collection of data commenced in both countries with the introduction of registration of deaths in the middle of the nineteenth century and of statutory notification of certain infectious diseases in the 1880s. While other sources of data have been developed in the UK, notably reporting from laboratories and information about hospital admissions, it is only recently that similar data have become avilable to a limited extent in Italy. As a result, notifications of clinical illness continue to be the fundamental instrument of surveillance in Italy, and effort for development has been directed towards improving the means by which these data are collected centrally, and the requirement for laboratory confirmation of viral hepatitis. The UK on the other hand has made little recent progress in improving the quality of notification, and data from other sources have played an increasing and complementary part in surveillance.[34]

Problems of communicable disease are similar in many respects in Italy and in the UK, and similar data are required for surveillance. However, there are differences in the sources of data and methods of analysis which reflect the struggle in each country to provide an integrated system which will fulfil the requirements of successful surveillance.

Mortality registration provides data for those diseases which led to death; however, it is only recently that every diagnosis mentioned on the death certificate has been coded in every country in the UK, while in Italy all causes are coded, but only the underlying cause analysed for publication, so that much valuable information is lost during analysis.

In both Italy and the UK there is considerable undernotification of infectious diseases. In both countries the list of diseases to be notified is long, sixty-five in Italy and twenty-nine in England and Wales, and includes some which are inappropriate at the present time. The system does allow the identification of trends, and in both countries data are now available and published within days of the end of the period to which they relate. In England and Wales, statutory notification has been supplemented by reporting from a sample of general practices of some common communicable diseases which are not notifiable, as well as some that are.

Reports from laboratories of proven infections are in some respects the basis of surveillance in the UK. In Italy there is no comprehensive network of public health laboratories comparable to that in the UK on which such a system could be based, and reporting is currently limited to a few laboratories which contribute to specific programmes such as those for influenza and legionellosis surveillance.

Hospital data provide useful information about those infections which usually require admission. Until 1986 only a 10 per cent sample was analysed centrally in England and Wales, but from the beginning of 1987 data on all discharges from hospitals throughout the UK will be reported and analysed centrally. In Italy the small sample available nationally is inadequate for the surveillance of communicable diseases.

Vaccination against certain infections is compulsory in Italy, but this is not the case in the UK. However, in Italy only the number of doses given is registered so that the number of people who are fully protected is not known. In the UK recipients who have completed a course are reported, allowing the uptake rate of satisfactory immunization against each infection to be estimated.

Both Italy and the UK have developed special programmes for the surveillance of individual diseases during recent years. In addition, other systems have been developed in the UK, such as reports of illness from a sample of boarding schools, and of outbreaks from medical officers for environmental health, which contribute data on incidents that are not necessarily identified from any other source.

Conclusion

During the development of surveillance systems, epidemiologists in Italy and the UK have independently reached similar conclusions. More than one source is necessary for communicable disease surveillance and co-ordination of data from different sources and from all parts of the country is a fundamental requirement which should be accomplished by a national centre.

The success of any surveillance system depends greatly on the quality of data collected. Quality improves if the number of infections to be reported is small and if the method of reporting is kept simple and easy. Standard definitions and clear, concise and unambiguous instructions are essential. The system should be designed to detect well-defined problems; the temptation to expect it to provide the answers as well as pose the questions must be resisted, because this inevitably makes any surveillance system unwieldy. Quick reliable and accurate analysis and timely publication of results in an acceptable format improves the link between the national centre and local health care workers, facilitating cooperation in other aspects of communicable disease control.

Although considerable success has been achieved in the past using manual methods of communication, processing, and analysis, advantage should be taken of the contribution that modern technology has to make towards an increasingly effective surveillance system.

Bibliography

1. La peste a Venezia, Venezia, Catalogo Mostra Rispoli (1978).
2. Legge sulla tutela dell' Igiene e della Sanità Pubblica del 22.12.1888, No. 5849.
3. Testo Unico delle Leggi Sanitarie, R.D. 27.07.1934, No. 1256.
4. Istituzione del Servizio Sanitario Nazionale, 23.12.1978, No. 833.
5. Santoro, R., Ruggeri, F. M., Battaglia, M. *et al.*, Measles epidemiology in Italy. *Int. J. Epidemiol.* **3**, 201–9 (1984).
6. Cislaghi, C., Morosini, P. L., Il medico come produttore ed utente di statistiche sanitarie: le denunce di malattie infettive, *Epidemiologia e Prevenzione* **1**, 56–9 (1977).
7. Greco, D., Verdecchia, A., Mariotti, S. *et al.*, The information system for the monitoring of communicable diseases. In *Health information system: the Italian approach* (M. Luzzana and M. Palumbo, eds). Proceedings of the IFIP–IMIA, Fourth World Congress on Medical Informatics. Amsterdam (1983).
8. Istituto Superiore di Sanità, SIRMI. Bollettino Epidemiologico Nazionale, 28 Guigno (1984).
9. Rosmini, F., Castellani Pastoris, M., Mazzotti, M. F. *et al.*, Febrile illness in successive cohorts of tourists at a hotel of the Italian adriatic coast: Evidence for a persistent focus of Legionella infection. *Am. J. Epidemiol.* **119**, 124–34 (1984).
10. Istituto Superiore di Sanità, Sorveglianza Nazionale della Legionellosi. Bollettino Epidemiologico Nazionale, 12 Maggio (1983).
11. Mele, A., Rosmini, F., Ganganella, G., and Gill, O. N., Integrated epidemiological system for acute viral hepatitis. Rapporti ISTISAN, Rome (1986).
12. Stroffolini, T., Le meningiti batteriche. Roma: Rapporti ISTISAN, Rome (1985).
13. Rezza, G., Ippolito, G., Marasca, G., and Greco, D., AIDS in Italy. *Lancet*, **ii**, 642 (1984).
14. Moro, M. L., Stazi, M. A., Marasca, G., Gresco, D., and Zampieri, A., The national prevalence survey of hospital-required infections in Italy. *J. Hosp. Inf.* **8**, 72–85 (1986).
15. Graunt, J., *National and political observations made upon the Bills of Mortality*. Martin, London (1662).
16. Births and Deaths Registration Act (1836) c. 86.
17. Births and Deaths Registration Act (1874) c. 88.
18. Notification of Infectious Diseases Extension Act (1899) c. 8.
19. Williams, R. E. O., *Microbiology for the public health*. Public Health Laboratory Service, London (1985).
20. Galbraith, N. S. and Young, S. E. J., Communicable disease control: The development of a laboratory associated national epidemiological service in England and Wales. *Community Med.* **2**, 135–43 (1980).

21. Reid, D., Communicable diseases (Scotland) unit. *Hlth Bull.* **28,** 30–2 (1970).
22. Ashley, J. S. A., Present state of statistics from hospital inpatient data and their uses. *Br. J. Prevent. social Med.* **26,** 135–47 (1972).
23. Tillett, H. E. and Spencer, I. L., Influenza surveillance in England and Wales using routine statistics. *J. Hyg. Camb.* **88,** 83–94 (1982).
24. Alderson, M. R., Bayliss, R. I. S., Clarke, C. A., and Whitfield, A. G. W., Death certification. *Br. med. J.* **287,** 444–5 (1983).
25. Galbraith, N. S. and Berrie, J. H. R., Statutory notification and surveillance of infectious diseases. *Hlth Trends* **10,** 32–4 (1978).
26. Goldacre, M. J. and Miller, D. L., Completeness of statutory notification for acute bacterial meningitis. *Br. med. J.* **2,** 501–3 (1976).
27. Clarkson, J. A. and Fine, P. E. M., The efficiency of measles and pertussis notification in England and Wales. *Int. J. Epidemiol.* **14,** 153–68. (1985).
28. Office of Population Censuses and Surveys, *Annual review of communicable diseases 1983*, OPCS (Monitor Series MB2 86/1), London (1986).
29. Fleming, D. M. and Crombie, D. L., The incidence of common infectious diseases: the weekly returns service of the Royal College of General Practitioners. *Hlth Trends* **17,** 13–16 (1985).
30. Hall, S. and Bellman, M., Reye's syndrome in the British Isles: First annual report of the joint British Paediatric Association and Communicable Disease Surveillance Centre surveillance scheme. *Br. med. J.* **288,** 584–5 (1984).
31. PHLS Communicable Disease Surveillance Centre, Surveillance of the acquired immune deficiency syndrome in the United Kingdom, January 1982–July 1983. *Br. med. J.* **287,** 407–8 (1983).
32. Gill, O. N., Sockett, P. N., Bartlett, C. L. R. *et al.*, Oubreak of Salmonella napoli infection caused by contaminated chocolate bars. *Lancet* **1,** 574–7 (1983).
33. Stanwell-Smith, R. E. and Ward, L. R., An international point source outbreak of typhoid fever identified by epidemiological method. *Bull. WHO* **64** (2), 271–8 (1986).
34. Galbraith, N. S., Communicable disease surveillance. In *Recent advances in community medicine* (ed. A. Smith) pp. 127–41. Churchill Livingstone, Edinburgh (1982).

15

Surveillance of occupational health

E. LYNGE

Introduction

Occupational surveillance systems focus on registration of hazards or diseases or on both. They are either public or private.

The hazard surveillance system includes registration of chemical substances, physical demands, ergonomic conditions, noise levels, etc. The disease surveillance system extends from biological monitoring of body samples to epidemiological data on mortality and morbidity in selected occupational groups.

The ideal occupational surveillance system is a combined hazard and disease surveillance system. Hazard surveillance is directed towards exposures known or suspected to be associated with adverse health effects, while disease surveillance operates as the 'security net', aiming at picking up health problems that may occur despite the operation of a hazard system.

Unlike public surveillance systems which are concerned with prevention of disease in the population in general and with nationwide preventive measures, surveillance systems in private companies focus on selection and surveillance of the company's own work-force.

The crucial point for any surveillance system is whether it offers a valid basis for action and priority setting. A precondition for this is that the data collected give a reliable picture of the realities as experienced in the workplace. It is outside the scope of this chapter to evaluate the reliability of occupational data used in the surveillance systems. However, four examples have been selected for discussion, all originating from public surveillance systems in Denmark, Finland, and the US.

Accidents at Work

Surveillance of accidents at work is described in detail in Chapter 16. Here it is discussed from the point of view of data quality in occupational surveillance systems. Protection against accidents at work has been an issue of concern for factory inspectors for a long time. Reliable statistics are a precondition for effective intervention. Registration of accidents at work should cause few problems in this respect, they are well defined in time and space and also from a diagnostic point of view. Nevertheless, it appears that the compilation of reliable accident statistics is not a straightforward task.

In Denmark accidents at work causing three or more days of absence were registered from 1960 to 1972 in connection with the system of payment by the employer of statutory daily allowances.[1] In 1973 all employees were given the right to daily allowances from the first day of absence from work, independent of whether the absence was due to accident, sickness, or childbirth.

In order to continue the registration of accidents it therefore became compulsory in 1974 for employers to notify accidents causing more than one day's absence to the National Board of Labour Protection.[2] This change in the notification criteria was followed by a drop in the registered number of accidents at work from 68 000 in 1972 to 25 000 in 1974, despite the fact that an increase was expected.

In 1983 the right to daily allowances on the first day of absence from work was abolished, except in those cases where it was caused by an accident at work. This change was followed by an increase in the registered number of accidents at work from 35 000 in 1982 to 47 000 in 1983.[3]

Surveys carried out by the National Board of Labour Protection in 1975 and 1981 estimated the number of accidents at work to be around 125 000 per year.[3] A linkage study of data on notified accidents at work in 1981 and hospital discharges in 1981 showed that 3100 persons were found to have been hospitalized for their injuries from notified accidents at work, but an additional 2300 persons were found to have been hospitalized for injuries caused by accidents at work that had not been notified.[4] The fluctuations in the registered number of accidents at work indicate that the outcome of a surveillance system depends on its organization and on the financing. The efficiency increases when notification causes 'money to change hands'.

In a country like Denmark it seems reasonable to consider alternative data sources for registration of accidents at work. All hospital discharges are registered by making use of a personal identification number. An increasing number of hospitals also register their out-patients by personal identification numbers, as well as all services provided by general practitioners outside the Copenhagen area. When relevant codes for the place of the accident, etc. are included it would become possible to establish a reliable registration system for all accidents at work that need treatment.

Occupational Cancer

In contrast to many other diseases that may be related to exposure in the workplace, such as neurological disorders caused by solvent exposure, cancer is a well defined entity from a medical point of view. Furthermore, according to IARC, epidemiological evidence for a causal association between cancer and exposure to specific agents now exists for thirty chemical compounds or groups of chemicals and for nine industrial processes. Examples are asbestos and pleural mesothelioma and lung cancer, wood dust and nasal cancer, vinyl chloride and liver angiosarcoma, and 2-naphthylamine and bladder cancer. Another 14 chemicals or groups of chemicals are considered to be potentially carcinogenic to humans with a high degree of probability based on combined human and animal data, and further 49 chemicals with a lower degree of probability. For a total of 115 chemicals or groups of chemicals there is moreover sufficient evidence for their carcinogenicity in experimental animals without corresponding evidence in humans.[5] The IARC considers it reasonable for practical purposes to regard these chemicals to be a carcinogenic risk to humans too.

In 1981 Doll and Peto estimated that approximately 4 per cent of incident cancer cases in the US could be attributed to occupational exposures.[6] Estimates of this kind are necessarily crude as the data are limited and independent exposures may act in a multiplicative way, for example with tobacco and asbestos, whereas non-smoking asbestos workers have a fivefold greater risk of lung cancer compared to non-smoking non-asbestos workers, while smoking non-asbestos workers have a tenfold greater risk, asbestos workers who smoke have a fiftyfold greater risk.[7]

In Denmark physicians and dentists are requested to notify to the National Board of Social Security and/or to the National Board of Labour Protection all cases of proven and suspected occupational diseases of which they become aware. In 1983 and 1984 the National Board of Labour Protection only received notifications from about 20 per cent of general practitioners and practising specialists, and half the notification came from 3 per cent of the physicians.[9] A total of 84 cancer cases were notified in 1984, of which half were lung cancers, and asbestos was the most frequently reported exposure.[10] If we use the 4 per cent estimate of Doll and Peto[6] on the Danish data, 920 of the 23 000 incident cancer cases in Denmark in 1982[8] would be caused by occupational exposure.

Persons who develop a disease included in the official list of occupational diseases or other diseases considered to be caused by their work are entitled to compensation. The list includes diseases caused by exposure to, for instance, arsenic, chromium, and nickel; skin cancer related to exposure to soot, tar, and mineral oils, and lung cancer and mesothelioma linked to asbestos exposure. In 1982–83 eleven cancer patients were compensated for an occupational cancer.[11] This figure should be compared with the annual number in Denmark of 55 mesothelioma cases and 37 nasal cancer cases[8] for both of which an occupational aetiology would be highly likely.

In 1986 a standard notification form for the National Board of Social Security and the National Board of Labour Protection was introduced, thus making it easy for physicians to fulfil their obligation to notify. Moreover, in addition to the clinic for occupational disease at the central state hospital in Copenhagen, occupational clinics have now been established in seven counties. This will improve the possibilities for examination of the occupational and exposure history of cancer patients.

Exposure to Carcinogens

Occupational mortality statistics are able to identify those occupational groups exposed to carcinogens many years previously. However, other surveillance systems are required to identify persons actually being exposed to carcinogens. In 1979 a registration system was implemented in Finland in order to provide data on 'known carcinogenic substances used in particular plant departments and all the available exposure data for the specific employees for their periods of work at hazardous jobs.[12] The system, called ASA, is based on annual notifications from the employers to the Regional Labour Protection Offices. Data from the regional offices are combined in a central computerized register. From 1979 to 1985 a list of 50 carcinogens was in use; a new list of 162 substances will come into effect in 1986. The number of employees exposed to at least one of the 50 carcinogens on the list increased from 3767 in 1979 to 10 815 in 1984. The main occupational groups reported to ASA in 1984 were 'machine and engine mechanics', 'welder and flame cutters' and 'laboratory assistants'. These groups together constituted 40 per cent of the notified employees. Exposure to chromates and to nickel and its inorganic compounds were equally common and together constituted half of the notified exposures. Other quantitatively important exposures were asbestos, polycyclic aromatic hydrocarbons, cadmium and its inorganic compounds, and benzene.[13]

Based on data available from the ASA register in 1984 the following conclusion was drawn:

ASA register is the first systematic attempt to register exposure to a wide range of carcinogens in Finland. Comparable information is not available from other countries either, so that the coverage of the registration is hard to determine. Nevertheless, the strong annual growth indicates that the register may not be close to full coverage. Separate studies have also shown that the relative proportion of employees reported to ASA within an industry varies by geographic area. The variation appears to be too large to be explainable by the real differences in exposure.[13]

Exposure to Chemical Substances in general

Attempts have been made to construct job-exposure matrices of potential chemical exposure within given jobs. Most of these have been based on literature reviews of for example textbooks of industrial hygiene, in some cases limited to specific carcinogens,[14,15] and in some cases including both carcinogens and chemicals with other chronic or acute effects.[16,17]

Only one attempt has been made to identify all potential chemical exposures from an actual survey of randomly selected workplaces. This was the US National Occupational Hazard Survey (NOSH) carried out by NIOSH in 1972–74.[18]

A total of 5200 industrial facilities in 67 metropolitan areas representing all non-agricultural business covered under the Occupational Safety and Health Act of 1970 were included in the survey. Each plant was visited by an engineer. All material utilized for more than thirty minutes per week or three full eight-hour workdays per year were recorded. Three types of exposure were notified:

1. *Potential exposure* which include any substance for which there is an intended control other than natural. Registered as exposed to these substances are those employees who have worked directly with the operation as well as those others who have come in contact with the substance.
2. *Actual exposures* include mists, dusts, vapours, gases, or liquids, and all employees exposed were surveyed.
3. *Inferred exposures* were an observable accumulation (dusts or mists) which directly indicated that the substance was present in the air; in such an instance employees working in the immediate area of the accumulation were surveyed.[18]

A total of more than 9000 different potential hazards were discovered and more than 85 000 trade name products were listed in the survey. In a further stage more than 10 500 manufacturers of these trade name products were contacted and the chemical ingredients for about 60 000 products were identified.

Based on the survey, estimates were made on the number of workers in the US exposed to given chemical substances. Examples given were 1 500 000 workers exposed to benzene. When these estimates were used as a basis for calculation of the expected number of cancer cases attributable to these exposures,[19] it was argued that both actual, potential, and inferred exposures had been included in the estimates, that exposure levels were higher in the past, and that it might be inappropriate to group certain exposures together, nickel refining with other exposures to nickel for example.[20]

Quantification of Occupational Hazards

The weakness in the existing disease-surveillance systems have led to construction of a hazard-surveillance system based on computerized data on work force, use of chemicals, exposure levels, and data on dose–response relationships. The method has been applied to industries in Los Angeles County, classified by the Standard Industrial Classification (SIC).[21]

Four indices of the hazard profile of each industry (SIC) have been calculated:

1. An *industrial risk index* (*IRI*), where each chemical is rated on a potency scale using toxicological data and weighted by a NOSH estimate of how many workers are potentially exposed. The results are summed for all chemicals in the SIC.
2. An *OSHA Weighted Index* (*OWI*) calculated as IRI but taking into account only those 450 chemicals regulated by OSHA.
3. An *Inspection Based Exposure Ranking* (*IBER*), based on the results of 60 000 industrial hygiene test samples registered by OSHA in 1979–1982. A summary IBER rank has been calculated for each industry (SIC) based on the measured severity-level (= concentration/permissible exposure level) and number of substances for which test samples were registered from the industry (SIC).
4. The *number of persons* employed in the industry.

If an industry appears at the top of several lists, it indicates that there is a history of documented overexposure to certain chemicals (IBER-list) and of potential exposures to a number of other highly toxic substances, and that a significant number of workers are thought to be exposed (IRI and OWI-lists). Eight SICs were in the top 20 per cent of SICs in all three ranking methods. These were plastic, resins (SIC 2821), paints, allied products (SIC 2851), miscellaneous pottery products, NEC (SIC 3269), metal cars (SIC 3411), metal coating (SIC 3479), truck trailers (SIC 3715), shipbuilding (SIC 3731) and repair services NEC (SIC 7699). A total of 34 000 persons were employed in these eight industries in Los Angeles County; a number which should be seen in relation to 129 000 persons employed in hospitals (SIC 8062), and 102 000 persons employed in eating places (SIC 5812).[21]

Conclusion

The purpose of governmental occupational surveillance systems is to obtain a basis for priority of regulations and preventive measures. It is evident from the examples discussed above that there is a striking contrast between the quality of information in some existing governmental surveillance systems and the potential quality of information, considering the possibilities for linkage of computerized data. In Denmark a work classification system (AKM) is now in operation where the employment status and workplace of each citizen are registered annually, based on data from taxation forms and various other administrative data sources.[22] A product register (PR) is in operation to which manufacturers and importers are requested to give information on certain chemical compounds, mainly those labelled as dangerous according to Danish and EEC regulations.[23] As described above for the

US, in Denmark there is also a computerized registration of all industrial hygiene test samples.[23] Improvements are desirable in all these systems, but it is important to point out that combination of these data sources provides a potential for a thorough registration of chemical exposure for each individual employee. Similarly, the registration of work-related diseases could be much improved by combination of existing disease registers. Thus, technically, we have the possibilities today for much better occupational surveillance systems than those that are actually in operation.

Bibliography

1. Sikringsstyrelsen, *Rapporter fra Sikringsstyrelsen, 1960*. Copenhagen (1972).
2. Danmarks Statistik, *Statistiske Efterretninger 1975/77*. Copenhagen (1975).
3. Arbejdstilsynet, *Arbejdsulykker. Aarsstatistik 1982–1983*. Copenhagen (1986).
4. Nielsen, S. and Ørhede, E., *Samkøring af landspatientregistret og registret over arbejdsulykker*. Arbejdstilsynet. Rapport No. 18. Copenhagen (1985).
5. Vainio, H., Hemminki, K., and Wilbourn, J., Data on the carcinogenicity of chemicals in the IARC monographs programme. *Carcinogenesis* **6**, 11, 1653–65 (1985).
6. Doll, R. and Peto, R., The causes of cancer: Quantitative estimates of avoidable risks of cancer in the United States today. *J. Natl. Cancer Inst.* **66**, 6, 1191–308 (1981).
7. Selikoff, I. J. and Hammond, E. C., Asbestos and smoking. *J. Am. Med. Ass.* **242**, 5, 458–9 (1979).
8. Danish Cancer Registry, *Cancer incidence in Denmark 1981 and 1982*. Copenhagen (1985).
9. Sundhedsstyrelsen, *Meddelelse til laeger og tandlaeger om anmeldelse af arbejdsbetingede sygdomme og dødsfald*. Copenhagen (1986).
10. Arbejdstilsynet, *Anmeldte arbejdsbetingede lidelser. Aarsopgørelse 1984*. Copenhagen (1986).
11. Sikringsstyrelsen, *Arbejdsskadeforsikringen. Beretning for aarene 1982, 1983 og 1984*. Copenhagen (1986)
12. Herva, A. and Partanen, T., Computerising occupational carcinogenic data in Finland. *Am. Ind. Hyg. Ass. J.* **42**, 7, 529–33 (1981).
13. Työterveyslaitos, Katsaukia 83. ASA 1984. Helsinki (1986).
14. Macaluso, M., Vineis, P., Continenza, D., Ferrario, F., Pisani, P., and Andisio, R., Job exposure matrices: Experience in Italy. In *Job exposure matrices*. Scientific Report No. 2. MRC Environmental Epidemiology Unit. Southampton (1983).
15. Coggon, D., Pannett, B., and Acheson, D. E., Use of job exposure matrix in an occupational analysis of lung and bladder cancer on the basis of death certificates. *J.Natnl. Cancer Inst.* **72**, 1, 61–5 (1984).
16. Hoar, S. K., Morrison, A. S., Cole, P., and Silverman, D. T., An occupation and exposure linkage system for the study of occupational carcinogenesis. *J. Occupational Medicine* **22**, 722–6 (1980).
17. Siemiatycki, J., Richardson, L., Gerin, M., Goldberg, M., Dewar, R., Desy, M., Campbell, S., and Wacholder, S., Associations between several sites of cancer and

nine organic dusts: Results from an hypothesis-generating case-control study in Montreal, 1979–1983. *Am. J. Empidemiol.* **123,** 2, 235–49 (1986).

18. NIOSH, *National occupational hazard survey.* DHEW Publication No. (NIOSH) 74–127. Cincinatti, Ohio (1977).

19. NIOSH, Estimates of the fraction of cancer in the United States related to occupational factors. National Cancer Institute (1978).

20. American Industrial Health Council, *Estimates of the fraction of cancer in the United States attributable to occupational factors.* New York (1978).

21. Froines, J. R., Dellenbaugh, C. A., and Wegman, D. H., Occupational health surveillance: A means to identify work-related risks. *Am. J. publ. Hlth* **76,** 1089–97 (1986).

22. Danmarks Statistik, *Registerfolkestaellingen 1981. Folke- og boligtaellingen 1. Januar 1981. L1. Landstabelvaerk.* Copenhagen (1984).

23. Arbejdstilsynet, *Introduktion til brug af Arbejdstilsynets edbregistre om arbejdsulykker, arbejdsbetingede lidelser, arbejdspladsmaalinger, stoffer og materialer.* Copenhagen (1986).

16

Surveillance for accidents at work

A. DE BOCK

Introduction and Definitions

In order to gain insight into the occurrence of accidents at work and to analyse statistical data, it is necessary to define adequately the concept of accidents at work.

This is a difficult task. Almost all countries use different definitions. This reflects the varying degree of development of existing compensation systems which refund consequences of accidents at work and the national legislation for safety at work. This legislation, mostly under the jurisdiction of the Ministry of Labour and Employment and sometimes the Ministry of Social Affairs, describes the fields of human activity in which accidents at work may occur.

In the United Kingdom, OSHAW (Occupational Safety and Health At Work), a fairly recent legislation for safety at work, has decreed that these fields include all areas where human beings perform work, including the home.

In The Netherlands virtually no distinction is made between absence by illness and absence by accident at work. National statistics on accidents at work also vary enormously, depending on the criteria by which cases have or have not to be registered. In many countries only accidents that cause at least some days of disability are registered. A difference is also made between absence in terms of working hours lost and absence counted in calendar days.

In Belgium all accidents at work resulting in at least one day of absence, the day of the accident not being included, have to be reported.

The severity of accidents, expressed by the number of days of absence from work and by the degree of partial or total permanent disability, also depends on systems for the control of absenteeism based on compensation criteria and on the level of care provided by insurance companies.

It is well known that in small firms where a limited number of contractual workers are employed, accidents at work are less frequent, less severe and notably underreported. Pressure at work, personal interest, and pursuit of gain play a role. In the current economic climate, the fear of losing one's job leads to shorter and less frequent spells of absence due to accidents. In some industries management indeed postulates that accidents at work are nearly always caused by faulty actions which are then severely condemned. Moreover, a collective rewarding system for safety at work exerts group pressure upon each group member to avoid accidents at work, or when they occur, to obscure or minimize them. This particularly applies to multinational firms. As a result of the safety policy pursued, their statistics on accidents are the most favourable of all industries. Absence caused by an accident at work may not be notified, either because the victim is forced to take one or more days off, or because substitute work and travel facilities are offered to the employee.

Summarizing the discussion on the definition of an accident at work one can broadly say that all definitions state that accidents at work are directly concerned with the execution of work during which, because of an unexpected occurrence in the process of work, human injury suddenly appears, thus reducing the work capacity at short notice. In older definitions the term 'unpredictable' occurrence is used. But 'unpredictable' is often the synonym for 'overlooked' or 'neglect' due to lack of risk analysis. Modern methods of risk-analysis such as the MORT (Management Oversight and Risk Tree) rule out many of these 'unexpected' or 'unpredictable' causes. We also have to put 'unexpected' between brackets as the occurrence of an accident at work is usually preceded by a series of disturbances or occurrences which do not immediately cause injuries. In professional jargon they are called 'symptoms'. If a building worker has been hit on the head by a falling stone on an insufficiently protected building site and people are working without safe scaffolding or without steel helmets, one can hardly accept the 'unexpectedness' of the accident. Even the 'involuntary' character of the accident with regard to the victim could be questioned.

Finally it will be clear also that the borderline between the concepts of accidents at work, occupational diseases, and common diseases is often vague and difficult to interpret.

Data Collection and Analysis

National

Reporting accidents at work is generally uniform for a country and is duly observed. However, varying premium systems, the control system of work-inspectorates, the impact of the trade unions, the quality and authority of the safety and occupational health departments, and various *ad hoc* committees may influence the reported data. This also refers to the safety policy of the management.

The value of national statistics is very relative. In principle statistics should be a safety gauge to indicate concrete and precise situations. They should draw parallels between the industries belonging to the same sector and test the appropriateness of the legislation for safety at work, so that necessary legislative measures can be taken. The results do not always show what they should. This is due to variation in what should be reported and registered, and also variation in the way this information is actually reported.

In many countries statistical data are collected on standard report forms, often precoded, and statutorily registered. The maximum time period allowed for reporting is also strictly determined. There is little or no control on the correctness of the report, unless in case of serious or fatal accidents the work-inspectorate and the coroner carry out investigation in depth. The reports of less serious accidents are therefore often incomplete. If it is evident that the statutory regulations on safety have not been observed and are the cause of the accident, the employer exposes himself to prosecution. He will therefore do his best to disguise his responsibility. Often the victim is blamed for having acted incautiously or having neglected the safety regulations.

On the other hand, due to the short time allowed for reporting, an accident report in Belgium, for example, is drawn up in three phases. The first report contains the minimum compulsory information required for official notification (mostly to the work inspectorate). A second report includes information on the medical condition of the victim. This is of importance to the insurance company which has to cover the damage. The real and most valuable report can often only be drawn up a long time after the accident when the final evaluation has been done. Accident investigation is time-consuming, for instance it may be that the victim is in such a condition that it is impossible to question him.

Thorough analysis of all the elements that could contribute to the real causes of the accident also takes up a lot of time. Often imperfections in management and organization are discovered. These findings are not systematically published although they could lead to fundamental improvements in safety at work. In our opinion this shortcoming is one of the main reasons why enforcement of the legislation for safety at work does not produce the expected results.

International

The relative importance and weakness of national statistics on accidents as a useful and appropriate instrument of a national prevention policy are illustrated in the previous chapter. The analysis of international statistics is even more disappointing. Except in very broad terms they are very difficult to compare.

We have already mentioned that the organization of national statistics differs from country to country; this makes precise intercountry comparisons almost impossible. Of course, there are definite trends, for example, in all countries accident figures are highest in the building and agricultural sectors. Breaking down national statistics by degree of risk and type of management one can see that in all countries, in large industries with serious risks (petrochemical, chemical industry) safety is well organized and accidents at work are minimized through a strict prevention policy. The very severe accidents that infrequently occur mostly affect the surrounding population. Closer control and stricter preventive measures are then imposed by the political and managerial authorities, such as the compulsory licences and the duty to report serious risks such as have recently been laid down in the SEVESO guidelines.

Safety is not only implemented for the prevention of injuries, but also to control and minimize damage, both human and material. Personal accidents frequently go together with material damage, though there are more accidents causing material damage than injuries to people. The money involved in material accidents far exceeds the compensation paid for human injuries. Material accidents and accidents to people have the same causes. Prevention of the former positively affects prevention of the latter and vice versa.

Accidents at Work in Some EEC Countries

Belgium

The frequency rate is lower in large companies than in middle-size ones but the severity rate is significantly higher. Since 1979, the frequency rate as an overall gauge for occupational safety has considerably decreased for all industries, whereas the severity, i.e. time lost by accidents, has gradually increased and stabilized during the last few years. The leader in the field of accidents remains the construction industry but in 1984 the figures were shifting towards shipbuilding yards and ship-repair shops (frequency 135·51 per thousand exposed employees) and the metal industry (frequency 100·34), whereas construction works yielded a frequency rate of 95·09.[1] This is probably due to factors related to the lasting crisis in the construction industry. This ranking order also stands for the severity rate. Shipbuilding yards rank highest (5·97) followed closely by construction works and the metal industry. In Belgium, agriculture, forestry, and the fishing industry are grouped together and score 57·57 for frequency but 2·74 for the severity rate. All figures refer to 1984 and severity rates are expressed as 'total', i.e. including the time lost for permanent partial or total disability. It should be borne in mind that these figures are not of equal importance since they cover an estimated sample of the sector considered as follows: agriculture, forestry, and fishing 26 per cent, metal products 80 per cent and construction 55 per cent. The greatest total severity rate is found in the road transport sector: 6·07 (frequency 76·76) and a representative sample fraction of 20 per cent only. The overall figures for all industrial and commercial sectors in 1984 are: frequency 42·00, total severity 1·34 and this applies to an overall estimated 75 per cent of the total working force involved.

The average cost of occupational accidents in Belgium increased from 3 053 100Bfr. (about £42 404) in 1979, to 4 312 800Bfr. (about £59 900) in 1984, for fatal accidents. For accidents causing permanent disability the figures are 716 900Bfr. (about £9956) (1979) to 1 007 000Bfr. (about £13 986) (1984) and for accidents causing temporary disability or no disability: 17 200Bfr. (about

£239) (1979) to 25 100Bfr. (about £349) (1984) for blue-collar workers. There is only a slight difference for accidents to white collar employees.

The Netherlands

As in most other industrialized countries accidents rank fourth among causes of death in The Netherlands. The Central Statistical Office (CBS) supplies the data. As is the case with most other national offices, published material is delayed by two to three years with regard to the year in which the accidents occur. As in other European countries the number of victims of fatal accidents in the private sector is ten times higher than the number of victims of accidents at work.[2] Accidents at work are regarded as accidents that occur during the execution of a labour contract and cause inability to work. These accidents have to be notified to the Directorate General of Labour. Since 1968 the statistical processing has been done by the above mentioned CBS. There is no obligation to report accidents occurring on the way to or from the work-place. In an excellent analysis[3] the shortcomings of the Dutch statistics on accidents in comparison with those of the Federal Republic of Germany are described.

In The Netherlands, until 1967, precise data on accidents at work existed through notification, in accordance with the health insurance act, but since the act was amended in that year, there is no longer any difference between absence from work due to illness or due to an accident. Employers are obliged to notify accidents at work separately to the Directorate General of Employment, but in practice this is often neglected.

Comparing The Netherlands and Germany—both countries being about equally industrialized—shows that in The Netherlands only two-thirds of the accidents at work causing absence are registered as such or appear in the national statistics. The recent 'Arbo-law' (Arbeidsomstandighedenwet) will probably lead to favourable improvements, in that complete and correct notifications, providing a better external control, is complemented by better internal supervision (through employee representatives and the occupational safety and health departments).

During the period 1974–81 the frequency of accidents at work decreased, which according to CBS is due to better prevention, increased automation of dangerous work, and shifting of the active occupational population to less risk-holding occupational branches (and to service sectors). Therefore frequency, in this case the number of accidents at work per 1000 exposed employees, decreased from 29·8 in 1978 to 20·7 in 1981.

In 1981 10 out of 1000 exposed persons younger than 30 years of age sustained an injury. This number should be evaluated in relation to the age distribution of the active population. In order of importance the building industry heads the list of all sectors followed by mining and agriculture/fishing. One quarter of the accidents occur with mechanical tools (utensils, machines).

It is astonishing indeed that only one-fifth of the accidents are due to slips and falls, where in other countries these total one-third of all accidents at work.

As to the average duration of disability at work, in 1982 half of the cases lasted one to three weeks, a quarter was limited to one week, the other quarter had longer periods of disability. This is roughly the same as the Belgian total average of fourteen days of absence per accident at work.

Federal Republic of Germany

Data have been drawn from a booklet[4] which for many years has been published annually and which refers to about 90 per cent of the active professional population, i.e. about 20 million fully employed persons (here also there is a lapse of about two years between occurrence and publication).

It seems that the frequency (= number of accidents per 1000 exposed persons), after a drastic decrease between 1965 and 1975, remained stable till 1980 and from then on has decreased steadily. Probably this is attributed to the same causes as in The Netherlands, but also to the improved organization of safety and the improved training of safety personnel in these industries.

In 1981, the building industry remained in the lead, followed by mining and quarrying. Expenditure for prevention and compensation of accidents has steadily increased. Also here the highest frequency of accidents is in the age group up to 35: there is an even distribution from 35 to 50. The most frequent accidents are due to slips and falls and these represent about 17·5 per cent of all accidents. Approximately 12 per cent of accidents result from the use of tools and machines. Accidents in agriculture have not been included in the above mentioned figures.

Interesting details on the nature and cause of injuries can also be found in Dr Wolfgang Abt's *Unfall Analyse*.[5]

Lack of completeness of the German statistics is due to the fact that agricultural accidents are recorded in separate statistics and that accidents only have to be notified after a minimum of three days of absence from work.

An abstract on comparative statistics for 1980, published by the EEC, shows conspicuous inconsistencies. For instance, if we compare the figures for Belgium and The Netherlands, for Germany, France, and Great Britain (table published as annex in a proposal for resolution: EEC, second programme of action for safety and health at the working place) (Table 16.1).

Despite the relative value of these statistics for international comparison, we have reservations about their reliability. By examining the French published data for 1983,[6] we find the same accident figures as in columns 3 and 5, but for employees (column 1) the figure of 14 075 205 instead of 23 000 000. Therefore columns 4 and 6 in the EEC table have to be corrected to respectively 69 and 10.

Table 16.1 Comparative accident statistics in the EEC—1980

Country	IRL	L	B	NL	DK	I	GB	F	FRG	GR
1. Employees × 1000	224	130	2000	5300	1440	19 600	20 700	23 000	22 300	1310
2. Enterprises	20 000	10 000	150 000	500 000	139 000	2 000 000	1 200 000	1 800 000	1 800 000	207 000
3. Number of accidents at work 1980	4330	16 530	210 000	90 000	33 900	1 600 000	400 000	971 300	2 158 000	47 500
4. Frequency of accidents/ 1000 employees	19	127	105	17	23	82	19	42	98	36
5. Fatal accidents	30	17	250	80	75	2200	700	1423	3998	250
6. Frequency of fatal accidents 100 000 employees	13	13	13	2	5	11	3	6	18	19

France

From French publications[7] we learn that:

1. An accident at work is registered as such if it results in at least one day of absence, not including the day of the accident (the same as in Belgium).
2. From 1979 to 1983 the number of accidents has steadily decreased from 37·4 to 33·5 (expressed in number of accidents per million hours of work: i.e. the frequency rate).
3. Here again the most unfavourable results continue to come from the building sector (frequency-rate 73 to 76). Agriculture has not been mentioned separately in the French statistics.
4. The severity of accidents, expressed as the number of working days lost per 1000 hours of work, remains almost constant and fluctuates around 1 (in the building industry 2·5 to 2·8) for temporary disability, whereas for accidents causing permanent disability it has decreased from 38·2 to 34·6 (building sector: 100·5 to 103·8, thus showing an increase).

The duration per accident at work amounts to thirty days, notably higher than in other countries.

Italy

The following data for 1979 and 1980 have been derived from an Italian study.[8]

No. of employees	T_f time	T_f persons	Death	Total T_f
Agriculture:				
1979: 6 053 580	14.43	2.03	0.10	16.56
1980: 5 968 404	14.81	2.23	0.09	17.13
Industry:				
1979: 14 235 411	60.70	1.55	0.09	61.34
1980: 14 461 258	58.60	1.72	0.09	60.41
Total:				
1979: 10 288 991	75.13	3.58	0.19	78.90
1980: 20 429 662	73.41	3.95	0.18	77.54

Remarks:

T_f is the degree of frequency of accidents expressed in numbers per 1 000 000 hours of work; it is usually called frequency rate.

T_f time is the degree of frequency of accidents causing more than three days of work disability and/or a permanent disability of less than 11 per cent.

T_f persons is the same, but for accidents with more than 11 per cent of permanent disability.

T_f total is the total of the previous plus the degree of frequency of fatal accidents.

Except in agriculture, we notice a declining trend in industry in general as well as in the sector with the greatest risk, i.e. the building sector.

Yet there is an increase in the frequency of accidents with a high degree of permanent disability. Perhaps this is due to better reporting because of improved social compensation. Here again it is striking that these figures do not correspond with those mentioned in the EEC table for this country.

Metal industry (Figs 16.1 and 16.2, Table 16.2)

In the annual report of SIDMAR (a Belgian steel plant) there is a good graphical representation of accident statistics based on comparable steel-works in EEC countries. It would be interesting to produce similar graphs of accident figures comparing other industrial or commercial activities.

Conclusion

In each country, accidents are defined and registered differently. Complete-ness of statistics and good comparability between countries are thus imposs-ible.

On first analysis it would appear that big differences in degrees of safety exist among countries with a comparable pattern of work organization and industrial development. The figures are doubled in certain countries. Such differences emphasize how diverse the registration of accidents at work is and thus the figures obviously give a false picture.

In order to make comparisons possible, the authorities of the European Community are attempting to eliminate differences between the national statistics. This will be a difficult and almost impossible task. A member of the 'Bundesministerium für Arbeit und Sozial Ordnung' in Bonn has made a re-

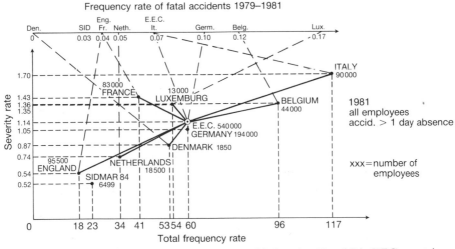

Fig. 16.1. Comparative accident figures in steel industries. F and S in EEC countries (excluding Ireland).

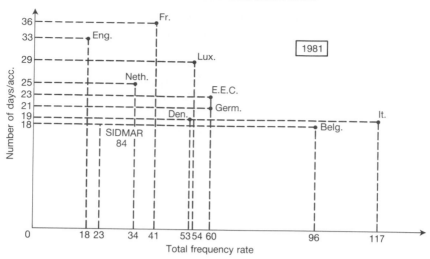

Fig. 16.2. Other data: relation F to number of days of absence at work per accident in EEC countries.

Table 16.2 Other comparative figures

Country or industry	Total No. employees	Frequency rate	Severity rate	No. of days/ accident
Sidmar 1984	6 499	23	0.42	18
Solmer 1981	6 200	23	1.10	48.7
Usinor 1981	± 30 000	27	1.21	45
IJmuiden 1981	± 18 500	34	0.86	25.3
Steel-industry Belgium 1983	± 41 500	84	1.37	16.4

markable analysis on the possible difficulties and has published a noteworthy contribution.[9]

National statistics indicate yearly trends in accidents at work according to frequency and severity. These trends can be compared among the different countries. In general the situation is evolving favourably. The severity is influenced on a national level by the ruling social legislation with regard to compensation for absence from work, the degree of care and rehabilitation of victims of accidents at work and the economic crisis weighing upon absence from work, making employees afraid to lose their jobs.

Frequency and severity are influenced by tighter selection of employees, by better working conditions and by quicker tracing and correction of disturbances in the process of production. On the other hand in large-scale industries having a high pace of production and using many new products and processes, severe accidents can occur especially when the health risks have not yet been recognized. The list of dangerous products used is growing steadily. Legally required notification gives only a limited and very incomplete picture of the circumstances and causes of accidents. There is a danger that on the basis of such imcomplete data wrong conclusions may be drawn that could lead to unnecessary statutory regulations. A positive sign is that as a result in some countries attention has been paid to better organization and supervision of safety in the work-place.

It is essential that in the future, using information from positive national experiments, the responsible authorities of the EEC partners should create a better co-ordinated international organization for safety at work, with a more homogenous and quicker statistical processing of accidents at work, defined in a standardized way. The delay by which statistics are still being published is not acceptable any more in view of the current possibilities for data processing.

Besides the European Communities, the International Labour Office (ILO) in Geneva also publishes relevant statistics annually. This office uses uniform definitions for reporting frequency and severity of accidents at work. However, a large number of countries only partly follow these definitions so that comparisons are difficult to make.

Bibliography

1. De Lange, H. and Schoenmaeckers, M. B., Statistieken van arbeidsongevallen en beroepsziekten. Promosafe 5, NVVA, Brussels, 453–67 (1985).
2. Stichting Consument en Veiligheid: cijfers ongevallen in Nederland. Veiligheidsheids instituut, Amsterdam (1984).
3. Prins, R. and Geurts, L., Statistics on accidents as instruments for research and management. *Safety* **59**(4), 183–8 (1983).
4. Arbeitsunfallstatistik für die Praxis. Hauptverband der gewerblichen Berufsgenossenschaften e.v., Bonn (1983).
5. Abt, W., Unfall Analyse. Schriftenreihe des Hauptverbandes der gewerblichen Berufsgenossenschaften e.v., Bonn (1980).
6. *Statistiques techniques d'accidents du travail, année 1983*, Caisse Nationale de l'Assurance Maladies des Travailleurs Salariés, Paris (1985).
7. *Statistiques nationales d'accidents du travail, années 1981, 1982, 1983*, Caisse Nationale de l'Assurance Maladies des Travailleurs Salariés, Paris (1985).
8. *Notaziario Statistico*, Istituto Nazionale per l'Assicurazione contro gli infortuni sul lavoro 1 (1982).
9. Mertens, A., Probleme mit der europäischen Unfallstatistik. *Die Berufsgenossenschaft* 434–8 (1984) and 124–7 (1985).

17

The Home Accident Surveillance System

GEOFFREY FRANCE AND MALCOLM BARROW

Introduction

In England and Wales some 5000 people die each year from accidents in the home, about 40 per cent of all fatal accidents; about 100 000 are admitted as in-patients; nearly 2 million receive out-patient treatment at hospitals; and a further 800 000 are treated by general practitioners. Home accidents involve numerous and wide-ranging causes and to identify these the Home Accident Surveillance System (HASS) was introduced towards the end of 1976. It provides a level of detail not previously available in the UK and is used in conjuction with other, existing, sources, for example statistics provided by the Office of Population Censuses and Surveys on fatal accidents (compiled from death certificates), general information from the Hospital In-patient Enquiry and Fire Brigade statistics.

Administration of HASS

The Home Accident Surveillance System is run by the Safety Research Section of the Consumer Safety Unit of the Department of Trade and Industry. It covers the mainland of Great Britain. The Safety Research Section has a complement of nine posts, including five specialist research scientists, two administrators, and two sandwich students. About half of the total effort of the Safety Research Section is devoted to the administration of HASS, whilst the remaining effort is deployed on other activities, principally related research and, more recently, the introduction of the European Home and Leisure Accident Surveillance Scheme (EHLASS) (see below).

A commercial market research agency (the British Market Research Bureau) is employed to recruit, train, and supervise the clerks who collect the data; to check report forms and monitor quality prior to the further quality controls operated by the Safety Research Section. The total cost of running HASS in 1985 was of the order of £300 000 which must be seen in the context of the £200 million medical costs of treating some 3 million home accident victims, the concomitant 20 million days of incapacity, the 2·5 million working days lost, and 5000 deaths.

Objectives of HASS

The objectives of the accident surveillance system are that it should

(a) provide reliable, comprehensive, and nationally representative information;
(b) enable accidents which are amenable to action to be identified and allocated priorities;
(c) monitor the accident problem so that new hazards may be identified and new trends in known hazards investigated;
(d) aid the evaluation of the effectiveness of preventive action; and
(e) provide a basis for estimating the costs of different types of accidents.

Both accident and home are clearly defined for the clerks completing the forms.

In order to find out exactly how the accidents have occurred, more detailed information than that provided by the surveillance system may be required. Because of the complex nature of accidents, involving the interaction of the person, the product, and the physical and social environment, this level of detail can often only be gained by a follow-up study, investigating the nature of the accident in depth. These studies may be done either by the staff of the Safety Research Section or contracted out to research agencies. Where it is warranted, this typically includes visits, telephone calls, or the use of postal questionnaires. However, it must be stressed that all information collected is strictly in confidence and neither the Consumer Safety Unit nor its appointed researchers can ascertain the identity of any patient other than by use of a bridging code which can only be linked to an individual by the participating hospital. No approach is made to an individual unless he or she has specifically agreed to this at the time of the first hospital visit; and then only with the further agreement of the hospital.

Hospital Participation

Information on home accidents is collected from 20 major Accident and Emergency (A & E) departments throughout England and Wales. The twenty hospitals are selected by a random sampling procedure. The sampling frame includes approximately 270 hospitals which fulfil the following criteria:

1. The hospital receives over 10 000 new A & E attendances each year, (figures obtained from the Department of Health and Social Security).
2. The hospital offers a 24-hour A & E service.
3. The hospital has a *major* A & E department, i.e. generally classified as one that receives ambulance cases.

The HASS uses a rolling sample. The sampling procedure is based on geographic location and size of hospital (as determined by the number of new A & E attendances each year). Each hospital remains in the system for four years and five hospitals are replaced each year.

Data

A standard form is used for data recording; it includes details of:

(a) date of treatment
(b) time of attendance
(c) where in house or garden the accident occurred
(d) the product(s) involved
(e) the accident—a brief description
(f) time of accident
(g) employment
(h) age and sex of patient
(i) injury type
(j) body part injured
(k) outcome of visit to A & E department; for example, sent home, admitted as in-patient

Home accident report forms are generally completed by a trained HASS clerk, but when not on duty other reception staff may initiate the forms or at least mark the casualty register; HASS clerks are also responsible for coding the forms. Computing is handled centrally on the Departments's ICL 2900 computer.

Use of HASS

Although a report is produced annually, there are several specific reports (such as BMX bikes, chain saws, and electric blankets) and reports on other topics (such as 'accidents to babies under 1 year old' and 'personal factors in domestic accidents'), the intent has always been that HASS should be an information system capable of interrogation. As such it is used extensively by the Department of Trade and Industry and other government departments, by local authorities and by organizations such as the British Standards Institution, The Royal Society for Prevention of Accidents and the Consumers' Association. The following examples illustrate the uses to which the system has been put.

1. *Legislation.* The Consumer Protection Act 1987 received Royal Assent on Friday 15 May 1987. A vital element of this new legislation is the 'General Safety Requirement' making it an offence to supply unsafe goods. This measure was proposed in the July 1984 'Safety of Goods' White Paper; and follows the enactment of some of this White Paper's proposals relating to increased powers for enforcing safety legislation in the Consumer Safety (Amendment) Act 1986 which entered into force on 8 August 1986. Extensive use of both the HASS and the associated follow-up research carried out by the Safety Research Section was made in drafting both the White Paper

and the associated legislation. In 1987 the Government will prescribe the use of Child Resistant Packaging for the most hazardous DIY, household, and gardening chemicals; and this action is also based on an evaluation of HASS data and detailed research based on HASS carried out within the Safety Research Section.

2. *Discussions with suppliers.* HASS data revealed some 2500–3000 accidents a year that involved tins and tin-openers; nationally this approximates to around 40 000 cases a year. Most of the injuries are, fortunately, not severe but they do, in total, impose a considerable burden on limited health service resources. Half of all these accidents involve corned beef tins and whilst the proportion of corned beef tins to others in use is not precisely known it has been estimated by the Canned Foods Advisory Service as approximately 0·1 per cent. On this basis if the tin being opened is of the corned beef type then the probability of an accident occurring is *1000 times higher* than if it is not. Discussions are currently being held with suppliers. An example of the HASS Print-out is shown in Fig. 17.1

3. *Medical research.* The Medical Commission on Accident Prevention is planning a study of spinal injuries and HASS data are being used to help quantify the problem. Detailed summaries have been provided with case-listings.

4. *Teaching.* A teaching pack prepared by the Safety Research Section in collaboration with school teachers, is now in use in many junior schools in the UK. It aims not at direct teaching of home safety, but at providing real data as a basis for teaching basic numeracy, assessment of information, and the use of micro-computers. The intent is that by incorporating such data into an existing curriculum, the children will gain awareness of the potential hazards to be found in the home.

The European Home and Leisure Accident Surveillance System (EHLASS)

The Commission of the European Communities has decided to introduce an accident surveillance system similar to HASS in all Member States of the European Economic Community. This system is known as EHLASS, and is similar to HASS but with the addition of information on leisure accidents. Eleven of the twelve member States are basing EHLASS on collection of accident data at hospitals in the same way as HASS in the UK. The Federal Republic of West Germany is basing its implementation of EHLASS on an existing system of collecting accident statistics from insurance companies whilst retaining the option of switching to a more compatible hospital based system at a later stage. The United Kingdom has introduced EHLASS at seven of its twenty HASS hospitals in England and Wales, with the intention

	24/09/84	17/09/84	19/09/84	2/07/84	22/04/84	20/04/84
DATE						
DAY	MONDAY	MONDAY	WEDNESDAY	MONDAY	SUNDAY	FRIDAY
TIME ATTENDED	1900 HRS	2300 HRS	0600 HRS	1900 HRS	1500 HRS	1200 HRS
CLERK PRESENT	NO - MEDICAL RECORDS	NO - RECEP INTERVIEWED	NO - MEDICAL RECORDS	YES - INTERVIEWED	YES - INTERVIEWED	YES - DID NOT INT'VIEW
AMBULANCE	AMBULANCE NOT USED	AMBULANCE NOT USED	AMBULANCE NOT USED	AMBULANCE NOT USED	AMBULANCE USED	AMBULANCE NOT USED
INFORMANT	PATIENT NT INFORMANT	PATIENT NT INFORMANT	PATIENT NT INFORMANT	PATIENT NT INFORMANT	PATIENT NT INFORMANT	PATIENT NT INFORMANT
BUILDING	UNKNOWN	UNKNOWN	UNKNOWN	HOUSE	HOUSE	FLAT
RESIDENCE	UNKNOWN	NORMAL RESIDENCE	UNKNOWN	NORMAL RESIDENCE	NORMAL RESIDENCE	NORMAL RESIDENCE
LOCATION	OTHER (UNSPECIFIED)	YARD/DRIVEWAY/PATH	OTHER(UNSPECIFIED)	KITCHEN	OTHER(SPECIFIED)	BEDROOM
ACTIVITY	OTHER(UNSPECIFIED)	CHILDREN PLAYING	OTHER(UNSPECIFIED)	CHILDREN PLAYING	CHILDREN PLAYING	RESTING OR SLEEPING
TIME OF ACCIDENT	UNKNOWN	EVENING	LATE EVENING	EVENING	AFTERNOON	MORNING
DAY OF ACCIDENT	1 DAY PRIOR	SAME DAY	1 DAY PRIOR	SAME DAY	SAME DAY	SAME DAY
ACCIDENT TYPE	FALL BETWEEN 2 LEVEL	FALL BETWEEN 2 LEVEL	FALL BETWEEN 2 LEVEL	FALL BETWEEN 2 LEVEL	FALL BETWEEN 2 LEVEL	FALL BETWEEN 2 LEVEL
FIRST ARTICLE	CHAIR (NOT FOLDING)	BICYCLE(CHILD)	BED	KITCHEN UNIT	CHILD (UND 16) NOT PT	BED
1ST FUEL SOURCE	NEVER POWERED	NEVER POWERED	NEVER POWERED	NEVER POWERED	NEVER POWERED	NEVER POWERED
FIRST FEATURE	NK	NK	NK	BREAKFST BAR	BROTHER	NK
SECOND ARTICLE	------	------	------	SOFA/COUCH/OTTOMAN	LAWN/GRASS AREA	FLOOR UNSPEC COVERNG
2ND FUEL SOURCE	------	------	------	NEVER POWERED	NEVER POWERED	NEVER POWERED
SECOND FEATURE	------	------	------	SETTEE	UNEVEN	BEDROOM
FOLLOW UP	UNKNOWN	FURTHER INTERVIEW	UNKNOWN	FURTHER INTERVIEW	FURTHER INTERVIEW	UNKNOWN
EMPLOYMENT	OTHER(UNSPECIFIED)	PATIENT UNDER 16 YRS	PATIENT UNDER 16 YRS	PATIENT UNDER 16 YRS	PATIENT UNDER 16 YRS	NOT EMPLOYED
AGE	20 YRS	4 YRS	4 YRS	3 YRS	11 YRS	85 YRS
SEX	MALE	MALE	MALE	FEMALE	FEMALE	FEMALE
1ST INJURY	SPRAIN/STRAIN	BRUISES/CONTUSIONS	TENDERNESS/SWELLING	BRUISES/CONTUSIONS	TENDERNESS/SWELLING	TENDERNESS/SWELLING
1ST INJURED PART	TRUNK - LOWER PART	TRUNK - LOWER PART	TRUNK - LOWER PART	TRUNK - LOWER PART	HIP	TRUNK - LOWER PART
2ND INJURY	------	------	------	TENDERNESS/SWELLING	TENDERNESS/SWELLING	------
2ND INJURED PART	------	------	------	TRUNK - LOWER PART	TRUNK - LOWER PART	------
DISPOSAL	G.P./OUT-PATIENT	HOME	HOME	HOME	IN-PATIENT	HOME
INPATIENT	------	------	------	------	2 DAYS(S)	------
SEC DISPOSAL	------	------	------	------	G.P./OUT-PATIENT	------
ACCIDENT DESCRIPTION	FELL BACKWARDS OFF A CHAIR YESTERDAY	FELL OFF BICYCLE-BRUISED LOWER BACK	FELL FROM BED-HURT LOWER BACK	CHILD CLIMBED ONTO BREAKFAST BAR FELL ONTO SETTEE THEN ONTO FLOOR INJURING BACK	PUSHED BY BROTHER OF FOUTHOUSE ROOF FELL 20 FEET TO BUMPY GRASS - HURT BACK	FELL OUT OF BED SAME MORNING-NOW HAS CONSTANT PAIN IN LOWER SPINE - CAN WALK

" 1 " INDICATES A CHANGE IN SORT-KEY 1 : ACCIDENT TYPE

Fig. 17.1. Example of HASS print-out for back injuries.

206

that eventually there will be eleven EHLASS hospitals in the UK. It is anticipated that hospitals in Northern Ireland and Scotland will be brought into
both HASS and EHLASS in due course. By late 1986, data collection for
EHLASS was under way at hospitals in all the eleven participating Member
States. Following the lead set by the UK ten years ago, the Commision of the
European Communities intends to supplement EHLASS with more detailed
follow-up research into specific hazards.

18

Surveillance for road accidents

Y. TOUNTAS AND D. TRICHOPOULOS

Introduction

In the course of human history, the fatalistic acceptance of disease and death has often been one of man's dominant beliefs. In some areas, even in developed countries traces of these old beliefs survive. Accidents are among them. The average person considers an accident as something due to change over which the individual has little, if any, control. Besides, accident is defined in many dictionaries as something that happens unexpectedly and by chance, usually something unpleasant.

In the sphere of health, the term accident has been used to denote unexpected physical and chemical injuries to the body. Today it is recognized that from the scientific point of view this definition is not applicable in a variety of cases. It is, therefore, gradually being replaced by descriptions of the injuries themselves and the physical and chemical agents or conditions which are responsible for their occurrence.

As far as the use of the term 'injury' is concerned, it must be noted that there is no fundamental scientific difference between injury and disease. In some cases the aetiological agents are identical and in others there is no biological distinction between injury and disease.

Road accidents, fatal and non-fatal, constitute a major part of all accidents. The daily life and economic growth of every country depend on certain factors, among which transportation is one of the most important. However, the development of transportation has also caused a series of undesirable side-effects. Some of these, such as pollution, noise, and traffic congestion, are immediately noticeable. Others, such as road accidents and their effects on human health and life, may be demonstrated only through aggregated statistics and epidemiological studies.

In many developed countries, road accidents today remain one of the main causes of morbidity and mortality despite the fact that both the general public and the authorities have become more sensitive to the issue. The size of the problem has made the reduction of road accidents and the control of the consequences an urgent priority. However, the multiplicity of factors responsible poses a variety of obstacles. It is therefore important to view the question of road safety from many angles and to look at all the determinants of the road accident, be they related to a road network, the vehicle or to human factors.

The effectiveness of such an approach depends to a great extent on the proper surveillance of road accidents. The continuous and systematic collection of data, the formulation and use of suitable indicators, and the substantial and in-depth analysis of the different determinants, are the essential steps for a study of the aetiological factors in road accidents and for the implementation of a comprehensive road safety policy.

In order to satisfy these needs, epidemiologists must become much more involved in the surveillance and control of road accidents. Without their active participation, neither data collection and analysis nor policy design, implementation, and evaluation can be satisfactorily achieved.

Data Collection

In most countries, responsibility for the collection of data and information relating to road accidents is in the hands of the public transport services. The police usually submit summary reports which make up basic material for annual statistics. The findings of a study carried out by the WHO show that public health services play a limited role in the collection and utilization of health-related data on road accidents.[1]

The main drawback of this methodology is that is does not generate sufficient material for the study of the effects of road accidents on human health and life. Since most road casualties are not hospitalized, the only available sources of information are police and insurance company records, but neither of these sources deals directly with health-related data. On the other hand, even hospital statistics make an inadequate contribution. The morbidity rates that are usually based on these statistics do not allow for evaluation of changes in the incidence and severity of the various forms of injuries.

Another set of problems concerning the collection and utilization of data relates to the lack of commonly accepted definitions. This is most apparent in the case of death as a result of a road accident and in the assessment of the severity of the injury. The United Nations has suggested that among deaths due to road accidents be included only those persons who are killed immediately or die within thirty days. With regard to injuries the definition for 'severe injury', put forward by the Economic Commission for Europe of the UN, does not provide adequate clinical criteria for the designation of severity.[2] WHO recommends that a new definition of 'severe injury' should be adopted, based on the duration of hospitalization and the expected degree of disability.[1]

For most of the other terms related to road accidents, the International Classification of Diseases provides a single frame of reference which satisfactorily covers a large part of the problem. In this WHO publication definitions are included for all kinds of vehicles, road users and conditions of accident.[3]

Because of the inherent problems in data collection, various measures should be taken in each country depending on the local conditions. Health-related data should be integrated into police reporting, which should indicate the exact site and nature of the injury. Commonly accepted definitions of all related terms should be used at national and international level. Recorded data should include the physical circumstances of the accident, the features of the vehicles involved and their movements, the characteristics (age, sex, etc.) of the road users, the nature and severity of the injuries, and related health data with a bearing on the aetiology of the accident. These data and eventual findings should be properly treated in order to become comprehensible and readily available to the general public and to all interested workers. The data should be presented in such a way as to facilitate assessment of the costs of accidents and of the benefits to be expected from their reduction, allowing an overall evaluation of the cost-effectiveness and cost-benefit of road safety measures. All approaches should be conceptually and methodologically multifactorial, taking into account such factors as the rate of change in the number of vehicles per inhabitant, the number of dead and injured per inhabitant or per vehicle, the size, the composition and the density of the population, the number and type of vehicles, the severity indicators of the accidents, etc. Futhermore, the evaluation of the problem should not be static; it should also include the monitoring of changes in time and the study of norms and deviations.

The successful implementation of these proposals requires a limit to the number of authorities involved, so as to avoid extreme division and overlapping of responsibilities. Preferably, one authority should have the main responsibility and the power required to execute a central policy. The role of the health services should not be restricted to the medical care of road casualties, but should cover other sectors as well, including the epidemiological investigation of accidents and the drafting of administrative and legislative regulations and standards. For example, epidemiological analysis would allow the comparison of the marginal effectiveness of speed limit imposition at various levels taking into account the road network function and overall productivity parameters.

Health Indicators

The effects of road accidents are felt throughout a broad spectrum of human activities. Road accidents reduce production forces, increase medical care expenditures and impede transportation. They also often cause problems that arise from the conflicting interests of insurance companies, from the associated legal problems and from the increased workload they impose on the courts. Nonetheless, injury, disability, and death are the most dramatic consequences of road accidents. For this reason the study of health indicators such as the resulting numbers, proportions, and rates of deaths, the loss of expected life and the numbers, proportions, and rates of persons injured are of particular importance for the surveillance of road accidents. Among the possible denominators a trade-off must be made between desirability and feasibility. Passenger-kilometres is attractive and widely used in other situations (i.e. air traffic accidents) but it is difficult to calculate and takes no account of the lack of independence of numerator events and network and driving conditions; time-weighted denominators are both difficult to conceptualize and estimate but are particularly useful for risk equivalence exercises. Traditional population based denominators have several shortcomings but they can be readily calculated and generate figures comparable to those referring to other causes of morbidity and mortality. Of the above indicators the mortality rate is considered to be the most valid, since the comprehensiveness of the statistical recording of accidents and injuries varies according to time and place and is significantly affected by the criteria used for classification.

Mortality

Fatal accidents today constitute one of the main causes of death in developed countries. In the EEC, more than 50 000 people are killed annually in road accidents. Cardiovascular disease and cancer may be ahead on the list as causes of death, but as far as the loss of expected life is concerned, road accidents take precedence over the other main killers, since they are the main cause of death in men 15–24 years of age. In women road accidents are less important as a cause of death at a ratio of about 2:5 for each age group.

Deaths from road accidents do not include only drivers or passengers of transport vehicles. Pedestrians, of whom the very young and the very old form a considerably exposed group, are particularly vulnerable. It has been found that deaths among pedestrians correspond to two-fifths of total road accident deaths.[4] The number of deaths among pedestrians depends more on the size and density of the population than on the degree of motorization. Indeed, fatality as against the risk of injury is greater for pedestrians than it is for the remainder of road users.[2] This risk is particularly great among children, who are slow in adjusting to the changing traffic environment.[5]

The probability of death from road accident is ten times greater for motor cyclists than it is for users of other motor vehicles.[6] In England and Wales the number of deaths in this category corresponds to one-eighth of total road accident deaths, with the 15–19 age-group being particularly affected. Motor cycle casualties increase every year at a rate greater than the general increase of traffic and other indicators. In the same areas, deaths among pedal cyclists correpond to one-twentieth of total road accident deaths.[7] The same trends have been noticed in the Federal Republic of Germany, where deaths among motor cyclists amount to 1500 annually, serious injuries to 14 000 and minor injuries to 23 000.[8]

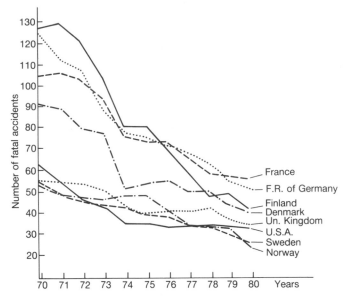

Fig. 18.1. Fatal road accidents per 100 000 vehicles, from 1970 to 1980, in developed countries. (Source: United Nations, Commission Economique pour l'Europe (1983): Aspects Techniques et Economiques de la Division Internationale du Travail dans l'Industrie Automobile.)

The majority of road accident deaths are due to head injuries and multiple fractures. Contrary to what people believe, a minority of fatal accidents occur on motorways or expressways. Most of them happen in built-up areas and on surrounding minor roads.

Mortality from road accidents is associated with the number of vehicles per inhabitant but is also affected by many other factors. Indeed, in many developed countries there has recently been a reduction in the number of deaths per 100 000 vehicles (Fig. 18.1). A similar association applies to the severity indicator, which expresses the proportion of fatal casualties and which is calculated by dividing the number of deaths by total casualties. The severity indicator decreases with the improvment of medical care and increases with an increase in the proportion of motor cyclists and pedal cyclists.[9]

In most EEC countries (Table 18.1), there has been a reduction not only in deaths per vehicle but also in absolute figures. The actual reduction is even more important if the unfavourable secular trends in many of the population determinants of road accident mortality (number of cars, proportion of new drivers, etc.) are taken into account.[10] The Federal Republic of Germany, The Netherlands and Denmark show the greatest reduction. The other countries show a smaller reduction, with the exception of Spain, Greece, and Ireland which have shown an increase. For 1980, Belgium and France show

Table 18.1 Age-adjusted mortality rates from road accidents in 1970 and 1980 in 10 EEC countries

Countries	Mortality rates (per 100 000)		
	1970	1980	Percent change
Belgium	27.2	24.8	− 9
Denmark	24.8	13.3	− 46
France	23.5	20.5	− 13
F.R. Germany	31.3	18.2	− 42
Greece	11.6	15.2	+ 31
Ireland	16.3	18.9	+ 16
Italy	24.3	18.3	− 25
Spain	13.0	17.7	+ 36
The Netherlands	24.4	12.2	− 50
United Kingdom	14.2	11.7	− 18

Sources: WHO (1976): *The Epidemiology of Road Traffic Accidents.*[1]
WHO (1983): *World Health Statistics. Annual*, Vol. 1.[10]

the highest mortality rate, which exceeds 20 deaths per 100 000 inhabitants, whereas the lowest rates, not exceeding 15 deaths per 100 000 inhabitants, are shown by the United Kingdom, The Netherlands and Denmark. Not included in Table 18.1 are Luxembourg and Portugal, for which recent statistical data are not yet available.

Morbidity

The number of non-fatal road accidents and their effects on human health are difficult to estimate. Many non-fatal accidents are not recorded by the authorities, while for others there is inadequate reporting. Moreover, not only does the reporting underestimate the true facts, it also frequently contains misleading inaccuracies. These problems are more marked in the less protected categories of road-users, mainly among pedestrians and pedal cyclists who run the greatest risk.

In the USA it has been estimated that there are about 50 to 100 injuries for each fatality. In the EEC countries more than 1.5 million people are injured in road accidents every year. Many European countries use up to 10 per cent of hospital beds for the hospitalization of these cases. The resulting economic burden of hospitalization exceeds 0.5 per cent of GNP.[11]

The number of road accident casualties is related to the number of vehicles and to the population. For the measurement of the relationship various formulas have been proposed. The number of casualties may be predicted by the following formula:

$$0.003 \, (NP^2)^{1/3}$$

where N stands for the number of vehicles and P for population.[12]

Mortality from motor-vehicle accidents may be also estimated by multiple regression equations taking into account vehicles per inhabitant, length of road network, population in large towns, young population, old population, and private cars and taxis.[13]

One important indicator over a prolonged period of time is the change in the morbidity rate per vehicle; the general trend is towards a gradual decrease.[14]

Another important observation concerning industrialized countries is that a positive correlation exists between accident risk level (and injury severity) and the engine capacity of motorcycles, for riders in this category.[15]

Surveillance of Determinants

The main determinants of road accidents can be classified into three categories: the physical environment (i.e. the road network), the vehicle, and the human factors. The surveillance of these determinants is a fundamental aspect of every policy aiming at the prevention and control of road accidents. Despite the fact that the aetiological importance of each determinant varies from accident to accident, the interaction among them is always important in shaping the final result. Therefore, in addition to the surveillance of the different determinants, the surveillance of their mode of interaction and of the resulting effects are of great importance for the promotion of road safety.

Physical environment

The characteristics of the physical environment (road network) contribute to accidents in many ways. The physical conditions of the road, including structural features, curvatures, width, unidirectional or omnidirectional traffic, intersections, resistance to braking, road maintenance, weather conditions, and physical obstacles may contribute, sometimes decisively, to the causation of an accident and to its final outcome.[16] Information factors including visibility, road signs, and timely communication, play an especially important part. Another important factor stems from the degree of segregation of certain classes of road users, particularly pedestrians and pedal cyclists. Part of the physical environment which can also be considered in an indirect way is the driver's compliance with traffic regulations.

For the surveillance of these factors which collectively determine road network safety, several techniques are currently in use in EEC countries, while others are at an experimental stage. A fully automated incident detection system has been tried in the UK, with microprocessors constantly examining the output from a series of detectors, whereas a specially developed algorithm is used to detect the disturbances to traffic flow that invariably follow an incident.[17] In The Netherlands, data on density and speed of traffic are sent to a central computer which in turn supplies the peripherals with the appropriate signals after calculating the correct sequence. This system has been able to reduce by half the number of secondary accidents which form up to 50 per cent of those occurring on some motorways.[18] Control of vehicle speed has proved very important. In the USA, occupant deaths dropped from about 43 000 in 1973 to 36 000 in 1974 after enactment of the national 55 m.p.h. speed limit.[19] Recording and analysing traffic behaviour in detail by using video-systems may give a good deal of information about the functioning of several road design elements, and may help the study of the behaviour of road users.[20] Roadside telephones, detectors, television surveillance, and vehicle recovery facilities have been found to reduce road network problems whilst increased lane widths, marginal strips, and hard shoulders may improve road safety. Systems for surveillance against icy road conditions use road surface sensors covering air temperature, humidity, and precipitation, plus wind speed and direction sensors where necessary.[21]

Vehicle

The proper design and construction of a vehicle, especially of a motor vehicle, contribute to the reduction of road accidents and to the alleviation of the severity of injuries. In the United Kingdom and in France it was reported that 8 per cent and 7 per cent respectively of road accidents had as primary cause mechanical or technical failures and faults in the vehicle.[22]

The main factors that determine the safety of a vehicle concern: the maintenance of the steering system, the condition of the tyres, the lighting, the fitting of safety belts, overall visibility, cruising properties, and interior design. In the USA, it has been estimated that nine out of ten of road injuries in urban areas and three out of nine in rural areas occur at an impact speed of under 40 m.p.h. At such speeds the protection afforded by the safe design and construction of a vehicle is very important, and may ensure a substantial reduction in deaths and injuries.

Part of a safe design is the provision of occupant restraint systems. These systems have been associated with reductions in crash injuries.[23] Ideally, proper design should automatically protect the occupant of a vehicle. That is why preference should be given to 'passive' measures such as airbags and automatic seat-belts which do not require individual co-operation in order to be effective.[24]

In practice, although automatic protection is improving, occupants must still manually co-operate by using seat-belts. Lap belts reduce the chance of death or serious injury to front seat occupants by about 30 to 60 per cent.[25]

Australian legislation requiring the use of restraints in cars resulted in an increase in use to as much as 75 per cent in commuter traffic. A 25 per cent decrease in deaths was reported in New South Wales and a 21 per cent decrease in urban areas of Victoria.[25]

For all these reasons, the surveillance of a motor vehicle, whether this concerns the standards of construction or adherence to the standards of use and maintenance, is a crucial issue for road safety promotion. Police authorities may contribute substantially to the surveillance of motor vehicles, as well as to the surveillance of the road network and some of the human factors. It has been observed that increased police surveillance frequently results in the reduction of accidents. Police traffic surveillance in the Federal Republic of Germany includes measurement of distances between vehicles, noise measurement, emission measurement, testing of headlamps, measurement of axle loads, and the carrying out of breath tests.[26]

Human factors

Human behaviour is the major cause of most road accidents. It contributes to 95 per cent of injury-producing accidents and is solely responsible for almost two-thirds of accidents.[15]

The surveillance of driver behaviour allows the evaluation of certain factors, such as individual responses to a variety of situations and events, changes in these responses, their deeper causes, etc. Within the context of this effort it has been observed that, except for children and the aged, the main failure is not in sensory or motor ability but in the acceptance of too narrow safety margins. This faulty threshold for subjective risk leads to acceptance of hazards, some of which, as a statistical consquence will produce accidents.

The surveillance of road behaviour takes on a greater importance in certain categories of road users. It has been suggested that some people are more prone to accidents than others. Special psychological tests have supported the existence of personality traits that correlate with accident proneness. However, the concept of accident proneness, because of a number of methodological difficulties, has not yet proved useful as a basis upon which susceptible individuals may be recognized in advance of their accidents.

Another high risk category are said to be people who suffer from disease such as diabetes, epilepsy, cardiovascular diseases, and psychiatric disorders. The incidence of road accidents is twice as great among drivers suffering from the above diseases.[27] In the Federal Republic of Germany it has been estimated that of the various pathological conditions of drivers who had been involved in road accidents, 25 per cent concerned cardiovascular diseases, 25 per cent sensory disorders, 25 per cent metabolic disease, 15 per cent neurological disorders and the remaining 10 per cent various other diseases.[28] There is, however, no consensus about the overall contribution of medical disabilities to road accidents.[29] The issue should be further explored and a case-control study should be conducted in order to estimate how much these diseases contribute to road accidents. Moreover, scientifically based screening tests with adequate specificity and sensitivity are not available. Except for very high risk groups, it has been argued that the medical resources needed for screening and special surveillance could be more usefully deployed elsewhere.[19,30]

The necessity of surveillance, on the other hand, is not questioned in the case of drivers who are under the influence of alcohol. One-half of all motor accidents fatal to the occupants, more than one-fifth of accidents in which occupants experience serious injury, and one-third or more of the accidents that are fatal to adult pedestrians are related to the prior consumption of alcoholic beverages.[31] In most countries legislation provides regulations for the control of the problem which emerges when blood ethanol concentration exceeds 50 mg/100 ml. Risks increase considerably when concentrations exceed 80 mg/100 ml and concentrations of 100 mg/100 ml or higher are presumptive evidence of intoxication.[32]

The consumption of drugs, mainly psychotropic ones, may also impair driving ability, particularly when the drugs are taken in combination with alcohol. Psychotropic drugs in this category include hypnotics, analgesics, antidepressants, anorexiants, and anxiolytics. Stimulants also, usually consumed by professional long-distance drivers, are included in the above category. Cough sedatives, muscle relaxants, antispasmodics, antihypertensives, and antidiabetic drugs may also impair driving ability.[32]

Although the human factors and conditions described above are undoubtedly responsible for a considerable number of road accidents, they do not seem to affect to any great extent the creation of international variations in the level of mortality from motor vehicle accidents. In a study of factors related to mortality from motor vehicle accidents in European countries, a relatively high figure (0·8) was estimated for the multiple correlation coefficient of mortality with demographic and transport factors. This finding indicates that the unknown factors, and those which were not measured (behaviour of drivers, psychosocial conditions, etc.) are not as significant as is sometimes assumed in predicting trends and deviations across different countries.[13]

Comment

As a closing remark, it is important to stress that the collection and analysis of data, the surveillance of health indicators, and the surveillance of the determinants of road accidents should not be confined within the frontiers of each country. The increasing development of international highway networks and the growth in the volume of inter-country traffic render necessary the tackling of road accidents at international level and the drafting of a common policy framework. This need is particularly evident among neighbouring countries that have developed important trade and other bonds, such as the countries of the European Economic Community.

Bibliography

1. WHO, *The epidemiology of road traffic accidents.* Report on the Vienna conference of 1975. WHO, Regional Office for Europe, Copenhagen (1976).
2. United Nations, Economic Commission for Europe, *Statistics for road traffic accidents in Europe, 1973. Annex 1: Definitions and general notes,* UN–ECE, New York (1974).
3. WHO, *Manual of the international statistical classification of diseases, injuries and causes of death,* 2nd edn. WHO, Geneva (1977a).
4. United Nations. *Statistics of road traffic accidents in Europe, 1975,* Geneva (1976)
5. WHO, *The prevention and control of road traffic accidents.* Report on the Third European Liaison Meeting, Copenhagen 8–10 December 1976. WHO, Regional Office for Europe, Copenhagen (1977b).
6. Andrew, T. A, A six month review of motorcycle accidents. *Injury* **10,** 317 (1979).
7. Department of Transport, *Roads to safety.* Department of Transport, London (1978).
8. Federal Minister of Transport, *Limits of use of cycle tracks on two-laned roads outside urban areas.* Federal Minister of Transport, Bonn (1979).
9. Transport and Road Research Laboratory, Report LR 546. Transport and Road Research Laboratory, London (1973).
10. WHO, *World health statistics.* Annual, vol. 1, WHO, Geneva (1983).
11. Henneberg, G, *Communication to a medical workshop on road traffic accidents.* Commission of the European Communities, Brussels (1978).
12. Smeed, R. J, The usefulness of formulae in traffic engineering and road safety. *Accid. Anal. Prevent.* **4,** 303 (1972).
13. Trichopoulos, D., Tsachageas, A., Papadakis, J. Kalapothaki, V. and Koutselinis, A, Factors related to mortality from motor vehicle accidents in European countries in 1970. *Accid. Anal. Prevent.* **7,** 9 (1975).
14. Council of Scientific Affairs, Automobile related injuries: components, trends, prevention. *J. Am. Med. Ass.* **249,** 3216 (1983).
15. WHO, *Road traffic accidents in developing countries.* Report of a WHO meeting. Tech. Rep. Ser. 703, WHO, Geneva (1984).
16. Doege, T. C. and Levy, P. S, Injuries, crashes and construction on a superhighway. *Am. J. publ. Hlth* **67,** 147 (1977).
17. Anonymous, Incident detection prevents multiple motorway pile-ups. *Surveyor* **163,** 8 (1984).
18. Greeman, A, Motorway control turns to computer. *New Civ. Eng.* **624,** 20 (1985).
19. Haddon, W. and Baker, S. P., Injury control. In *Preventive and community medicine,* 2nd edn (eds D. W. Clark and B. MacMahon) Little Brown, Boston (1981).
20. Van der Horst, A. R. A, *The analysis of traffic behaviour by video.* Proceedings of the Third International Workshop on Traffic Conflicts Techniques. Institute for Road Safety Research. Leidschendam, The Netherlands (1982).
21. Edwards, B. D, Ice detection system for roads could save money and lives. *Munic. J.* **92,** 1626 (1984).

22. Sicard, A, Accidents de la route. *Bull. Acad. Nat. Méd.* **166,** 841 (1982b).
23. Robertson, L. S, State and federal new-car safety regulations: Effects on fatality rates. *Accid. Anal. Prevent.* **9,** 151 (1977).
24. Haddon, W. Jr, Strategy in preventive medicine: Passive versus active approaches to reducing human wastage. *J. Trauma* **14,** 353 (1974).
25. Robertson, L. S, Estimates of motor vehicle seat belt effectiveness and use: Implications for occupant crash protection. *Am. J. publ. Hlth* **66,** 859 (1976).
26. Anonymous, The role of the police: Its coordinating and educational activities. In *Penal and penitentiary aspects of road traffic.* L. Wyckmans, Brussels (1977).
27. Waller, J. A, Chronic medical conditions and traffic safety: A review of California experience. *New Engl. J. Med.* **273,** 1413 (1965).
28. Sicard, A, Endémiologie des accidents de la route. *Bull. Acad. Nat. Med.* **166,** 727 (1982a).
29. Baker, S. P. and Spitz, W. U. Age effects and autopsy evidence of disease in fatally injured drivers *J. Am. med. Ass.* **214,** 1079 (1970).
30. West, I, The impaired driver: a critical review of the facts. *Calif. Med.* **98,** 271 (1963).
31. Jones, R. K. and Joscelyn, K. B, *Alcohol and highway safety: A review of the state of knowledge.* Report UM-HSRI-78-5. University of Michigan Highway Safety Research Institute. Ann Arbor, Mich. (1978).
32. WHO, *The influence of alcohol and drugs on driving.* Report on a WHO *ad hoc* technical group. Euro Rep. 38, WHO, Copenhagen (1981).

19

Surveillance of physical and chemical hazards in the environment

L. MASSE

Introduction

Hippocrates when writing on disease occurrence made a distinction between the steady state, the endemic state, and the abrupt change in incidence, the epidemics. Regarding the environment he made a distinction between the basic permanent state or *catastasis* and the sudden change in environmental conditions, the popular Greek concept of *catastrophe*.

Surveillance of physical or chemical components of either 'catastasis' or 'catastrophe', can be done at various levels:

(a) source surveillance;
(b) environmental and exposure surveillance;
(c) health effects surveillance (biological surveillance).

Sometimes environmental and exposure surveillance are considered together for practical purposes.

Source surveillance

The best historical example of surveillance of source is the 1952 London smog episode which led to systematic surveys of both industrial and domestic sources of air pollution and resulted in such effective control measures that the traditional London smog has disappeared and mortality rates for respiratory diseases decreased.[1,2] Similar studies were performed with good results in the water pollution problem of Lake Annecy in France.

Environmental and exposure surveillance

The main agents considered for surveillance of the environment or of exposure can be physical or chemical agents or complex environmental entities. A list of the main agents is given in Reference 3.

Physical agents The main physical components of the environment which are recognized to have some bearing on health can be classified as follows:

(a) *General*: physical trauma, pressure, humidity, temperature;
(b) *Vibrations*: subsonic vibrations, noise, ultrasound;

(c) *Electro-magnetic radiations*: infra-red radiation, optical radiation and lasers, ultraviolet radiation, magnetic fields, radiofrequencies, microwaves;
(d) *Ionizing radiations*.

This list is not exhaustive but covers the most important physical agents that have an impact on human health.

Chemical agents   It is not possible to list all the chemical agents that show some evidence of adverse effect on the experimental animal or in man and thus deserve some form of surveillance. Two international periodicals systematically review these chemicals (see below 'Surveillance at international level'). In Chapter 13, on cancer, some other examples are quoted.

Complex environmental entities   These can be roughly classified under the following headings:

(a) *Land*: geology, soils, solid waste disposal;
(b) *Fluids and gases*: the weather, air, outdoor and indoor environmental hazards, fumes and other emanations of toxic substances, potable and non-potable water supplies (surface water, ground water, recreation water: surface or coastal), sewage disposal, and other effluents;
(c) *Man-made environmental entities*: clothing, housing, public buildings, urbanism

Fumes, emanation of toxic substances, sewage disposal, effluents, and solid waste disposal are entities covered by a 'source monitoring' type of surveillance.

Air and water supply require the more complex type of surveillance described below.

Methods for Environmental Surveillance

For chemical agents there are several methods of surveillance which will be briefly reviewed. This includes rapid assessment, routine surveillance, automatic surveillance, *ad hoc* surveillance, sentinel surveillance, and historical monitoring.

Rapid environmental assessment can be used in two different circumstances, in a developing area and in an emergency situation.[4]

In developing areas rapid assessment methods have essentially been initiated during the last ten years to cope with the environmental problems of rapidly industrialising urban areas. They cover, on the one side, monitoring of industrial activities (such as air emissions from stationary combustion sources and from mobile combustion engine sources, solid waste disposal, effluents), and on the other side, domestic sources (air pollution, solid waste disposal, and effluents). The total burden to the environment can then be estimated.

Although in most industrialized countries sophisticated plans exist in order to cope with most of the problems, in emergency situations it appears that the principles of rapid assessment are complementary to these plans. Four aspects are looked after: source release, environmental impact, population exposures, and possible immediate health effects.

Routine environmental surveillance is the most frequent type of environmental surveillance. Routine 'source monitoring' is aimed at evaluation and controlling solid waste disposal, effluents, fumes, and emanation of toxic substances.[5]

Routine 'environmental monitoring' aims at air and water quality control. For air, the main targets are the urban areas in the vicinity of industrial locations. When sampling air the following elements play a role: the density of human settlement, the emission cycle both for fixed and mobile sources, the dominant winds, and other specific meteorological features.

The main variables to be sampled (and suggested frequencies) are sediments (monthly), dust, sulphuric acid, oxidants, nitrogen dioxide (all daily), gravimetry (three times a day), fumes (hourly) and as a continuous process, methane, nitrogen monoxide, carbon monoxide. Other gases, like ozone and sulphur dioxide, may be surveilled continuously or daily.

For water supply two different systems have to be developed, one for river basins and another for water supply networks. For river basins the sampling system should be decided upon according to sources of industrial and domestic pollution, frequency of peaks, needs for surface water, resources available in personnel, equipment, finances, and the capability of the surveillance unit to analyse and make use of the data collected.

Regarding the water supply network, sampling should be based on a complete chemical examination when a new supply comes into service, when a new catchment area is used or when a major change occurs in the water supply. On the other hand routine sampling for chemical components is usually needed less frequently than for microbiological components.

Two types of chemical components should be considered:

1. *Type I chemicals* (arsenic, chloride, cyanide, fluoride, pesticides, selenium, sodium, sulphate, total dissolved solids and hardness) are unlikely to vary in the water distribution network and are in fact dependent upon the source of water so that only at the water supply plant is sampling needed.
2. *Type II chemicals* undergo some change in the water distribution network and include aluminium, benzene, chlorinated alkalenes, benzenes and phenols, iron, manganese, benzopyrene, cadmium, chromium, copper, lead, and zinc.

These Type II chemicals should be checked on samples collected from the consumer's tap although the collecting method differs with the chemical considered.

Automatic surveillance is an advanced routine surveillance process used for continuous assessment of the environment and for systematic feedback.[5]

One of the first automatic monitoring systems for surface water was the Ohio river basin surveillance programme, organized in the early 1960s in Cincinnatti.

In 1962, a continuous air monitoring programme (CAMP) was instituted in six major cities in the US.

The first example of a completely automatic air pollution surveillance system was the Rotterdam area system, in operation over the last twenty years: as soon as the level of sulphur dioxide and other related variables reach a given level, an alarm is triggered and some of the industrial activities stopped. There are several 'degrees of alarm' and a number of legal requirements for stopping activities.

Similar systems for air pollution have been developed for other industrialized areas; for example, in the western part of Germany and the northeastern part of France, and in some cities in Scandinavia, the Mediterranean countries, and Japan.

The most comprehensive automatic air quality monitoring system at a national level, which covers not only urban areas but rural areas also, operates in The Netherlands. One hundred monitoring stations are located in a grid pattern and a hundred others in the main urban areas. This system allows an immediate appraisal of the origin of the pollutants, and compliance with air quality standards. It also allows the effects of air pollution on man and the effectiveness of control measures to be assessed.

This system requires fully automatic monitoring with automatic data transmission and management of the network by regional centres and a national control centre that coordinates actions to be taken.

Some environmental problems are not fully covered by the routine surveillance system and require *ad hoc* studies.[6] Many such studies have been undertaken in areas with high lead exposure. Some of these studies cover the whole environmental field (soil, grass, vegetables, air, sediments, and fall out) and several biological markers (blood and teeth) and consider the various aspects of an environmental control programme.

The classic example of an *environmental sentinel* is the miner's canary which has been used from the eighteenth century until comparatively recently as an alarm system to warn the miner of the accidental spread of odourless natural gas (methane) in the mine. Nowadays garden vegetables such as spinach are used as sentinels. The observation of pets allows the assessment of exposure to pollutants and also gives some idea of the biological response. As was shown in the case of the occurrence of bladder cancer among dogs in highly industrialized areas of the US, a biological response was noted before evidence in man became apparent.[7,8] Another example was the systematic use of military dogs in the US armed forces. In this example post-mortem necropsy findings served as a sentinel surveillance system for the human population living near army air fields where these dogs were employed. This system was essentially for surveillance of the use of pesticides in rural areas.

Historical surveillance is the use of available environmental material to make assumptions on past environmental situations and compare them with the present status. The most common elements studied are: sediments, ice and snow, peat, tree rings, paper, soil, museum specimens, guano, and human remains such as hair, teeth, bones, organs.

Sediments are essentially being studied in lakes in North America and in Europe. One in-depth study did make it possible to trace the environmental amount of mercury, lead, arsenic, cadmium, copper, and some organic compounds over the last 200 years in North America and to follow up the effects of successive phases of the industrial revolution.

Ice and snow have essentially been analysed in Antarctic, Arctic and European glaciers in relation to the development of the atomic energy industry over the last forty years. Peat cores can be dated by using ^{14}C, ^{210}Pb, ^{133}Cs, to follow up conditions at the local level. Tree rings have been used for relatively short historical records of pollution (last fifty years). It started with the study of lead in trees near main roads.

As zoological specimens, mainly fluid-preserved fish and dried specimens of bird feathers are used for detecting alkylmercury, and herbarium specimens such as mosses and lichens for alkyllead.

Old hair samples are commonly available and are used for studying lead concentration, teeth for lead and fluoride. Dried umbilical cords, used in traditional medicine, have been used to record the increase of methyl-mercury in the Minamata area in Japan since 1930.

Biological banks (essentially serum banks) have now been developed in some parts of the world and could become an effective means of keeping records of existing pollution as a basis for future comparisons.[9]

Surveillance at International Level

Man-made physical and chemical agents in the environment tend to increase both in the levels observed and in diversity and complexity. Chemical agents cross political barriers through air and water. To cope with all these agents is becoming an increasingly difficult task, requiring highly sophisticated methods that few countries, if any, are capable of setting up on their own. International co-operation started between countries sharing the same resource: the Rhine river basin, or the air pollution area between the UK and Western Germany.

Ionizing radiation: Another important area of international co-operation concerns the surveillance of ionizing radiation.[10,11] As early as 1966 the International Atomic Energy Agency (IAEA) issued a 'manual on monitoring in normal operations', completing the safety series on various topics concerning the handling of radioactive products (safety series Nos. 1, 5, 9, 10, and also FAO[10] and WHO[12] guides). This manual deals essentially with the surveillance of the production, handling and use of radioactive material *under normal conditions* (monitoring of sources) without considering accidents. For each type of release, it reviews carefully the various aspects of the natural history of the released nuclide, all the way from its release along its path to man by direct contact, contact after migration of the material into soil, sediments, beaches, ground water, surface water, plant roots, plants, animals, milk, egg, meat, etc.

In 1969, in co-operation with the International Reference Centre for Radioactivity in Le Vesinet, a network of 8 national centres started collecting data from some 140 sampling stations on radiation levels in the air, in rain and in milk. In 1975, as a result of a joint meeting betwen WHO and IAEA, a more extensive and detailed guide was issued. The following points have been considered[11]:

(a) the need and the objectives for environmental monitoring under normal conditions ('Planned release'), and also in case of emergency situations ('unplanned release').
(b) the design of an environmental monitoring programme utilizing procedures and systems at both local and international levels.

The essential objectives were the assessment of the adequacy of release control systems, estimation of the upper limit of exposure acceptable for man, compliance of the operators with existing regulations, detection of trends of change in the environment, better information to the general public, and to all those involved in the production in order to be able to deal better with emergency situations.

In planned release, field measurements can be made through direct measurement: scintillometric explorations are made and dosimeters installed at well defined points. Samples of air, rainwater, sediments, soil, foodstuff, and vegetation are collected according to a locally designed sampling procedure. Laboratory analyses are made at three different levels: gross radioactivity, detailed analysis of specific radionuclides, and isolation of specific radionuclides for quantitative estimates of radioactivity.

In case of 'unplanned release' of limited size, the design described above is sufficient. However, in the event of a real emergency situation 'the cooperation of laboratories and organizations at international level' should be sought in order to aid in the assessment of the environmental impact. A recent catastrophe shows how badly this type of international co-operation is needed.

The first information about the 'unplanned release' to reach the surveillance system should come from the operator. If not, one should rely upon continuous measurement of radioactivity at fixed stations, as close as possible to the discharge point, hopefully linked with a chart recorder and some sort of alarm system. Surveillance efforts should then be aimed towards the determination of the nature and the extent of the contamination, a mapping of the main routes of dispersion through air and water. Rapid surveys should be made with additional instruments, *'as many as necessary'*, to cover a wide field that can quickly be replaced in case of failure and that are ready to use, periodically inspected, robust, reliable, portable, and simple to operate. These rapid surveys should be followed by analyses of samples performed by samplers trained quickly on the spot.

This guide for surveillance of ionizing radiation in the environment can serve as a model for better surveillance of other physical and chemical agents.

International surveillance systems among others include the health related monitoring programme started by WHO in the early 1970s as a response to the rise in cost and complexity of the problems linked with physical and chemical agents in the environment. The 'United Nations Environmental Programme' (UNEP) was initiated in 1972. WHO and UNEP started to work together through the 'Global Environment Monitoring System' (GEMS) in close cooperation with other UN agencies such as FAO, IAEA, UNESCO, and WHO. The air monitoring project started in 1973 and focused on SO_2 and suspended particles. There are now 170 air-monitoring sites located in 50 countries. The monitoring of water quality started in 1976 and 450 stations in 59 countries are now participating. Heavy metals, pesticides, and fluorides are the major concern in these programmes.

Surveillance of Health Effects (Biological Surveillance)

The methods used in surveillance of health effects in industrial workers often differ from those used when looking at general population groups.

In *occupational medicine*, a topic considered in more detail in Chapter 15, the main critical assessment system since James Lind and Sir George Baker, of the relationship between an agent and some health effect has been the analytical epidemiological approach. During the last thirty years retrospective cohort studies have lead to some estimate of the dose–response relationship. This is 'epidemiological evidence'.

In the *general population*, however, the true epidemiological findings of long-term effects of physical and chemical agents, apart from a few historical examples, are not so common, and, in many cases 'experimental evidence' is considered sufficient.[3]

Experimental evidence is based on several steps:

1. The agent is demonstrated to be harmful to experimental animals, with a measurable dose–response relationship.
2. Man is at risk of being exposed to this agent.
3. On the basis of the observed animal response, some computation is made of a possible threshold limit for man, even in the absence of any epidemiological finding.
4. A safety margin of two or three orders of magnitude, depending on the size of the risk, the size of the exposed population, and often on some economic consideration, is applied and a critical limit for the environment accepted and legally enforced.

'Experimental evidence' is not proposed as an ideal model. It is simply the method used at present for action when there is no reliable epidemiological evidence.

The Global Envrionment Monitoring System (GEMS) within the framework of 'exposure monitoring' has recently started a pilot project monitoring biological fluids and tissues, including lead and cadmium levels in blood, and cadmium levels in the kidneys of accidentally deceased persons in ten different countries. Another project involves the measurement of organochlorine pollutants (PCB and DDT) in human milk, and a further project the use of personal monitors carried by volunteers over a period of time while they keep a diary of their activities.

The GEMS-HEAL (Human Exposure Assessment Location) will undertake comprehensive environmental and exposure programmes incorporating climatic data and life-style data.

The health effects of physical and chemical agents are evaluated by two international bodies:

1. In 1971, the International Agency for Research on Cancer (IARC) initiated a programme on the evaluation of the carcinogenic risk of chemicals to humans, which concentrated on individual chemicals and did not accept any conclusive evidence unless at least one reliable epidemiological study could demonstrate the carcinogenic effect on man. Most of the positive findings, however, come from occupational medicine and from iatrogenic medicine and not from environmental data from the general population. The IARC monographs are now an essential reference series.[12]
2. In 1976, WHO with UNEP started a publication: '*Environmental health criteria*', 60 issues are now available. In these series individual physical and chemical agents, and their health consequences, are reviewed, as well as surveillance and control aspects relying—when epidemiological evidence is absent—on experimental evidence.

Conclusions

Surveillance of the physical and chemical environmental determinants of health is an increasing need; it started in urban areas of industrialized countries with occupational environmental conditions; but there are now growing reasons to develop surveillance in the general population and to extend it to rural areas and developing countries.

Source monitoring should be more systematically developed, using routine statistical data on industrial production and human settlements, or in cases where such data do not exist, rapid assessment methods.

For environmental monitoring, past trends should be evaluated through historical methods; present situations should be assessed through automatic monitoring in very advanced areas and through routine surveillance everywhere else. As far as possible data used should be made compatible with the level of the continent as a whole.

For exposure monitoring several techniques should be developed; environmental sentinels, exposure registries, biological banks—not only in the field of occupational medicine (in that instance exhaustively) but also for the general population, with appropriate sampling frames. *Ad hoc* studies should be pursued whenever possible in circumstances not covered by routine exposure surveillance systems.

Health effects monitoring provides reliable epidemiological evidence concerning occupational hazards but much less is ascertained about the general population. Again, environmental sentinels, exposure registries, and biological banks might help to increase our knowledge within the framework of proper follow-up studies.

Various recent catastrophic natural or man-made events occurring in several continents had, at least, the marginal advantage of emphasizing the growing relative impact of physical and chemical environmental determinants of health; these determinants are more often 'catastic' and consequently less obvious, but the type of surveillance they require is now an essential part of current epidemiological and public-health practice.

Bibliography

1. Ministry of Health, Report on public health and medical subjects No. 95. Mortality and morbidity during the London fog of December 1952. HMSO, London (1954).
2. Royal College of Physicians, *Air pollution and health*. London (1970).
3. WHO, *Environmental health criteria*, IPCS series. WHO, Geneva (60 issues since 1976).
4. WHO, Rapid assessment of sources of air, water and land pollution. WHO Offset Publications No. 62 (1982).
5. WHO, Regional publications, European series No. 1. Manual on urban air quality management, Copenhagen (1976).

6. Eylenbosch, W. J., van Sprundel, M., and Clara, R., Lead pollution in Antwerpen, Belgium. *Ann. Acad. Med.* **13**, No. 2 (1984).
7. Green, L. A., A North-American sentinel practice system: Progress, problems and potential. In *Environmental epidemiology* (eds P. Leaverton, L. Masse, and S. Simchez) pp. 141–147. Praeger, New York (1982).
8. Karhausen, L. R., Health sentinels, early warning systems and related activities in the EEC. In *Environmental epidemiology* (eds P. Leaverton, L. Masse, and S. Simchez) pp. 111–19. Praeger, New York (1982).
9. Bosson, P., Coudurier, N., Massé, L., and Merieux, Ch., Geneva county serum bank. 12th Anglo-French meeting, Bischenberg, April 1986).
10. FAO, Atomic Energy Series. Methods of Radio Chemical Analysis, No. 1 (1959). Organisation of survey of radio nuclides in food and agriculture, No. 4 (1963).
11. International Atomic Energy Agency.
    −*Safe handling of radio-isotopes* (Safety series No. 1).
    −*Radioactive waste disposal into the sea* (Safety series No. 5).
    −*Basic safety standards* (Safety series No. 9).
    −*Radioactive waste disposal into fresh water* (Safety series No. 10).
    −*Manual of environmental monitoring in normal operations* (Safety series No. 16).
    −*Objectives and design of environmental monitoring programmes for radioactive contaminants* (Safety series No. 41).
12. WHO. IARC monographs on the evaluation of the carcinogenic risk of chemicals to humans, IARC, Lyon.

20
Surveillance of mental illness
D. WALSH

Introduction

Psychiatric illness accounts for approximately 30–40 per cent of all occupied hospital beds in the countries of the Commission of European Communities and since it is estimated that there is a sizeable psychological component in up to 20 per cent of all cases consulting general practitioners, the surveillance of mental illness, its extent and characteristics, becomes an important issue in the planning, not only of mental health services, but also of health services generally.

Problems of Definition

Over a century ago matters of definition in relation to mental health and illness were relatively simple. People were classified as either mad or insane and the policy of caring for the insane was simple. The nineteenth-century ideal for the treatment of the mentally ill was to send them to large lunatic asylums which were plentifully provided. Nineteenth-century surveillance consisted in providing data on the numbers of persons admitted to and resident in lunatic asylums and, in addition, in many countries, in estimating the number of lunatics 'at large'. Based on the numbers 'at large' additional asylums were built to provide places for those lunatics currently in the community. At least the Victorian policy was clear; lunatics should be in lunatic asylums and therefore sufficient places must be provided. Thus it was that the numbers of lunatics in asylums throughout Europe increased progressively during the nineteenth century.

The main form of surveillance therefore was the observation of trends in numbers of admissions and numbers of residents. We should not think lightly of psychiatry in this regard but reflect that these data from lunatic asylums were among the earliest and most complete health-surveillance data available. In fact in some countries of the European Commission it is the case that complete information about the activities of general hospitals is still not available whereas that for psychiatric hospitals has been available for well over a century and a half.

Surveillance of nineteenth-century hospital data, which showed progressive increases throughout the century of numbers of patients being admitted to psychiatric hospitals, was interpreted as indicating a constant increase in the extent of mental illness. Even today the meaning of these data is still being debated. There are those who maintain that the increase in numbers was entirely due to nosocomial influences rather than to an increase in the amount of serious mental illness and there are others who maintain that the increase in numbers may in fact have reflected a real increase in the incidence of mental illness, and in particular what we now call schizophrenia, in the nineteenth century.[1] With the twentieth century, and particularly after the Second World War, wider concepts of what constitutes mental illness have expanded the meaning of the term and created greater diagnostic and logistic difficulties.

Attempts to overcome these are mirrored in widely accepted classifications of psychiatric disorder. The first of these, the ninth edition of the *International Classification of Diseases* (ICD) devotes its section five entirely to psychiatric disorders. This classification is widely used for administrative and research purposes. More recently the Classification of the American Psychiatric Association which is provided in its *Diagnostic and Statistical Manual*, now in its third edition and colloquially referred to as DSM III, embodies much current thinking in the field of mental health (and disease). The DSM III is a step forward in psychiatric classification in that it provides specific and explicit inclusion and exclusion criteria for each diagnostic category. This is a great help to the clinician which enables the diagnostic procedure to become more objective than, for example, in the case of ICD 9 which, although it gave in its Glossary brief descriptions of various conditions, did not lay down any rules for their diagnosis. Computer programs have been made available for conversion of DSM categories to those of ICD 9 and we can expect an even closer compatibility btween DSM 4 and ICD 10.

As well as encompassing the usual diagnostic categories a wide variety of conditions are included that would not, until comparatively recently, have figured as psychiatric disorders. These are to be found under headings such as personality disorders, disorders of impulse control, somatoform disorders, substance abuse disorders (including nicotine), and such 'conditions not attributable to a mental disorder that are the focus of attention or treatment as borderline intellectual functioning, academic problem, occupational problem and uncomplicated bereavement'.

In the face of these considerations it becomes difficult to draw the line at what constitutes psychiatric disorder, when, for whom and under what circumstances. Even in relation to illnesses which may broadly be thought of as being dimensional, such as depression, decisions have to be made as to what level of severity constitutes a case. The concept of 'caseness' is one that has preoccupied workers for some time now and the matter is discussed at some length, and differences between community psychiatric illness and that encountered by psychiatrists outlined, in Williams.[2]

In the 1950s WHO reviewed the position of psychiatric nosology internationally and found that there were almost as many classificatory systems as there were countries. Aware of the hindrance this posed to international scientific communication and research major WHO Resources were devoted in the 1960s to a programme of standardization of classification and diagnosis. One of the outcomes of this programme was the setting up of the International Pilot Study of Schizophrenia[3] in which ten centres around the world differing greatly in economic and social background used the same diagnostic instrument, the Present State Examination of psychiatric status, to identify major functional psychotic disorders. Another collaborative comparative symptom rating and diagnostic exercise between English-speaking countries was the US/UK project.[4] The exercise explored the differing frequencies with which schizophrenia and affective disorder were being diagnosed between US and British psychiatrists. The broad general conclusion of the project was that the differences between the US and Britain lay in the diagnostic practices of psychiatrists rather than the clinical differences in their patients.

In epidemiological research, standardisation of diagnosis increasingly has become important. Because psychiatric illness, unlike much of physical illness, lacks biological markers, it has been necessary for psychiatrists to become better diagnosticians to overcome subjective judgements and to use internationally accepted classificatory nosologies. To this end many standardized interview procedures, leading to objective data which can be computerized to yield meaningful diagnostic categories or equivalents, have been devised. These include the Present State Examination as already mentioned, the Schedule for Affective Disorders and Schizophrenia (SADS), the Diagnostic Interview Schedule (DIS), and the Structured Clinical Interview for DSM III (SCID).

Gross Indicators of Mental Illness—Extent and Trends

Useful as the diagnostic instruments mentioned above are in specific studies of epidemiological or clinical psychiatry, they are of limited value in the general surveillance of the trends, location, and characteristics of mental disorders generally. Thus information systems more sophisticated and extensive than those merely relating to hospitals are necessary. This is because, increasingly, mental-health care is delivered outside hospital settings. The most useful instrument for this purpose is the psychiatric case register which provides extensive and comprehensive data on illness treated by psychiatric services of all kinds, and not just within the hospital. Some psychiatric case registers even provide information about psychiatric illness that makes contact with general practitioners and social work agencies. In Europe, at least, psychiatric case registers have been growing in number and, among the countries of the Commission of the European Communities, now exist in Denmark, the

UK, Italy, Ireland, The Netherlands, and Germany. These registers form the most useful basis for the surveillance of mental illness for administrative and planning purposes as well as for more purely epidemiological and scientific uses.

The extent and characteristics of mental illness treated in general practice are notoriously difficult to derive, not only because of inherent difficulty in some countries of obtaining any data from general practice but also because of varying clienteles of practices which makes it difficult to obtain a representative sample. However, there have been some successes[5] and some more recent work has highlighted the characteristics of mental illness seen in general practice and points out that there are substantial differences between mental illness encountered in general practice and that seen by the specialist psychiatric services.[6]

Health Services Research—Surveillance of Need

Adequate data for planning purposes may be obtained by a community survey and an estimate of unmet need may be obtained from this approach. In fact fairly precise data concerning the incidence and prevalence of the more serious mental illnesses have come from epidemiological studies. Thus we know that in a community of about 100 000 people we can expect approximately 15–20 new cases of schizophrenia each year. This is important for planning purposes and surveillance of the needs, met and unmet, of this group of people, and is of vital importance for delivering an appropriate mental-health service quantitatively and qualitatively. Similarly, fairly reliable data are available about the extent of the prevalence of dementia in the elderly; approximately 5 per cent of those over 65 and 20 per cent of those over 80 will suffer from severe dementia. Since European populations generally are ageing, notably those aged 75 and over, dementia, particularly Alzheimer dementia, will be one of the most common illnesses of the next century. Institutional and community service planning is greatly helped by epidemiological surveillance that has led to data of this kind.

In assessing the qualitative aspects of health care it is possible to arrive at some idea of how developed these are by looking at gross indicators. Thus the ratio of patients to the population base, the numbers of hospitals with over 1000 patients, and other gross indicators of this kind such as the number of day places and hostel places to the catchment population are also highly relevant. Similarly, staffing ratios per head of population are also useful in surveying the extent of services.[7]

The surveillance of particular treatments such as drugs used by the health services in treating psychiatric disorders is also valuable in helping towards evaluation of a service. Recent surveys of the extent of electroconvulsive therapy (ECT) treatment, for example have been coming out and make some interesting comparisons between countries.[8]

High Risk Groups

Clinical experience as well as epidemiological and ecological surveillance indicates that certain groups are particularly at risk for mental illness. Thus, persons with a family history of psychotic disorder have themselves a risk of psychotic disorder that is greater than that of the general population. This is seen at its most extreme in the children of two schizophrenic parents, for example, where the risk is as high as 40 per cent.[9] Young married women of lower social class are particularly at risk for depressive disorder and the elderly elderly (i.e. those over 75) run high risk of dementia, particularly Alzheimer's disease. The value of such knowledge derived from surveillance enables the deployment of resources that are adequate and appropriate to need. This is nowhere more apparent than in the field of child psychiatric services where working-class areas, with large families and often unsatisfactory housing conditions, are particularly in need of comprehensive services.

Persons working in particular occupations or exposed to particular environmental hazards are known to have high susceptibility to particular disorders, whether by selection or otherwise. Examples include an unduly high proportion of alcohol abusers in the catering and drink industry and the relationship between lead levels in the environment and mental handicap.

Suicide and Attempted Suicide

The quality of data on suicide varies from country to country and is vitiated by the strictness of legal definitions of suicide in countries where the coroner system operates. Nevertheless, study of suicide rates by age and sex groups may well indicate groups at risk although it is difficult to draw any general conclusions about the mental health of whole communities from suicide rates. In general suicide rates tend to fall in face of community adversity and there is some evidence to suggest that rates of depression may also do so. However, suicide rates are particularly high among the elderly, the widowed, the physically ill, the schizophrenic, and drug and alcohol abusers. Indeed long-term changes in, for example alochol consumption, are often positively associated with rises in suicide rates.[10]

Attempted suicide has been predominantly a late twentieth-century phenomenon and has been particularly common among younger women. The extent to which attempted suicide reflects disorganization, unhappiness and incoherence in society, as distinct from individuals, is debatable, but at least there are reasons for thinking that the consequences of attempted suicide may not all be negative. Thus the majority of acts of attempted suicide are not repeated in individuals. Many suicide attempts bring about change in what has hitherto been an undesirable or intolerable situation and even when they do not, they ensure greater attention to and assistance with difficulties that may be ongoing or unresolvable.

Surveillance of Psychiatric Disorders in Childhood

Ideally, the early detection and treatment of any disorder is most likely to yield results. This principle presumably holds good for mental disorder as well. Therefore the surveillance of the extent of mental disorder in childhood becomes important. The disorders most easily detected in childhood are those which cause most social or behavioural disruption. These are neurotic disorders or personality disorders in early life rather than psychosis which is uncommon in childhood. There is, inevitably, a close correlation between the detectable conditions of childhood and general socio-economic deprevation which is relevant to the disposition of services. Conditions like these and mild moderate mental handicap will be picked up by the child psychiatric services pre-school or by school services later on. So far child psychiatric services cannot be said to be adequately provided in the community as a whole and since information on the extent of child psychiatric disorders is still fairly rudimentary, it is impossible to make any time trend comparisons. Surveillance for any psychiatric disorder in childhood is still literally in its infancy.

Conclusion

In conclusion, although surveillance of mental illness, at least from hospital data, has been in operation for over a century and a half no firm conclusions can be drawn about trends in incidence and prevalence of the major mental disorders. Apart from the obvious disappearance of the psychiatric consequences of neurosyphilis, conquered by penicillin and all but vanished from psychiatric hospitals, the disappearance of the psychiatric complications of dietary insufficiency such as beriberi, the late complications of encephalitis lethargica and the gradual disappearance of hysterical conversion and other symptoms in the developed world, there would appear to be little or at least questionable change in the frequency of major psychiatric disorders.

Psychiatric disorders related to alcohol consumption have of course, waxed and waned over the years correspondingly with the rises and falls of consumption of alcohol itself. Increasing adventure-sport participation and road accidents have led to an increase in chronic brain syndromes resulting from cerebral damage. Whether these should be classified as psychiatric disorders is a debatable question and, in any case, chronic incapacitating neuropsychiatric disorders of these kinds will increasingly find specialized accommodation outside of psychiatric services.

For the future, surveillance of psychiatric disorders will probably proceed along the lines already indicated. More sophisticated information systems and more refined epidemiological, and to some extent clinical studies, designed to answer more specific questions relating to the causation and outcome of psychiatric disorder are likely to become the surveillance measures of the future. Surveillance of outcome based on different prevalences in the face of constant incidence may also be valuable in highlighting the efficacy of different treatment approaches and, indeed, the whole field of the cost-effectiveness of contrasting therapeutic approaches is one of considerable importance in psychiatry where many treatments are often available for the same condition with little evaluation of their respective efficacies. In like manner the cost effectiveness of using professional and even lay personnel of different degrees of training and skill in expensive treatment programmes is a fascinating question for the future.

Bibliography

1. Hare, E., Was insanity on the increase? *Br. J. Psychiat.* **142,** 439–55 (1983).
2. Williams, P., Tarnapolsky, A. and Hand, D., Case definition and case identification in psychiatric epidemiology: Review and assessment. *Psychol. Med.* **10,** 101–14 (1980).
3. WHO, *The international pilot study of schizophrenia,* vol. 1. WHO, Geneva (1973).
4. Cooper, J. E., Kendell, R. E., Gurland, B. J., Sharpe, L., Copeland, J. R. M., and Simon, R., *Psychiatric diagnosis in New York and London.* Oxford University Press (1972).
5. Shepherd, M., Cooper, B., Brown, A. C., and Kalton, G. W., *Psychiatric illness in general practice.* Oxford University Press (1966).
6. Goldberg, D. and Huxley, P., *Mental illness in the community.* Tavistock Publications, London (1980).
7. WHO, *Mental health services in Europe: 10 years on.* Regional Office for Europe, Copenhagen (1985).
8. Latey, R. H. and Fahy, T. H., *Electroconvulsive therapy in the Republic of Ireland.* Galway University Press (1986).
9. Gottesman, I. I. and Shields, J., *Schizophrenia—The epigenetic puzzle.* Cambridge University Press (1982).
10. International study of alcohol control experiences, in collaboration with the World Health Organization Regional Office for Europe, *Alcohol, society, and the state,* vols 1, 2 and 3. Addiction Research Foundation, Toronto, Canada (1981).

21

Surveillance for alcohol abuse

D. WALSH

Introduction

In a sense the title 'surveillance for alcohol abuse' is incorrect, because what is meant here is keeping an eye open for alcohol use in an attempt to spot signs of abuse. For alcohol, surveillance can take place at either the community or individual level and there is good evidence that there is a link between the two. The ultimate value of surveillance in the health field must be to enable appropriate preventive or curative measures to be undertaken.

What constitutes alcohol abuse is variable between countries and even in the same country at different times. To some extent what constitutes a problem is defined by the eye of the beholder. Thus middle-class persons will regard noisy public drunkenness as a social outrage, but will be less concerned by cirrhosis mortality deaths. Commonly used indicators of alcohol problems include prosecutions for public drunkenness, admissions to psychiatric hospitals for alcoholism, drunk-driving prosecutions, family violence, suicide, and attempted suicide. Of these it is obvious that prosecutions for public drunkenness and drunk driving are influenced by staffing levels of police forces and by the vigour with which prosecutions are bought by the police. Obviously these extraneous factors have considerable bearing on the statistical indicators provided by alcohol-related prosecutions. In a similar fashion admissions to psychiatric hospitals, although they may be of some value in the short run and in the same jurisdiction, are of doubtful value over time and for data comparison between countries. Evidently the promulgation of the belief that alcohol is a disease which can be cured by medical intervention must have substantially increased the number of admissions to psychiatric hospitals, independently of the extent of alcohol dependence or other alcohol-related psychiatric pathology. The same 'softness' and susceptibility to 'nosocomial' influences is true of other indices of alcohol abuse that may be open to surveillance.

The relationship between alcohol consumption and alcohol abuse

While it is obvious that there can be no abuse of alcohol if there is no consumption of alcohol it is, perhaps, surprising that it was not until after the Second World War that attempts to examine the relationship between the extent of alcohol consumption in a community and the extent of problems that are believed to be related to alcohol in the same community were made. In the 1950s a French demographer, Ledermann, examined the levels of alcohol consumption among individual members of selected populations. He found that individual levels were smoothly and continuously distributed in his sample populations, and that levels of alcohol intake from the lowest to the very highest existed without any discontinuity between the very heavy drinkers, the heavy drinkers, moderate drinkers, and light drinkers. This result challenged the age-old belief that drinkers of alcohol could be divided into those who were problem drinkers, or 'alcoholics', and those who were 'normal' drinkers. It indicated that there was no basis for belief in a qualitative difference between the two but rather that such differences as there were, were quantitative. A further important Ledermann assertion was that there is a positive relationship between community levels of alcohol intake and the extent of alcohol-related problems. This gives the 'Ledermann model' a plastic and mobile quality indicating that at community level the proportion of heavy drinkers can be influenced by lowering or raising mean consumption levels. In terms of the individual it also means that persons who are drinking at levels of intake which create problems for themselves or others, have the capacity to continue drinking, but at reduced levels of intake which do not result in personal physical damage to themselves or cause social problems to their families or the wider community. This ability to change from problem to harmless social drinking was first observed by Davies [1] in a follow-up survey of formerly problem drinkers, but the implications have been vigorously resisted by therapists of traditional mould.

The extent of the distribution about a particular mean may vary greatly. The various points of view about this topic have been brought together in a collection of papers entitled the Ledermann Curve.[2] In the light of this, surveillance of national levels of alcohol consumption is of great importance, but should not be relied on as the only indicator of alcohol abuse.

Surveillance of Alcohol Consumption Levels

Because of the fiscal interest of governments in alcohol production and consumption data are available in all EEC countries on the amounts of home-produced alcohol' retained for home consumption'. Similar data exist for imported alcohol. These data are complete in every country and therefore comparable between national jurisdictions. Of course, alcohol that is taxed as soon as it is released from bond onto the home market or alcohol that is imported and released from bond is not always consumed immediately afterwards. So the amount of alcohol that is registered as being taxed is not the same as the amount of alcohol that is being consumed during a given period. Thus alcohol may be bought and stored for some considerable time before consumption; this may happen, for example, in anticipation of a change in levels of alcohol taxation in a forthcoming budget. Furthermore, there is an unregistered amount of alcohol consumed from time to time that is illegally produced and therefore not taxed. More recently, especially in countries with high alcohol taxation levels, there has been a growth in the legal home production of alcohol with the availablility of wine and beer-producing kits. There may also be considerable illegal importation of alcohol because of favourable price differentials. An example would be in the large scale clandestine importation of spirits from Northern Ireland to Ireland during the early 1980s and, on a lesser scale, from Luxembourg to the Federal Republic of Germany. Despite all these provisos, national levels of annual alcohol consumption are fairly accurately reflected in EEC countries by excise returns.

The surveillance of changes in national alcohol consumptions both in total alcohol and in the various types of alcohol as between beer, wine, and spirits, is of considerable utility from the point of view of surveillance, as fluctuations in total consumption are likely to be reflected in the extent and typology of problems.

Unlike national consumption data which cost nothing at the micro level community surveys are expensive to carry out, but can make available much more useful additional information. Thus consumption by age or sex, quantity, and frequency as well as by rural/urban and social class indicators may be obtained.

From the use of 'consumption', data provide fairly clear information of the European alcohol scene. Overall alcohol consumption has increased since the 1950s in the countries of the Commission of the European Communities. There was a wide range of consumption levels with, in general, the northern European predominantly beer and spirit drinking countries consuming less alcohol than the wine drinking countries of the EEC such as France and Italy. This difference was as great as twofold but it has generally decreased between 1950 and 1980. This is because the lowest consuming countries in the Commission such as Ireland and the United Kingdom have substantially increased their national consumptions. One of the heaviest consuming countries, France (and more recently Italy) has greatly reduced its national per capita consumption since 1960 (Table 21.1). Consumptions are presented per head of population aged 15 and over rather than for total population because of the considerable variation in the number of persons aged under 18 in EEC countries.

Analysis of alcohol consumption patterns by beverage type indicates a growing 'internationalization'[3] of drinking patterns with a shift away from traditional beverages in each country towards the other types (Table 21.2).

Survey data from most European countries indicate that there are many fewer abstainers from alcohol than previously, that more young people are drinking than before and that women, particularly young women, are less likely to be abstainers than hitherto. Time-series data, age-specific, on alco-

Table 21.1   Alcohol consumption at age 15 and above in EEC countries

Country	Alcohol consumption Per capita (Litres of pure alcohol)		Percentage change
	1950	1979	1950–79
Belgium	8.0	14.4	+80
Denmark	4.9	12.2	+149
France	22.1	20.5	−7
F.R. of Germany	3.8	16.0	+321
Ireland	4.6	11.3	+146
Italy	12.4	16.1	+30
Luxembourg	8.5	16.8	+98
The Netherlands	3.0	12.2	+307
United Kingdom	6.3	10.3	+63

This table has been adapted from Davis and Walsh.[8]

Table 21.2   Alcohol consumption patterns in the EEC Spirits, beer and wine

Country	Spirits (%)		Beer (%)		Wine (%)	
	1950	1979	1950	1979	1950	1979
Belgium	13.0	26.8	74.4	51.2	12.6	22.0
Denmark	15.9	15.6	72.2	64.5	11.9	19.9
France	14.6	15.8	5.6	14.0	79.8	70.2
F.R. of Germany	34.4	26.3*	49.5	51.1*	17.0	22.6*
Ireland	20.0	29.5	72.4	62.9	7.6	7.6
Italy	7.4	16.4	1.8	7.0	90.8	76.6
The Netherlands	71.0	36.8	25.6	45.8	3.4	17.4
United Kingdom	13.2	24.1*	79.7	57.4*	4.1	15.1*

* = estimate
Source: Brewers Association of Canada, Ottawa. Alcoholic beverage taxation and control policies, 4th edn 1980. Mavis W. Brown and Paul Wallace.

hol consumption will be of considerable interest to see whether the younger cohorts will carry into later life the heavier consuming patterns that they are showing compared to younger people of early generations. If they do then we can expect higher levels of alcohol-related problems for these cohorts.

Surveillance of Alcohol-Related Problems

The surveillance of alcohol-related problems is a necessary corollary to the surveillance of alcohol consumption. Problems that are alcohol-related form a very wide spectrum of physical, psychological, and social pathologies. The degree to which alcohol contributes to these problems must, in an individual or in a community, be conjectural, but time-series epidemiological data comparing levels of alcohol consumption with levels of these problems strongly inculpate alcohol as one, but an important, element in a multi-factorial causality. The surveillance of these problems, and particularly their early identification, is an important aspect of preventive work on the alcohol field.

Surveillance of Alcohol Damage

It is now necessary to mention the more common and the more easily mensurable of these problems. Mortality from cirrhosis of the liver, although it may be caused by other antecedents such as the prevalence of hepatitis B carriers, is the most thoroughly valid and reliable index of alcohol damage and the one most closely related to levels of alcohol consumption. There is a very close temporal relationship between changes in alcohol consumption levels and changes in cirrhosis mortality. It is reasonable to suppose that at any point in time there are a number of individuals who are teetering on the brink of liver failure but who are redeemable if only their alcohol intake is abolished or drastically curtailed. This points to the importance of having reliable biological markers which identify individuals at risk and therefore makes individual surveillance a more meaningful undertaking. Search for such markers is essential. One has already been developed in relation to cirrhosis of the liver in that individuals whose HLA make-ups are B8 or B40 are more susceptible to liver damage than those of other antigenic constitution.

Surveillance of inter-regional differences within a country has sometimes been useful. Higher per-capita alcohol intake regions in France are also those with highest alcohol-related pathology. Northern regions, such as Brittany, have higher cirrhosis mortality rates than lower alcohol consumption regions such as Provence.[4]

The discovery, or perhaps more accurately the twentieth century rediscovery, of alcohol-related fetal damage has stimulated great interest in this problem. Not least has been the relationship between moderate degrees of alcohol consumption during pregnancy and pregnancy outcome. Surveillance of the incidence of congenital malformations by such means as 'Eurocat' (see Chapter 10 and glossary) may not yield as useful information as direct case-control studies and intervention procedures during pregnancy on the possible role of alcohol in a multi-factorial aetiology of fetal damage which does not amount to the full fetal alcohol syndrome.

In interpreting the data available for surveillance of alcohol-related problems it is important to keep an awareness of the influence of socio-cultural factors. This is because what constitutes a problem is strongly determined by prevalent national attitudes and, even within countries, by different social class expectations and practices. Thus it had long been believed that the Scots were a more 'problem' group of people than the English in relation to alcohol. This view, perhaps a predominantly English one, largely sprang from the much higher levels of hospital admission for alcoholism for Scotland compared to England and the greater susceptibility to prosecution for drunkenness of Scots. Recent work comparing the extent of alcohol-related problems of all kinds between English and Scottish communities has not sustained this view and, in line with the almost similar consumption levels of two countries, has identified very similar problem levels in the two communities.[5]

Comment

Most of the surveillance systems that operate currently in the alcohol field are oriented towards detection of alcohol problems that are well established, and scientific evaluation of intervention of treatment programmes with such individuals have not been shown to be conspicuously successful.[6] There is a generally agreed necessity to establish sensitive detection methods to pick up early cases where intervention already seems to show some promise. An example would be the screening by nursing staff of patients in general, medical, and surgical wards for incipient problem drinking and, following their identification, a simple session of advice which appears to have some effectiveness.[7] Other examples include the Centres d'Hygiène Alimentaire in France where routine gastroenterological screening is used to detect persons drinking at the problem level and counsel them accordingly. Individuals who have been convicted of a drinking/driving offence are also often referred to these centres by the courts.

In general, there should be a movement towards earlier community rather than institutional detection of those embarking on a problem drinking career so that intervention with a better prospect of success can be undertaken. However, it has to be borne in mind that there are limitations to the degree to which community intervention can take place, particularly in those countries where great emphasis is placed on the freedom of the individual. In Sweden citizens can report to their local temperance board persons they believe to have a drinking problem or to be using alcohol immoderately. The boards may then compel individuals reported in this way to undergo treatment.[8] However, such an approach would not be feasible in many countries, an illustration of the susceptibility of intervention and even surveillance procedures to socio-cultural influences.

Bibliography

1. Davies, D. L., Normal drinking in recovered alcohol addicts. *J. stud. Alcohol* **23**, 94–104 (1962).

2. Alcohol Education Centre, *The Ledermann curve*. Alcohol Education Centre, London (1977).
3. Makela, K., Room, R., Single, E., Sulkunen, P., and Walsh, B., *Alcohol, society and the state: 1. A comparative study of alcohol control*. Addiction Research Foundation, Toronto (1981).
4. Caro, G. and Bertrand, Y., Yec'Hed Mad, *A votre santé*. Editions Le Signor. B.P. 23, 29115 Le Guilvinec (1981).
5. Latcham, R. W., Kreitman, N., Plant, M. A., and Crawford, A., Regional variations in British alcohol morbidity rates: A myth uncovered? I: Clinical surveys. *Br. med. J.* **289,** 1341–3 (1984).
6. Pattison, E. M., Nonabstinent drinking goals in the treatment of alcoholism. In *Research advances in alcohol and drug problems*, Vol. 3 (eds R. J. Gibbins *et al.*). John Wiley, Chichester (1976).
7. Chick, J., Lloyd, G., and Crampsie, E., Counselling problem drinkers in medical wards: A controlled study. *Br. med. J.* **290,** 965–967 (1985).
8. Davis, P. and Walsh, D., *Alcohol problems and alcohol control in Europe*. Croom Helm, London (1983).

22

Surveillance for adverse reactions to drugs (ADR)

K. H. KIMBEL

Why undertake surveillance for adverse reactions to drugs?*

At a first glance the surveillance of a commodity, which is handed out to the customer by well-trained experts, does not seem one of the urgent problems of consumer protection. More than half of all drugs bought in the European Community (EEC) have been prescribed by a physician and could not have been obtained otherwise than at a pharmacy. This may be different in some southern regions of the EEC. The patient (or his or her dependants), who in most cases has been instructed by the physician on why and how to take the drug, could get further advice from the dispensing pharmacist or from the package insert, mandatory in most EEC countries.

Except for herbal and some other home remedies most non-prescription drugs are available only in licensed pharmacies where the advice of a university-trained pharmacist on the safe use of the drug is given or may at least be sought. In addition to that there is an abundance of popular brochures and booklets (admittedly only few of scientific standard) on the use and risks of drugs written for the lay population. So why spend scarce manpower and finances in a field where use and risk information seems to be much more abundant than, for example, for alcohol or motor vehicles?

In contrast to many risks of daily life which are sometimes taken for rather irrational reasons (e.g. alcohol, 'recreational' drugs, speed driving) the risk of taking a drug (better 'medicine') is traded for the benefit of mitigating or curing an ailment. Taking a medicine involves, consciously or unconsciously, a risk/benefit appraisal by the physician and/or the patient. With presently available information this is, however, not possible for many even commonly used drugs for which the risks have never been measured. Thus, despite the personal and formal conditions to convey it, quantitative information on both benefit and risk of most drugs prescribed or bought by the patient himself is still far from optimal. The exchange of toxicity data by poison control centres may serve as an operational model.

There are many reasons for this lack of information. Up to now, no legislative body has seen fit to compel manufacturers to provide *quantitative* data

*This includes vaccines and diagnostic agents but not ADRs caused by other therapeutic and diagnostic procedures.

on the occurrence of ADRs, their severity and sequelae after a sufficient number of patients have been treated with a drug. Nor have they asked the manufacturers to identify populations especially at risk because of concomitant medication, impaired excretory or inactivating capacity, or of specific immunological conditions. The reason may well be that the clinico-pharmacological as well as epidemiological institutions which could provide such data are not yet fully developed. Within the scope of this article, we shall concentrate on considering the epidemiological aspects of the present situation.

In the majority of European countries there are almost no voluntary schemes which can reliably determine the incidence and severity of adverse drug reactions (ADR) for a specific medicament. Some company sponsored studies have been completed (for example, dealing with the adverse reaction of Histamine-H_2-Receptor blockers or Angiotensin Converting Enzyme (ACE) inhibitors) but none provided data which are useful to the general practitioner in his risk/benefit evaluation. The only breakthrough in this field seems to be W. H. W. Inman's Prescription Event Monitoring (PEM) system.[1] There are some other similar studies in the course of preparation or implementation; for example, with anxiolytics, neuroleptics and anti-depressants in the Federal Republic of Germany. However, in contrast to Inman's studies their efficacy has still to be proven.

It seems that most of the burden of developing and testing new systems for the quantitative evaluation of drug risks has been shouldered by academic institutions, regulatory authorities, professional organizations, or other benefactors. There is some willingness on the part of the pharmaceutical industry to help finance such enterprises, but some reluctance to engage in costlier projects still prevails. Consequently, the surveillance for ADR in Europe rests almost exclusively on voluntary (spontaneous) reporting systems (VRS) established according to the recommendations of the World Health Organization, 1972[2] and provided by the WHO with a Collaborative Research Centre at the Drug Regulatory Authority of Sweden in Uppsala.

Before dealing with the established methods of spontaneous drug monitoring in Europe and attempts to quantify the risks of at least the more frequently prescribed drugs, we shall look at data already available in routine health statistics and patient records in hospitals and physicians' practices.

Use of Standard Mortality and Morbidity Statistics for ADR Surveillance

A significant proportion of ADRs resemble, or are identical to conditions occurring without drug treatment during the course of illness or disability. This holds true especially for milder ADRs like nausea, vomiting, headache, etc., and even for more severe ADRs such as asthmatic attacks. This explains why the administration of a placebo, i.e. the dosage form of a drug without an active ingredient, may induce various symptoms of milder ADRs. On the other hand there are conditions which rarely occur without drug treatment, but which are rather common in patients given certain drugs. Examples are agranulocytosis, sudden hepatic failure or primary vascular pulmonary hypertension. The regional mortality figures for such severe conditions are sometimes known over many years. An increase could thus point to a new, not yet detected drug risk, provided other environmental causes could be excluded.

Studies from Sweden[3] on the incidence of agranulocytosis in the total population indicated, however, that the figure remained stable over a period of several years despite the withdrawal of an incriminated group of drugs. On the other hand, the experience with the oxiquinoline derivatives in Japan demonstrated beyond doubt that after they had been banned, no new cases of Subacute Myelo-Optico-Neuritis (SMON) were seen.[4] It seems therefore advisable to establish within the countries of the EEC uniform *mortality* statistics detailed enough to recognize an increase in symptoms commonly associated with the use of medicaments. It goes without saying that this would require physicians to complete a comprehensive death certificate not only to define precisely the cause of death but also to obtain as complete a medication history as possible. Currently, cause of death certification is notably unreliable.

Most countries in the EEC have not yet succeeded in establishing reliable *morbidity* statistics. This would contribute, even more than mortality data, to an earlier detection of yet unknown drug risks. For example, the sudden increase in the occurrence of a rare condition like priapism would have directed attention to a group of depressed patients receiving a certain antidepressant with a novel chemical structure. This is an excellent but rare example because most non-life-threatening ADRs occur during treatment with a large number of other drugs or even when no other drug is given at all: for example, haemorrhage, hyperglycaemia, or even aplastic anaemia, are much more common than priapism.

It should, however, be kept in mind that improving existing or previously established morbidity statistics could enhance the identification of new, possibly drug-induced, symptoms. This is even more relevant for drug induced malformations and malignancies. Statistics on both conditions are available in most European countries. Restrictions or regulations in compliance with data protection laws and the reluctance of physicians to report on malformations without the consent of the child's mother invalidate most statistics of this kind with respect to the true incidence.

A further, by no means less important, source of information relevant to drug surveillance are the statistics of the sick funds, government employee health schemes and the private health-insurance schemes. Here also data protection considerations have led to a rather crude classification of diseases and disabilities for which the patient has been given medicaments. In contrast data on drugs prescribed to the patient, paid in full or in part by the patient or by the sick funds, are readily available even if some problems of confidentiality exist.

In summary, one can say that morbidity and mortality statistics established for general public health purposes may be modified at relatively little cost to serve as a valuable indicator for new ADRs and the increase of those already known. This requires close co-operation with the statistical offices and the drug surveillance authorities.

Specific ADR Surveillance Systems in the EEC

1. Voluntary reporting systems (VRS)

It is often assumed that voluntary reporting systems (VRS) for adverse drug reactions (ADR) came into existence only after the thalidomide disaster. In fact, a committee established to investigate chloroform anaesthesia deaths in 1877 asked practising surgeons for relevant information.[5] The first organized enterprise of this kind seems to have been the Adverse Reactions Registry of the American Medical Association established in 1952.[6] Its primary aim was to assess the risk of drug-induced blood dyscrasias.

In Europe, in 1958, the Drug Commission of the German Medical Profession (Arzneimittelkommission der deutschen Ärzteschaft) was the first to call on the physicians of the Federal Republic to report all ADRs observed to its secretariat. It took, however, another three years, and the vigorous support of the German Society for Internal Medicine, before a sizeable number of reports was received. In the United Kingdom the Committee on the Safety of Drugs (CSD) was set up in 1964 by the Health Minister (changed to Committee on the Safety of Medicines (CSM) later). In contrast to the German system which is run with professional funds only, the CSD/CSM was financed by the Department of Health. One year earlier (1963) a country-wide VRS was started in the Netherlands, which developed into the present Netherlands Centre for Monitoring of Adverse Reactions to Drugs (NARD). Like the SCM it is affiliated to the Drug Regulatory Agency of the Government. Both institutions saw to it that despite their official character 'all reports or replies that the committee receive from doctors will be treated with complete professional confidence . . .'.[7] In Scandinavia pilot projects for voluntary reporting of ADR's started in Sweden and Norway in 1965. Finland followed suit in 1966 and Denmark in 1968. It took until 1982 before Switzerland established its own VRS, SANZ (Schweizerische Arzneimittel-Nebenwirkungs-Zentrale).

In 1963 the member states of the World Health Organization requested that WHO should arrange 'for the systematic collection of information on adverse drug reactions'. WHO became actively involved in drug monitoring

Table 22.1 Drug surveillance centres in the European Community

		Establ.	No. of MDs at the centre	Reports	Special studies
Belgium	Centre National de Pharmacovigilance, Cité Adminivstrative de l'Etat, Quartier Vesale, B-1010 Brussels		2 (Pharmac.)	600	
Denmark	Pharmaceutical Laboratories, National Board of Health, Frederikssundvej 378, DK-2700 Bronshoj	1968	1 MD (part-time) 2 Pharmacists	1 600	
France	Service de Pharmacovigilance, Ministère des Affaires Sociales, 1, Place de fontenoy, F-75700 Paris	1984	19	8554	
Federal Republic of Germany	Division of Drug Experience, Federal Institute for Health (BGA), P.O. Box 330013, D-1000 Berlin 33 and	1978	1	see below	AMÜP Psychiatry (Clinics) FAT Psychiatry (Private Pract.) GP-Program Heidelberg
	Arzneimittelkommission der deutschen Ärzteschaft, P.O. Box 4 10 125, D-5000 Köln 41	1958		6500	
Italy	Pharmaceutical Division, Ministry of Health, Viale della Civilta Romana 7, 1 00 144 Roma	1975	8 (Ancona)*		*Special research— group not involved in VRs

Table 22.1 *cont.*

Ireland	Adverse Reaction Section, Advisory Board, 63–64 Adelaide Road, IRL Dublin 2	1967	1	947	
The Netherlands	Adverse Drug Reaction Centre, Postbus 439, AK 2260 Leidscherdam	1963	2.5	1006	Hospital Monitoring System (selected drugs) BCD
Spain (Catalonia)	Divisio de Farmacologia, Clinica Universidad Autonoma de Barcelona, P. Vall d'Hebron s.n., E-08035 Barcelona	1982	6	468 (Catalonia only)	Expansion planned to 3 regions (Navarra-Centre, Cantabria, Catalonia)
United Kingdom	Committee on Safety of Medicines, Market Towers, 1 Nine Elms Lane, GB-SW8 5NQ London	1964	4	12 655	
	Drug Surveillance Research Unit, University of Southampton, Winchester Road, GB-SO 3 BX Botley	1980		150 000	Prescription Event Monitoring
Greece	Drug Surveillance Centres, Voulis 4, 10562 Athens, Greece				

249

activities in 1968, when a feasibility study into a collaborative international VRS was commissioned. Out of an internationally staffed co-ordinating unit first located in Alexandria, VA, USA, the Research Centre for International Monitoring of Adverse Reactions to Drugs of WHO in Geneva, grew by leaps and bounds and moved in 1976 to Uppsala (Sweden) and is now called WHO Collaborating Centre for International Drug Monitoring.

At present all member states of the EEC except Greece, Luxemburg and Portugal maintain VRS. They all co-operate as 'National Centres' within the framework of the WHO and maintain additional contacts with the VRS of most developed countries through diplomatic channels and personal relations. Currently data from twenty-three countries are stored at WHO's Collaborating Centre in Uppsala and are available upon request by the National Centres for confidential use. The WHO data base contains, as of 1 January 1986, 430 000 reports on ADRs. The crucial prerequisites for such a valuable exchange of information are, however, uniform drug dictionaries and identical adverse reaction terminologies. Unfortunately, WHO never succeeded in establishing a world-wide register of marketed drugs. The Collaborating Centre has thus to maintain a file on all drugs which are reported to induce an ADR.

Due to the abundance of combination drugs in most European countries, the correlation of trade marks to active ingredients is rather difficult and complicates the search for all drugs containing the same active ingredient. Similar terminology problems exist in so far as the office maintaining the International Classification of Diseases (ICD), closely affiliated with WHO headquarters in Geneva, has not yet succeeded in incorporating the WHO Adverse Reaction Terminology into ICD-9. Thus a separate ADR terminology has to be maintained at the WHO International Collaborating Centre in Uppsala. Its upkeep suffers from inadequate manpower and the lack of an advisory body. Nevertheless, the exchange of information between the National Centres is functioning well and fast, greatly helped by the annual meetings organized by WHO headquarters and its Collaborating Centre.[2]

Professional and public knowledge about VRS   In spite of the great interest of the public and the media in all aspects of drug safety neither seems to know much about the purpose, scope, efficacy, and cost of a VRS. Most physicians, unless they participate in the system, are not sufficiently informed and thus not adequately motivated. As a rule, VRS is a signal or hypothesis generator. The causal relationship between the suspected adverse reaction and the incriminated drug reported is rarely established; for example, by a positive rechallenge or a specific *in vitro* test. Independent observations from several sources and locations may strengthen the suspicion; a lack of identical reports over a longer period of time may dissipate it.

All proposals to assess the strength of a suspected causal relationship by means of algorithms or other schemes have proved misleading or unreliable. They may serve only as a logic guide for the efficient evaluation of individual cases. The investigation of a possible causal relationship between a drug and a ADR requires carefully planned epidemiological (prospective or case-control) studies. Past experience with such studies—for example, on reserpine and breast cancer[8] or clofibrate and certain malignancies[9] delineated the problems—but it also proved (for example, the studies on diethylstilboestrol and vaginal cancer)[10] the feasibility of such endeavours. Some authorities, maintaining VRS and basing their regulatory decisions on such systems, still have to be taught that VRS cannot, as a rule, give information on the causal relationship, the frequency or the outcome of ADRs. VRS needs to be complemented by suitable epidemiological studies to serve as a solid foundation both for the physician's risk/benefit evaluation and for sound regulatory decisions.

There is no doubt that VRS have recognized most impending drug disasters with a few exceptions—for example, the practolol syndrome[11]—an oculo-muco-cutaneous fibrosis. It was only the aforementioned softness of the signal which led the authorities to hesitate to arrive earlier at the decision which had to be made in any case in the long run. The reluctance to initiate the necessary epidemiological studies had to be paid for not only by avoidable loss of life and suffering, but also, and much more importantly, by a severe loss of public confidence in drug therapy.

The most important criticism leveled at VRS is that of the reluctance of most physicians to report at all and the ensuing 'under-reporting'. It is certainly true that most medical students never learn about VRS at medical school and look it up in vain in most textbooks on pharmacology and drug therapy.[12] It is one symptom of the growth retardation of Clinical Pharmacology in many European countries, that the average physician is neither well prepared nor motivated to participate in VRS. Nevertheless, it is not mandatory that every physician participates in a VRS as is often insisted upon by lay people. It seems preferable to deal with several thousands of highly motivated and interested physicians rather than force tens of thousands of busy practitioners to fill in their forms grudgingly.

The average physician sees more than a thousand patients per year. Five thousand reporting physicians thus represent observations covering 5 million patient years; these are quite sufficient for even very rare events related to rarely prescribed drugs, provided the physician recognizes and identifies the symptom as an ADR and the drug which may have caused it. The information on the ADR fed back from the Monitoring Centre may in turn sharpen attention for further events.

One of the main advantages of a VRS is the rather short time between the observation of the ADR and the evaluation at the Monitoring Centre. In order to set priorities for early warning a highly trained and experienced group of physicians must screen the incoming reports at once. A well-stocked library, a literature and case data bank, and direct access to a sufficient number of outside experts are indispensable for their efficient work. Important reports with lower priority may be dealt with at regular advisory committee meetings; it can, however, be disastrous if a crucial report is shelved until the next committee meeting to discuss causal relationships instead of communicating the suspicion to other centres or institutions treating similar patients with the same drug. The evaluating team should also have drug consumption data at its disposal, to estimate the population at risk in order to set the right priorities.

To summarize: a VRS or Spontaneous Monitoring System is best suited as a signal generator, i.e. an early warning system for ADR. Electronic data processing is therefore much less important than for example in comprehensive monitoring systems. Simple programmes to help with the *ad hoc* evaluation can, however, be of value, like WHO evaluating programmes 'New to the system' and 'Drug/ADR combinations of special interest'. Most important for fast and efficient functioning are:

1. High motivation and undergraduate and postgraduate education of the participating physicians to think always of the possibility of an unexpected symptom being drug induced and to deduce from the pharmacological and/or immunological mechanism of action of a drug which ADRs could be expected and
2. Capability and experience of medical staff at a VRS centre to recognize and follow up even improbable drug/symptom relationships.

Both prerequisites exist only in few European countries.

2. Comprehensive monitoring systems

As already stated, VRS serve, except where deliberate or inadvertent re-exposure proves positive, only as a hypothesis generator, where the causal relationship between the observed event and the drug given are concerned. VRS also yield no information on the frequency of an ADR in all exposed or in special patient populations, for example the elderly. Only rarely do they provide information on the severity of an ADR. It has therefore been pointed out quite early, that VRS needs to be complemented by studies not only to confirm or reject the hypothesis created by the VRS, but also to estimate the patient population afflicted and the frequency and special conditions under which the ADR may occur. The epidemiological methods by which that could be achieved may be divided in general into *prospective* and *retrospective* studies. The latter have the advantage that they may be performed on already existing data and thus yield results much earlier than with prospective studies. Practical experience with retrospective studies has, however, often been hampered by incompleteness and unsuitability of the patient documentation in hospital or private practice, data protection stipulations, and unforeseen biases invalidating totally or partially the results of the study. Most comprehensive drug monitoring studies are therefore prospective ones, preferably begun shortly after marketing a new drug (post-marketing studies, PMS) or on already marketed drugs exhibiting new, unexpected ADRs.[13,14]

The study must not, however, deal with a certain drug or group of drugs. It may also comprise a certain patient population exposed to a number of different drugs. The most comprehensive type is Record Linkage, i.e. the complete documentation of all health relevant data of a large population. This has been done in Scotland for example.[15,16] By means of electronic data processing those data can be searched for interrelations between drugs given and symptoms observed. To assess the type and frequency of ADRs these should have been already identified as such in the files. This is, however, not always the case. The Boston Collaborative Drug Surveillance Program is an example of a comprehensive drug surveillance system in which *all* patients of a Department of Internal Medicine and their physicians were asked by specially trained nurses if they had observed any adverse drug reactions.

Drug-related comprehensive surveillance studies are mostly undertaken by pharmaceutical companies; unfortunately, most of them are not published or, if so, serve mainly promotional purposes. The proposed amendments to the present German drug law provide therefore for such studies and their protocols to be submitted to the regulatory agency prior to implementation. The simplest, least costly, but, however, quite efficient type of drug related comprehensive monitoring is the Prescription Event Monitoring (PEM) devised by W. H. W. Inman.[1] In contrast to VRS it provides as denominator the number of patients exposed to the drug and thus at risk. The prescribing physician receives a computer-generated letter asking him to complete a non-structured questionnaire on the events he or his patient experienced during and after taking the drug. The return rate was unexpectedly high (around 70 per cent), but ADRs prone to occur in patients less frequently treated by GPs, for example very old, incapacitated patients in homes, were not identified. A similar experience occurred in the USA, where new ADRs were not identified even by large PMS but through individual reports from the VRS. The most efficient type of comprehensive surveillance, symptom-oriented, has not found much favour. Institutions where patients with severe ADR's attend to receive specific treatment or diagnosis could without great effort establish a drug history (for example, in patients presenting with agranulocytosis or pulmonary hypertension) in order to identify a common causative drug. The registry for ophthalmological ADRs in the USA is one example, another is the analysis of all drugs taken prior to admission for gastric bleeding at Bochum university hospital.

Optimal drug surveillance thus requires efficient coordination not only between hypothesis generating and proving systems but also between physician, patient, drug manufacturer, and regulatory agency.

Bibliography

1. Inman, W. H. W., *Monitoring for drug safety*. MTP Press, Lancaster (1986).
2. WHO, Technical report series 498: International monitoring, the role of national centres. Geneva (1972).
3. Boettiger, L. E. *et al.*, *Acta med. scand.* **205**, 457 (1979).
4. Soda, T., Drug induced sufferings, *Excerpta Medica*, Amsterdam, I.C.S. 513 (1980).
5. Anonymous, *Br. med. J.* **11**, 998 (1980).
6. Smiley, R. K., Cartwright, G. E., and Wintrobe, M. M., *J. Am. Med. Ass.* **149**, 914 (1952).
7. Dunlop, D., Letter to all British physicians and dental surgeons, 4 May (1964), Committee on Safety of Medicines.
8. Labarthe, D. R. and O'Fallon, W. M., Reserpin and breast cancer. *J. Am. med. Assoc.* **243**, 2304 (1980).
9. WHO, Study on clofibrate: A cooperative trial of clofibrate in men, *Br. Heart J.* **40**, 1069 (1978).
10. Herbst, A. L. (ed.), *Intrauterine exposure to methylstilbestrol in the human*, American College of Obstetrics & Gynaecology, Chicago, 45 (1978).
11. Pfeifer, H. J., Greenblatt, D. J., and Koch-Weser, J., Adverse reactions to practolol. *Eur. J. Clin. Pharmacol.* **12**, 167 (1977).
12. Dölle, W., Müller-Oerlinghausen, B., and Schwabe, U. (eds), *Grundlagen der Arzneimitteltherapie*. BI-Wissenschafts Verlag, Mannheim (1986).
13. Dukes, M. N. G., *Meyler's side effects of drugs*, 10th edn. Elsevier, Amsterdam (1984).
14. Dukes, M. N. G. and Kimbel, K. H., *Arzneirisiken in der Praxis*, Urban, Schevarzenberg, Munich (1985).
15. Gross, F. H. and Inman, W. H. W. (eds), *Drug monitoring*, Academic Press, London (1977).
16. Walker, S., *Monitoring adverse drug reactions*, MTP Press, Lancaster (1986).

23

Surveillance of poisoning—the role of Poison Control Centres

GLYN N. VOLANS AND HEATHER M. WISEMAN

Functions and History

Surveillance of poisoning is necessary in order to determine causal factors, methods of treatment, and measures for prevention. This increasingly important function of Poison Control Centres (PCCs) is examined in more detail in this article.

The principal functions of PCCs are shown in Table 23.1. Of these the primary role is the provision of a 24-hour emergency service for information and advice on the risks and the management of poisoning and suspected poisoning in man. Over the last thirty years these centres have become established in industrialized countries throughout the world and they are now also being set up in developing countries. Directories of centres are available through the World Federation of Poison Control Centres and the European Association of Poison Control Centres (see Appendix), two organizations which promote the exchange of information and collaboration in studies related to poisoning in man.

In the 1950s the first centres found little existing information on the toxicity to man of the majority of commonly available manufactured products.[1] To correct this deficiency many centres devised ways of monitoring the cases reported to them for information on toxicity, treatment, and outcome, to develop a database from which to answer future enquiries. Thus the monitoring of poisoning by PCCs was initiated for very practical reasons to meet an

Table 23.1 Functions of a Poison Control Centre

1. Provision of information relevant to diagnosis and management of acute poisoning in man.
2. Consultative clinical service for treatment of poisoned patients.
3. Laboratory service for analysis of drugs and poisons.
4. Epidemiological studies (Toxicovigilance).
5. Training and education of doctors and other health service personnel.
6. Participation in measures for prevention of poisioning including education of the public.

immediate need and was not originally considered as a surveillance scheme. With time, however, this monitoring has become increasingly sophisticated and toxicovigilance[2] has become established as a fundamental role of PCCs.[3] Analysis of PCC enquiries provides data not only to improve the quality and quantity of information available to physicians but also to determine the incidence and causes of poisoning. This information can be made available to manufacturers and to policy-makers in health services and government organizations and to others who are concerned either with the provision of facilities for treatment of poisoned patients or with development, implementation, and evaluation of measures for prevention.

Information on aspects of poisoning can also be obtained from national statistics of morbidity and mortality, and from local, usually short-term, hospital-based surveys of poisoning, but PCCs can be considered the principal organizations involved in surveillance as defined earlier in this book. Thus it is appropriate to start with a discussion of the value of data collected by PCCs.

Surveillance by PCCs

Methods of data collection

PCCs collect data about each case of poisoning that is the subject of a telephone enquiry, usually recording information in writing on a preprinted registration form (Fig. 23.1). The minimum information documented includes the identification of the substance implicated, the time, degree and route of exposure, the sex, age and condition of the patient, the treatment already given, and the identity of both patient and enquirer. Many PCCs also record additional information about previous medical history, and the circumstances of the accident, including more details about the suspected poison, such as its packaging. In some centres this information is stored in a computer database from which detailed analyses are available.[4] Over the last three years such a system has been extensively used by the National Poisons Information Service (NPIS) which is one of the major PCCs in the United Kingdom.[5]

Information about clinical course, management, and outcome of a case may be obtained during subsequent telephone conversations between the enquirer and the Poisons Centre. In some PCCs, particularly those centres in the USA which receive enquiries from the public, it is routine procedure to follow up each case by calling back at specified intervals to check on efficacy of treatment and the need for more advice. In most centres, however, only serious cases of poisoning are reviewed by telephone, so complete case histories and additional information which is required for monitoring programmes is obtained by sending the enquirer a questionnaire or request for a discharge summary or detailed case history.

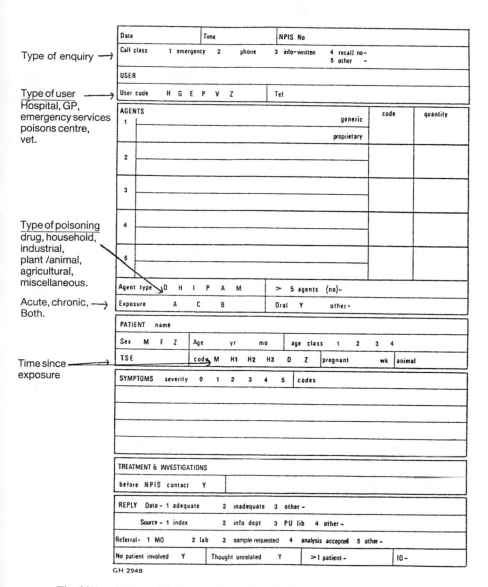

Fig. 23.1. National Poisons Information Service data collection form.

Most centres follow up only a proportion of the cases reported to them. In the early years of operation, our centre followed up every enquiry to obtain as much information as possible on the effects of poisoning with chemical products which at that time had only recently become widely available in the home, and which were of largely unknown toxicity to man. However, as the number of enquiries has increased it has become impossible to follow up every one, nor is it necessary as experience of poisoning is accumulated. There are also practical reasons why a process must be introduced to select those cases which are most likely to add to knowledge of product toxicity. The possibility of losing useful information by neglecting to follow up a case or including inaccuracies in analyses of call records which have not been verified by follow-up, must be weighed against the volume of work involved in sending out letters and processing the replies, the cost of postage especially when reply paid envelopes are used, and the possibility of alienating doctors who are sent too many questionnaires. Moreover, there is nothing to prevent a doctor from sending reports without being prompted by a questionnaire. However, in the experience of our centre few case histories are received spontaneously, although many enquirers promise to send a case history if the outcome is interesting. It is debatable how much this reflects the disinclination of doctors to participate in voluntary reporting schemes and how much it confirms the accuracy with which information staff select for follow-up most of the cases which will provide useful data.

Value and limitations of the data

Since the monitoring systems operated by PCCs are linked to information and advice services they have an advantage over totally voluntary systems such as the Committee on the Safety of Medicines (CSM) yellow card scheme in the UK,[6] in that the notification of cases does not depend entirely on the doctor's concern to report them to a monitoring centre. However, because the enquiries reflect the need for information, it is not usually possible to relate PCC case records to the total number of events in the community and the data are thus of limited value for epidemiological studies.

Several factors influence the doctor's decision to discuss a case of suspected poisoning with an information service. One factor is his familiarity with the substance implicated: less frequently occurring types of exposure are more likely to be referred and thus to be over-represented. Another factor is the severity of poisoning: advice is more likely to be sought when a patient has signs of serious toxicity or, at the other extreme, when the patient has few or no symptoms. The latter case was demonstrated by a hospital study which compared cases of childhood poisoning referred to a PCC with those that were not referred, and found that the children with minor symptoms were over-represented in the PCC sample, because doctors wanted to discuss the necessity of hospital treatment.[7] Distance of the doctor from the PCC is probably a factor in countries where the enquirer pays for the telephone call. For example, the NPIS in London serves the whole of England, but receives the majority of its enquiries from the surrounding south eastern area of the country.

In considering the value of data obtained by the PCCs it must be recognized that there are limitations inherent in data about suspected poisoning events. This is true not only for data available from PCCs but also for data available from other sources discussed below. First, the circumstantial evidence about both accidental and deliberate exposure may give inaccurate information about the nature of the substance taken. Secondly, the clinical picture can be complicated by exposure to more than one agent, making it difficult to attribute effects to one particular substance. Thirdly, the extent of exposure after accidental or deliberate overdose may be difficult to determine, so limiting the usefulness of the data for interpretation of dose-related toxicity. These inaccuracies can be minimized if appreciable numbers of reports are available for review. Furthermore, for many substances laboratory analyses of body fluids can be undertaken to confirm the link between clinical events and exposure to particular compounds, the extent of exposure or the concurrent ingestion of several products.

It can also be argued that data collected retrospectively from medical records are of variable quality, because significant information may have been omitted from the original records or from the history sent to the PCC. However, doctors who have been advised by a PCC about the signs and symptoms of poisoning are less likely to omit significant data from their records, and the PCC follow-up can prompt the selection of significant data from the case records if specific questions are asked. Most of the surveys carried out by our centre have used specially designed questionnaires which ask for specific data needed to assess the toxicity of one particular substance or group of substances. These are sent with covering letters explaining the purpose of the survey and including references or copies of relevant publications where appropriate.

Use of Poison Control Centre Data

Analysis of the information received at the time of the enquiry can show whether the relative incidence of suspected poisoning from different substances changes with time or between countries and can identify problems which might merit more intensive monitoring. PCCs which have computerized their enquiry records are able to undertake more detailed analyses and review more cases; an example of the use of such analysis is the investigation of acute poisoning in pregnant women.[8]

Intensive surveys of enquiries related to a single substance or group of substances using information obtained by follow-up as well as the initial case reports are able to establish acute toxicity, the efficacy of recommended treatment regimes, and the effect of changes in product safety. One such intensive monitoring survey which can serve as an example, was carried out in the UK to establish the acute toxicity of clonidine.[9] This was instituted after the NPIS noted an increase in the number of enquiries about suspected poisoning with this drug and found that there was disagreement in the literature about the clinical features and treatment of overdose. Clonidine is used for the treatment of migraine as Dixarit, a small, blue, sugar coated tablet containing 0·025 mg of active drug, and for the treatment of hypertension as Catapres, a large, white, uncoated tablet containing 0·1 mg or 0·3 mg. A survey of follow-up reports of 170 cases reported to the NPIS in 1976 and 1977 showed that 73 per cent involved children who allegedly ingested Dixarit and that this could cause severe and life-threatening symptoms particularly in young children. There were sufficient cases to give an adequate description of the clinical features and duration of clonidine poisoning, and an indication of the lowest dose which might cause poisoning. The difference in the number of enquiries about the two types of drug generated the hypothesis that Dixarit was stored less carefully, possibly because it was used for the relatively minor disease of migraine, and so was thought by the user to be less of a hazard than Catapres which was intended for the more serious condition of hypertension. In addition the sweet tasting, blue Dixarit tablets were attractive to children. Preventive measures were therefore recommended and implemented by the manufacturers with the aim of improving pack safety and labelling to increase parents' awareness of the need for safe storage of the drug.

Similar, more recent surveys have determined the acute symptomatology of β adrenoceptor blocker overdose reported in Sweden,[10] and the incidence and severity of ingestion of corrosives reported in The Netherlands.[11] From the UK, examples include surveys to determine the effects of the ingestion of Psilocybe mushrooms,[12] denture cleaners,[13] paracetamol in children,[14] non-steroidal anti-inflammatory drugs,[15] and to study the kinds of drugs taken in overdose by diabetic patients.[16]

The role of toxicological analyses

Surveys of acute toxicity carried out in conjuction with toxicology laboratories make it possible to confirm case histories by analysis of body fluids, and to assess toxicity of substances in relation to their concentrations in the body. In the UK, sodium valproate[17] and other non-barbiturate anticonvulsants,[18] chlormethiazole,[19] and 2,4-D[20] were all monitored in this way, by requesting blood and urine samples at the time of the enquiry to the centre. Another survey used laboratory analysis simply to confirm the nature of the solvents used in cases of solvent abuse reported to the NPIS, and demonstrate the variety of products used by 'solvent sniffers'.[21]

Post-marketing surveillance of drugs

PCC monitoring of the effects of drugs in overdose is an important aspect of Post-marketing Surveillance which can influence their use and availability. Many PCCs exchange information on drug overdoses and adverse reactions to their therapeutic use with agencies responsible for monitoring adverse drug reactions. In the UK the NPIS attempts to monitor all suspected overdoses of new drugs, and thus gathers information complementary to that collected by the CSM which conducts special surveillance for adverse reactions. As new antidepressants were introduced, the NPIS monitored suspected overdoses to establish their acute toxicity and compare them with tricyclic antidepressants and monoamine oxidase inhibitors. Trazodone,[22] mianserin,[23] and nomifensine,[24] were shown to be less cardiotoxic than existing drugs and were thus recommended as safer drugs for therapy of depression while maprotiline showed a similar toxicity to the tricyclics.[25] When regulatory authorities considered changing the status of ibuprofen from a medicine available only on prescription to one that was available without prescription from pharmacies, the NPIS was able to provide evidence of its low toxicity in acute overdose compared with analgesics already available for sale to the public to support the case for wider availability.[26] Work now in progress will assess the impact on the over-the-counter release of ibuprofen on analgesic poisoning in the UK. These activities in the UK show that there is scope for increasing co-operation between PCCs and Adverse Drug Reaction monitoring schemes.

Evaluation of treatments for poisoning

Information from PCC case reports is useful in assessing efficacy of treatment of poisoning and identifying problems resulting from specific treatment regimes. Surveys have evaluated the use of haemoperfusion for treatment of overdose with hypnotic drugs,[27] the use of naloxone in opioid poisoning,[28] the use of stellate ganglion block and active elimination techniques in treatment of quinine overdose,[29-31] of silibinin in Amanita poisoning,[32] and the treatment of hydrofluoric acid burns.[33] Such work can also detect unexpected problems associated with specific treatment regimes. In the course of surveying the morbidity and mortality of paracetamol overdose in adults, the NPIS received reports not only of adverse reactions to the acetylcysteine antidote but also of its administration in overdose resulting in similar, but more severe reactions. By reviewing these cases of iatrogenic poisoning the cause was identified as confusing labelling, resulting in errors in the calculations of dosage. It was thus possible to educate doctors by publication of these findings, and to recommend improvements in product labelling.[34,35]

There are many other examples that could be quoted to show the value of surveillance by PCCs. However, it must be accepted that the data from PCCs cannot be considered in isolation since only in exceptional cases can PCCs monitor all incidents that involve a specific substance occurring in a population. One such exception is the surveillance of paraquat poisoning by the NPIS with the co-operation of other UK PCCs and the help of the manufacturers. This aims at coverage of all cases of suspected paraquat poisoning occurring in the UK.[36] Since paraquat is relatively infrequently ingested, such an aim is feasible and necessary for the collection of sufficient data to evaluate the effectiveness of measures to improve product safety and effectiveness of treatment regimes. Generally however, to obtain information on the epidemiology of poisoning and monitor the incidence of poisoning in relation to defined populations, it is necessary to use sources other than PCCs.

Surveillance of Poisoning: Other Sources

Mortality and morbidity statistics

In looking at the value and limitations of these sources in health surveillance the aim is to show that they are complementary, each source contributing data which cannot be obtained elsewhere but which is by itself inadequate for surveillance.

Mortality statistics are collected by many European countries, and some can provide information on the incidence of deaths from poisoning or suspected poisoning by age and sex, with some broad categorization by type of substance involved.[37] However, the percentage of poisoning incidents resulting in death is relatively low especially in the under five-year-old group. In the UK between 1974 and 1980 poisoning resulted in 99 deaths in children under 5, which is a very low number compared to the 24 000 hospital admissions each year for suspected poisoning.[38] Thus there is a need to review morbidity. The availability of morbidity data, almost entirely related to rates of hospital admission and utilization varies between European countries.[39] Hospital Information Systems, such as Regional Hospital Activity Analysis in the UK from which the Hospital In-Patient Enquiry (HIPE) statistics are derived, are intended primarily to provide data for management and length of hospital stay classified by cause in broad terms. Information on location and other details of the circumstances of the accident is not found in such systems, but is recorded in the UK by the Household Accident Surveillance Scheme (HASS), which collects data on all patients who attend a sample of Accident and Emergency (A & E) departments as a result of home accidents, including suspected poisoning. There is very little information available about morbidity from poisoning in general practice.

Both mortality and morbidity statistics are subject to error which may arise from inaccuracies in diagnosis, patient information, or the population estimates which are required as the denominator. A useful summary by

Alderson[40] lists the causes of inaccuracies in clinical diagnoses recorded on death certificates. These can occur if laboratory analysis has not been used to confirm the history of exposure which, as already mentioned, can often be misleading. Also, in some countries, deaths can be certified by people without medical knowledge or by physicians who have not seen the body after death. Religious constraints on identifying suicides may introduce further inaccuracies. Some deaths from poisoning may escape registration because the poisoning goes unrecognized or because a complication of the poisoning is regarded as the cause of death. Errors have been found on death certificates even in the UK, where all deaths that are unnatural or where the cause is unknown are reported to the coroner, and where an autopsy is carried out in almost all cases of suspected drug overdose. Thus, by examination of past medical history, circumstantial evidence, post-mortem reports, and results of toxicological analyses Vale *et al.*[41] found that 24 per cent of deaths classified by coroners in 1979 as being due to the analgesic combination of paracetamol and dextropropoxyphene, were clearly the result of ingestion of another drug or drugs. The clinical data in hospital information systems are also subject to inaccuracy and imprecision.[42]

The value of national statistics on morbidity and mortality is that being representative and continuous samples of the population, they can provide information on the magnitude of the problem in terms of the incidence, severity, and socio-economic cost and information on trends in type of products implicated. Thus information about trends in incidence of products involved in accidental child poisoning, for example, can be obtained from HASS,[43,44] and from mortality statistics.[45,46]

Death certificates and coroner's records are a useful source for descriptive studies of poisoning. Craft,[38] for example, listed the substances commonly implicated in childhood poisoning deaths and found sufficient information in the coroner's records about the circumstances of the accident to make recommendations for preventive measures. In a similar study of fatal poisoning with tricyclic antidepressants it was possible to investigate the clinical events causing deaths in a larger number of cases than had been monitored previously through hospital-based surveys and also to identify the number of deaths occuring outside hospital. It was found that although death was assumed to be commonly the result of tachydysrhythmias, it was in fact more often a result of respiratory depression and convulsions. The observation that the majority of deaths occured outside hospital led to the recommendation that preventive measures were more important than improvements in clinical management in reducing mortality from tricyclic antidepressant poisoning.[47]

Occupational toxicology

Poisoning which occurs in the workplace is monitored by national and international organizations which are concerned with monitoring health and safety at work. In the UK, for example, the Health and Safety Executive collects reports of diseases related to work including those resulting from exposure to noxious agents, to monitor and help prevent ill-health at work. Manufacturers often monitor health and safety of people using their products or working in their factories, multinational organizations sometimes collate data at an international level. All these organizations are sources not only of data about individual people but also of information about incidents which may involve many people, such as accidents involving chemicals or mass poisoning incidents. Not every surveillance scheme provides information in a usable form however. The UK sickness absence reporting scheme provided information on incidence of industrial exposure to noxious agents, but data were collated in a form which was difficult to use for surveillance of occupational poisoning, and their use for this purpose has been abandoned since the regulations for reporting sickness absence have changed.

Epidemiological surveys

Although national statistics can provide some information on which to base prevention, more detailed analysis is necessary to investigate the factors contributing to accidental poisoning and to assess product toxicity. Epidemiological surveys based on smaller samples from one or two hospitals can provide such analyses. Retrospective surveys usually cover a longer time period than prospective studies. However, whereas the former are limited by the quality of information obtained retrospectively, the prospective studies can be more versatile and collect information which would not otherwise be recorded in the hospital notes about the social factors and causes of poisoning. Such studies can identify products implicated commonly, or in severe poisoning incidents, and suggest areas for prevention and evaluate measures already adopted. Information about patients attending hospital can be supplemented from other sources. For example, a one-year survey of childhood poisoning in Oslo included children examined at outpatients clinics,[48] and a concomitant survey of acute poisoning in adults provided a more accurate assessment of the incidence of self-poisoning by supplementing information on hospital admissions with information obtained from forensic records on those people dying outside hospital.[49] Calnan[50] investigated the use of all health-care services in an area by children with suspected poisoning and obtained more information by visiting childrens' homes and interviewing patients.

The size and representativeness of hospital based surveys is often limited by administrative resources. Multicentre studies can overcome the bias present in data collected form one centre by covering a wider geographical area. PCCs with their extensive knowledge of poisoning, have a role in planning and co-ordination of such surveys and they are currently an important part of the surveillance programme at our centre. In 1982 a multicentre survey was implemented to provide detailed information about analgesic overdose, including data about the patients' symptoms and treatment, with information about the relative involvement of different products and their packaging, and the place where the patient obtained them.[51] A second survey assessed the role of drug packaging in childhood poisoning accidents,[52] and a third is in progress investigating the incidence and severity of accidental poisoning occurring at work. The survey of childhood poisoning accidents was carried out at the same time as a survey of the availability of medicines in childrens' homes using home visits and interviews, so that the incidence of accidental poisoning with individual products could be compared with their availability in the home; a comparison which had been made previously in a study of childhood poisoning with household products.[53]

Although short-term surveys can provide useful information, continuous surveillance is needed. Christen *et al.*[7] have investigated the feasibility of a continuous surveillance system to collect epidemiological information about hospital patients with suspected poisoning to complement and be compatible with the information obtained from the continuous surveillance of cases referred to a PCC. Documentation was designed using their experience of a previous retrospective study, to facilitate routine case history documentation rather than to complicate it. This has been implemented to monitor childhood poisoning at the Luebeck paediatric hospital.

Epidemiological studies can identify poisoning cases from sources other than hospital records. Surveys which have sought to investigate factors related to the child and its environment rather than the substance involved, have used cohorts of children of the same age and compared children who have had accidents with those which have not. Sobell[54] looked at the psychiatric aspects of poisoning in a sample of children selected by inspection of the birth records from two areas of the USA for two years, and Wadsworth[55] investigated the interaction of family type and accidents, in a sample of children from a large national cohort of children born in Britain during one week.

Surveillance in Practice

In summary, no single source is by itself adequate for surveillance of poisoning. Nevertheless, one source may be able to provide information to make up the deficiencies in data available from another source as well as to aid in the assessment of the validity of that data. Thus hospital-based epidemiological surveys and analyses of PCC enquiries must be interpreted within the framework and perspective provided by national statistics, and these must themselves be interpreted with reference to the clinical data provided from other sources.

For example, when child-resistant containers were introduced in the UK for aspirin and paracetamol containing drugs, their effectiveness could not be demonstrated solely with reference to HIPE since this does not distinguish discharges for suspected poisoning from individual analgesics. An investigation of admissions to hospitals in Newcastle and South Glamorgan showed a decline in admissions for suspected childhood poisoning from aspirin, not paralleled by a change in admissions from paracetamol, benzodiazepines, or tricyclic antidepressants. This was good evidence of the effectiveness of child-resistant containers since the regulations for their use did not include anxiolytic drugs or liquid preparations which accounted for most of the paracetamol ingestions. The validity of using the results of these local studies as an indicator of national trends was justified by comparison with HIPE which showed an overall decrease in suspected child poisoning from medicines in the UK.[56]

Similarly, several sources were used to study analgesic poisoning in all age groups in England and Wales.[57] National mortality statistics showed that overall mortality from analgesic poisoning had increased between 1968 and 1980 and that opiates and opiate derivatives either alone or in combination with other analgesic agents were responsible for this increase. Deaths from paracetamol alone had risen less dramatically while deaths from aspirin had fallen. During the same period HIPE showed that hospital admission for suspected poisoning from analgesics had also increased. Information on admission for individual analgesics was obtained from a prospective survey of analgesic poisoning co-ordinated by the NPIS, involving five hospital Accident and Emergency departments. This showed that most patients took preparations which contained either aspirin or paracetamol alone rather than preparations in which these drugs were combined with opiates or other drugs. It also found that analgesics taken in overdose were usually obtained over the counter rather than on prescription. Comparing the incidence of poisoning with annual over-the-counter sales of tablets, showed that the use of paracetamol had increased while that of salicylate had decreased, and thus provided evidence that increase of mortality from paracetamol was largely due to increase in use of the drug.

Conclusions and Recommendations

Collaboration and co-operation within the limits of confidentiality are needed on an international scale. Action is needed at several levels to improve the quality and quantity of data available. Starting at the source of the data, improvements could be made to the precision of the medical data available from medical records. The following recommendations made by O'Gorman[42] are worth repeating:

1. Sustained educational campaigns geared towards winning the interest and active support of the medical profession for the concept of hospital discharge summary systems.
2. Restructuring of hospital medical records to facilitate the extraction of statistical data.
3. Provision of more adequate training for lay medical records staff.

The agencies involved in surveillance of poisoning also need to identify areas for improvement, for example, the monitoring of morbidity in general practice, of chronic and occupational toxicity, of environmental toxicity, and of the effects of preventive measures. They also need to discuss compatibility of data collected, with regard to its type and amount, and the way it is classified and coded, since this determines the precision and recall of data retrieval: information may be lost if classification is too broad. At a local level confusion of terminology may invalidate comparison of case histories received from different physicians, a problem noted by Van Heijst.[11] At an international level lack of compatibility may limit the possibility of comparison between different countries of incidence and trends in poisoning. There may be confusion, for example, about the scope of the category 'household product', or differences in the classification of patients' ages. Standardization of data is currently a topic of discussion between PCCs.[3]

Improvements in quality and quantity of data must be matched by improvements in methods to analyse and assess them. Poisons centres which are able to function effectively as surveillance centres do so by virtue of the large number of cases reported to them, so it follows that storage and retrieval of large amounts of data is a common problem. Efficient information retrieval systems can help to ensure that data on toxicity are made available quickly, when and where they are needed. Computers have been used in a few centres for several years, but PCCs have generally been slow to use information technology, and such systems that are in use are primitive compared with the sophisticated systems available in pharmaceutical companies for handling very similar data relating to toxicity and adverse reactions to their products. This undoubtedly reflects the difference in funds available to employ staff with expertise to design and implement computer information systems and to obtain the necessary equipment. However, it also reflects the different attitudes of managers in industry compared with those in the health service toward the importance of developing and maintaining efficient systems for information storage and retrieval. Outside pressures from drug regulatory-agencies have forced management of pharmaceutical companies to give this priority, but few such pressures have been applied to Poisons Centre managers, the majority of whom are physicians with little appreciation of the importance of information management. The contribution which information science can make to the efficient functioning of surveillance programmes has largely been ignored. Until there is a change in attitude by those who manage PCCs and those who fund them, the full potential of these centres to monitor poisoning cannot be realized.

Appendix

World Federation of Associations of Clinical Toxicology Centres and Poison Control Centres
Secretariat: Centre International de Recherche sur le Cancer, 150, Cours Albert-Thomas, 69372 Lyon Cedex 2, France
European Association of Poison Control Centres
Centre Belge Anti-Poisons, rue Joseph Stallaert, 15, B-1060 Brussels, Belgium.

Bibliography

1. Volans, G. N., Poisons information services. In *Monitoring for drug safety* (ed. W. H. W. Inman). MTP Press, Lancaster 2nd edition (1986).
2. Roche, L., Toxicovigilance. *Collection de Médecine Légale et de Toxicologie Médicale* **110**, 21–30 (1978).
3. Conference Report. Fourth general meeting of the World Federation of Associations of Clinical Toxicology Centres and Poison Control Centres, Geneva, 7–9 Oct. (1985).
4. Vincent, V., Computers in poisons information. *Hum. Toxicol.* **2**, 273–8 (1983).
5. Edwards, J. N., Volans, G. N., and Wiseman, H. M., Poisons information processing: the development of a computer database for case records. In *Current perspectives in health computing* (ed. B. Kostrewski). Cambridge University Press (1984).
6. Inman, W. H. W., The United Kingdom. In *Monitoring for drug safety* (ed. W. H. W. Inman). MTP Press, Lancaster 2nd edition (1986).
7. Christen, H. J., Zink, C., Zink, A., and Korporal, J., Childhood poisoning in a paediatric hospital: the Luebeck experience. *Hum. Toxicol.* **2**, 295–303 (1983).
8. Edwards, J. N. and Volans, G. N., A computerised case file for acute poisoning in man—the first year's experience. *Medical Informatics* **10**, 169–71 (1985).
9. Stein, B. and Volans, G. N., Dixarit overdose: The problem of attractive tablets. *Br med. J.*, 667–8 (1978).
10. Kulling, P., Eleborg, L., and Persson, H., β Adrenoceptor blocker intoxication: Epidemiological data. *Hum. Toxicol.* **2**, 175–81 (1983).
11. Van Heijst, A. N. P., The problem of the corrosiveness of products—a pilot study with a denture cleaner. *Hum. Toxicol.* **2**, 339–44 (1983).
12. Francis, J. and Murray, V. S. G., Psilocybe mushroom ingestion 1978–1981. *Hum. Toxicol.* **2**, 349–52 (1983).
13. Thompson, N. and Volans, G. N., Denture cleaner ingestion (abstract). Congress of the European Association of Poison Control Centres, Stockholm (1984).
14. Meredith, T. J., Newman, B., and Goulding, R., Paracetamol poisoning in children. *Br. med. J.* **2**, 478–9 (1978).
15. Court, H. and Volans, G. N., Poisoning after overdose with non-steroidal anti-

inflammatory drugs. *Adverse Drug Reactions and Acute Poisoning Rev.* **3**, 1–21 (1984).

16. Jefferys, D. B. and Volans, G. N., Self poisoning in diabetic patients. *Hum. Toxicol.* **2**, 345–8 (1983).
17. Volans, G. N., Berry, D. J., and Wiseman, H. M., Overdose with sodium valproate. *Br. J. clin. Pract.* **27**, Symposium supplement, 58–63 (1983).
18. Berry, D. J., Wiseman, H. M., and Volans, G. N., A survey of non-barbiturate anticonvulsant drug overdose reported to the Poisons Information Service (UK). *Hum. Toxicol.* **2**, 357–60 (1983).
19. Houston, A., Essex, E. G., Wiseman, H. M., and Flanagan, R. J., Acute chlormethiazole poisoning in patients notified to the Poisons Unit, Guy's Hospital, 1978–1981. *Hum. Toxicol.* **2**, 361–9 (1983).
20. Onyon, L. J., Liddle, A., and Flanagan, R. J., Acute toxicity of chlorinated phenoxy herbicides in man (abstract). British Toxicology Society Meeting, Oct. (1985).
21. Francis, J., Murray, V. S. G., Rupah, M., Flanagan, R. J., and Ramsey, J. D., Suspected solvent abuse in cases referred to the poisons unit, Guy's Hospital, July 1980–June 1981. *Hum. Toxicol.* **1**, 271–80 (1982).
22. Henry, J. A. and Ali, C. J., Trazodone overdosage: experience from a poisons information service. *Hum. Toxicol.* **2**, 353–6. (1983).
23. Newman, B. and Crome, P., The clinical toxicology of mianserin hydrochloride. *Vet. Hum. Toxicol.*, Suppl. 21, 60–2 (1979).
24. Ali, C. and Crome, P., The clinical toxicology of nomifensine: an update. The Royal Society of Medicine International Congress and Symposium series **70**, 121–3 (1984).
25. Crome, P. and Newman, B., Poisoning with maprotiline and mianserin. *Br. med. J.* **2**, 260 (1977).
26. Court, H., Streete, P. and Volans, G. N., Acute poisoning with ibuprofen. *Hum. toxicol.* **2**, 381–4 (1983).
27. Hampel, G., Wiseman, H. M. and Widdop, B., Acute poisoning due to hypnotics: The role of haemoperfusion in clinical perspective. *Hum. Vet. Toxicol.*, Suppl. 21, 4–6 (1979).
28. Jefferys, D. B. and Volans, G. N., An investigation of the role of the specific opioid antagonist naloxone in clinical toxicology. *Hum. Toxicol.* **2**, 227–31 (1983).
29. Dyson, E. H., Proudfoot, A. T., Prescott, L. F., and Heyworth, R., Death and blindness due to overdose of quinine. *Br. med. J.* **291**, 31–33 (1985).
30. Boland, M. E., Brennand Roper, S. M., and Henry, J. A., Complications of quinine poisoning. *Lancet* i, 384–5 (1985).
31. Bateman, D. N., Blain, P. G., Woodhouse, K. W., Rawlins, M. D., Dyson, M., Heyworth, R., Prescott, L. F., and Proudfoot, A. T. Pharmacokinetics and clinical toxicity of quinine overdosage. Lack of efficacy of techniques intended to enhance elimination. *Quart. J. Med.* **54**, 125–31 (1985).
32. Hruby, K., Csmos, G., Fuhrmann, M., and Thaler, H., Chemotherapy of Amanita phalloides poisoning with intravenous silibinin. *Hum. Toxicol.* **2**, 183–96 (1983).
33. Velvart, J., Arterial perfusion for hydrofluoric acid burns. *Hum. Toxicol.* **2**, 233–8 (1983).

34. Mant, T. G. K., Tempowski, J., Volans, G. N., and Talbot, J. C. C., Adverse reactions to acetylcysteine and effects of overdose. *Br. med J.* **289**, 217–19 (1984).
35. Henry, J. A. and Volans, G. N., Paracetamol poisoning. In *ABC of poisoning* (eds J. A. Henry and G. N. Volans). British Medical Journal, London (1984).
36. Whitehead, A. P., Volans, G. N., and Hart, T. B., Toxicovigilance for pesticides. Paraquat poisoning in the United Kingdom. *J. Toxicol. Med.* **4**, 51–53 (1984).
37. WHO, World Health Statistics Annual, 1982. WHO (1985).
38. Craft, A. W., Circumstances surrounding deaths from accidental poisoning 1974–1980. *Archs Dis. Child.* **58**, 544–6 (1983).
39. Roger, F. H., The minimum basic data set for hospital statistics in the EEC. In *Hospital statistics* (eds P. M. Lambert and F. H. Roger) pp. 83–111. Amsterdam, North Holland Publishing Co. (1982).
40. Alderson, M., *International mortality statistics*. Macmillan, London (1981).
41. Vale, J. A., Buckley, B. M., and Meredith, T. J., Deaths from paracetamol and dextropropoxyphene (distalgesic) poisoning in England and Wales in 1979. *Hum. Toxicol.* **3**, 135S–143S. (1984).
42. O'Gorman, J., Data accuracy and reliability. In *Hospital statistics* (eds P. M. Lambert and F. H. Roger) pp. 113–17. Amsterdam, North Holland Publishing Co. (1982).
43. Burgar, C., Analysis of child poisoning accidents. London: Consumer Safety Unit, Department of Trade and Industry, UK (unpublished report) (1984).
44. Hayward, G., Comparison of 6 years' data (1977–1982) on non-fatal suspected poisonings of infants in the home. London: Consumer Safety Unit, Department of Trade and Industry (unpublished report) (1984).
45. Fraser, N. C., Accidental poisoning deaths in British children 1958–1977. *Br. med. J.*, 1595–8 (1980).
46. MacFarlane, A. and Fox, J., Child deaths from accidents and violence. *Hlth Trends* **12**, 22–27 (1978).
47. Newman, B., Fatal tricyclic antidepressant poisoning. *J. R. Soc. Med.* **72**, 649–53 (1979).
48. Jacobsen, D., Halvorsen, K., Marstrander, J., Sunde, K., and Bakken, A. F., Acute poisonings of children in Oslo. A one year prospective study. *Acta paediatr. scand.* **72**, 553–7 (1983).
49. Jacobsen, D., Frederichsen, P. S., Knutsen, K. M., Sorum , Y., Talseth, T., and Odegaard, O. R., A prospective study of 1212 cases of acute poisoning: general epidemiology. *Hum. Toxicol.* **3**, 93–106 (1984).
50. Calnan, M. W., Dale, J. W., and de Fonseka, C. P., Suspected poisoning in children. *Archs Dis. Child.* **51**, 180–5 (1976).
51. National Poisons Information Service Monitoring Group, Analgesic poisoning: A multi-centre, prospective survey. *Hum. Toxicol.* **1**, 7–23 (1981).
52. Wiseman, H. M., Guest, K., Murray, V. S. G., and Volans, G. N., Accidental poisoning in childhood: a multicentre survey. 2. The role of packaging in accidents involving medications. *Hum. Toxicol.* **6**, 303–14 (1987).
53. Department of Prices and Consumer Protection, Child poisoning from household products. London: Consumer Safety Unit, Department of Prices and Consumer Protection (1976).
54. Sobel, R., The psychiatric implications of accidental poisoning in childhood. *Paediatric clinics of North America* **17**, 653–85 (1970).

55. Wadsworth, J., Brunell, I., Taylor, B., and Butler, N., Family type and accidents in preschool children. *J. Epidemiol. Commun. Hlth* **37**, 100–4 (1983).
56. Jackson, R. H., Childhood poisoning: perspectives and problems. *Hum. Toxicol.* **2**, 285–93 (1983).
57. Meredith, T. J. and Vale, J. A., Epidemiology of analgesic overdose in England and Wales. *Hum. Toxicol.* **3**, 61S–74S (1984).

Glossary

Acceptable risk A risk which has minimal detrimental effects, or for which potential benefits outweigh potential hazards.

Accident In the sphere of health, the term accident has been used to denote unexpected physical and chemical injuries to the body. Today it has been recognized that scientifically this definition is not applicable in a variety of instances. It is therefore gradually being replaced by descriptions of the injuries themselves and the physical and chemical agents or conditions which are responsible for their occurrence.

Accidents at work Sudden and unexpected events related to an activity, a condition or a circumstance, occurring to employees during a period covered by an employment contract and resulting in physical or mental harm.

Frequency rate
The number of accidents at work occurring during a defined period (usually one year) to all employees of a defined group, expressed per 1 000 000 hours of work done by the group.

Severity rate
The number of all lost days by a defined group of employees, during a defined period, caused by accidents at work. The days are counted as calendar days starting the first day after the disability or accident occurred, and ending the day before the injured takes up regular working hours. Usually expressed over a 1-year period and per 1000 hours worked by all members of the group.

Acute disease A disease having a short course, usually with sudden onset, compared with a chronic disease which may have a long course, or may be progressive over a long period, usually with gradual onset.

Age-sex register A list of all patients of a medical practice classified by age and sex, so that age and sex-specific rates for disease, consultations, etc. can be calculated (*see also* Register).

Amniocentesis The removal of amniotic fluid before birth by needle for laboratory examination.

Appropriateness Suitability for a purpose; in health the degree to which an interventive or other process is valid and acceptable for persons, circumstances, and place.

Association When two events occur more frequently together than would be expected by chance; the two events need not be directly related or causal.

Axis The direction of reference within a classification system. The ICPC Classification is bi-axial, with its primary axis representing body systems (chapters) and the other axis representing components.

Bias An effect that tends to produce a systematic error in the measurement of data—in surveillance, examples of bias would be the reporting of more severe disease, and the selective reporting by certain centres of diseases of special interest to them. Not the same as error, which is unsystematic.

Bias-recall Systematic error due to differences in accuracy or completeness of recall to memory of prior events or experiences.

Bias-reporting Selective suppression or revealing of information, an important cause of bias in surveillance systems.

Birth cohort *See* cohort.

Boarding schools Schools where children sleep for at least some nights during the week; in most boarding schools the children only go home at holidays.

BPA code The British Paediatric Association of the United Kingdom (BPA) have developed a specific classification of diseases for paediatric use.

Case fatality rate A measure of the severity of a disease which indicates the probability of death among diagnosed cases.

Chronic disease *See* Acute disease.

Classification Assignment to predesignated classes on the basis of perceived common characteristics.

Clinical trial An experiment on patients to determine the efficacy of a preventive or therapeutic agent or procedure.

Cluster analysis A set of statistical methods used to group variables or observations into strongly interrelated subgroups.

Clustering A closely grouped series of events, or cases of a disease or other health-related phenomena with well-defined distribution patterns in relation to time and place, or both. Usually describes an aggregation of a rare event.

Cohort A defined group of people studied over a period of time; often defined by birth (birth-cohort—those born in a single year or a five- or ten-year period) but sometimes by place.

Control group A comparison group, identified as a rule before the study is done, comprising persons who have not been exposed to the disease, intervention procedure, or other variable whose influence is being studied.

Coronary artery balloon dilation Percutaneous transluminal coronary angioplasty (PTCA).

Cusum Cumulative summation of the deviations from the baseline.

Denominator Population from which a sample has been taken.

Descriptive study A form of observational study which does not test a specific hypothesis.

Disability Temporary or long-term reduction of a person's capacity to function.

Disease severity A measure of the seriousness of a disease in a population, can be estimated by measuring; for example, the number of admissions to hospital compared with all cases, the complication rate or the case fatality rate.

Disease-specific register See Register

Diseases of affluence Those diseases whose prevalence is of major public health significance in many western nations, e.g. coronary heart disease.

Domesday book One of the very first registers, a survey of England executed in 1086 for William the Conqueror.

Drug utilization The marketing, distribution, and use of drugs in a society with special emphasis on the resulting medical, social, and economic consequences.

Encounter Any professional interchange between a patient and one or more members of a health care team. One or more problems of diagnosis may be identified at each encounter.

Episode A problem or illness in a patient over the entire period of time from its onset to its resolution.

Error A false reading obtained in a study; for example, a laboratory error. Surveillance data usually contain errors, which may be difficult or impossible to allow for in their analysis, and biases, which should be possible to allow for.

Eurocat A collaborative registration by EEC research workers, co-ordinated by the Commission of the European Communities using standardized methods of research on congenital abnormalities and twins.

Experimental epidemiology Often equated with randomized controlled trial.

Fax Facsimile transmission; the exact reproduction and transmission to another location of an original document by means of the ordinary telephone line—a long-distance photocopier.

Goal A specified state towards which intervention is directed, but it does not have to be quantifiable or meet a deadline, unlike targets and objectives.

Grid reference A reference to horizontal and vertical lines on a map so that a place can be identified.

Handicap Reduction in a person's capacity to fulfil a social role as a consequence of an impairment, inadequate training for the role, or other circumstances.

Health Care Services provided to individuals or communities by health services or professions or their agents for the purposes of promoting, maintaining, monitoring, or restoring health. Medical care is similar but narrower as it refers to therapeutic action by a physician. (*See also* Primary health-care.)

Health index A composite, usually weighted, of several indicators.

Health measure An individual activity which aims to alter, favourably, the natural history of a disease or to alleviate symptoms.

Health programme A set of health measures directed towards the attainment of specified health objectives.

Hospital Activity Analysis (HAA) A scheme in England and Wales sponsored by the Department of Health and Social Security and the Welsh Office in which information concerning patients in hospital is collected under nationally agreed headings, together with any items of local interest. Processing is on a regional basis to provide management and clinical information for health authorities.

Hospital In-Patient Enquiry (HIPE) A survey, based on a one in ten sample of National Health Service patients in England and Wales, excluding hospital beds designated for psychiatric disease. Extracted from the Hospital Activity Analysis. The sample is obtained at regional level and collected and coded by the Office of Population Censuses and Surveys (OPCS)

Indicators An objective measure; in health, a measure of health status or a health-related feature, used in planning and evaluating a programme.

In-patients Patients admitted to hospital for at least one night.

International Classification of Diseases (ICD) The classification of disease by an international group of experts who advise the WHO. The list is published by the WHO in the *Manual of the international statistical classification of diseases, injuries and causes of death*, and each disease is assigned a code number. The current edition is ICD-9.

International Classification of Health Problems in Primary Care (ICHPPC) A classification of diseases, conditions, and other reasons for attendance for primary care which may be used for labelling conditions in problem-oriented records. The classification is an adaptation of the ICD but makes allowances for the diagnostic uncertainty that prevails in primary care. Current revision is ICHPPC-2.

International Classification of Primary Care (ICPC) Formed by ICHPPC-2, ICHPPC-2-defined, IC-Process-PC and the International Glossary of Primary Care it is a comprehensive system designed to classify simultaneously three of the four elements of the problem-oriented record—*see* Chapter 8.

Longitudinal observation registers A register for collecting data on persons over a long time period, as for example in children in whom a congenital abnormality (such as deafness) may only be apparent some years after birth.

Medical care *See* Health care.

Minimum Basic Data Set For hospital data: 13 items recommended for recording hospital morbidity in the European Community. These are listed on p. 51, in Chapter 6.

Multifactorial Having more than one cause. Usually applied to aetiology.

MORT Management and Oversight Risk Tree, a logical diagram which facilitates the detection of organizational omissions or other deficiencies as basic causes for accidents.

Natural history of disease The course the disease would take in the absence of medical intervention.

Need A call for preventive, curative, rehabilitative care stemming from deficiencies of health determined by health professionals.

Notifiable disease Those diseases which are required to be notified statutorily to a local or other authority; steps taken to control a notifiable disease may have legal authority.

Occurrence A term describing the frequency of an event in a population without distinguishing between its incidence or prevalence.

Out-patients Patients who attend a clinic and are not admitted overnight.

Perinatal period From 28 weeks gestation to one week after birth.

Practice The organizational structure in which one or more physicians provide and supervise health care for a population of patients.

Solo practice (single-handed) A practice in which a single physician provides and supervises health care for a population of patients.

Group practice (co-operative practice in Denmark) A practice in which the patient population is cared for by a number of associated/affiliated physicians.

Single-speciality group A group practice in which all physician members belong to the same speciality.

Multi-speciality group A group practice in which the physician members belong to more than one speciality.

Prescription-Event Monitoring (PEM) Devised by W. H. W. Inman in England provides as denominator the number of patients exposed to the drug, and thus the risk. The prescribing physician receives a letter computer-generated from the prescription form asking him to complete a non-structured questionnaire on which events her or his patient experienced during and after taking the drug.

Prevention Hindering the occurrence as well as the progression of disease or disability in a community or individual.

(a) primary—*preventing* or postponing the onset of new cases;

(b) secondary—early *detection* of a disease while asymptomatic, while it is invisible, treatable, or possible to halt progression;

(c) tertiary—the *treatment* of a disease to prolong life or limit disability.

Primary health care The first level of contact with a health care system, usually a family doctor—*see also* Secondary, Tertiary health-care.

Problem A provider-determined assessment of anything that concerns a patient, the provider (in relation to the health of the patient), or both.

Problem-oriented medical record (POMR) A medical record in which the patient's history, physical findings, laboratory results, etc. are organized to give a cumulative record of problems rather than disease. The record includes subjective, objective, and significant negative information, discussions and conclusions and diagnostic and treatment plans with respect to each problem.

Process That which is done in the course of the management of a reason for encounter, problem or disease identified by a provider in a health care system.

Prophylaxis Measure taken to prevent infection.

Proportion A type of ratio in which the numerator is included in the denominator. The ratio of a part of the whole expressed as a 'decimal fraction' (e.g. 0·2) as a 'vulgar fraction' (e.g. 1/5) or, loosely as a percentage (20 per cent).

Provider A person to whom a patient has access when contacting the care system.

Quasi-experiment An experiment in which the investigator lacks full control over the allocation and/or timing of the intervention.

Reason for encounter The agreed statement of the reason(s) why a person enters the health care system, representing the demand for care by that person.

Record linkage A means of collecting, storing, and retrieving information contained in more than one record, so that the same individual is counted only once; it can also be used to collect together information on topics not predetermined or limited in their scope.

Register A file, book, list, or catalogue containing details of all cases of a particular disease or other important condition related to health in a defined population. Births and deaths registers and censuses are the most common types of register, but examples of disease specific registers include cancer, congenital malformations, and mental illness (see relevant chapters and also Part 1 of this book). *See also* Domesday book, Age–sex register.

Registry The organization and process involved in the support and maintenance of one or more registers.

Relative survival The observed mortality rate from certain diseases as a ratio of that expected in the population from which they come.

Relevance Applicability to or pertinence for a purpose; in health the degree to which an interventive or other process is applicable to or pertinent for persons, circumstances and place.

Resources The wherewithal—money, personnel, building, equipment, and technology—to provide a service.

Risk analysis Analysis of data to show the probability of an event occurring; can also be used to assess the amount that a given factor contributes to a disease or death (attributable risk) or increases risk of disease or death (relative risk).

Rubric A group of diseases, as in the ICD; a section or chapter heading.

Sandwich student A student who is given time off from an academic course to obtain work experience in the subject of study before returning to complete the course.

Scottish Morbidity Record A standard form completed for each patient discharged from or dying within a hospital. The form is then sent to a control agency for processing, analysis and publication (shown in Fig. 6.1, p. 53).

Screen The presumptive identification of unrecognized disease or defect by the application of tests, examinations, or other procedures which are usually more sensitive than specific and can be applied rapidly and usually cheaply.

Secondary health care Care provided through specialized services on referral from primary-care services.

Secular trend Changes over a long period of time; for example, years or decades rather than weeks or months.

Sentinel general practitioner A general practitioner who participates on a voluntary basis in a continuous registration programme on health problems and diseases of which the diagnosis or treatment is under his responsibility.

Severe injury The definition of 'severe injury' put forward by the Economic Commission for Europe of the UN does not provide adequate clinical criteria for the designation of severity. WHO recommends that a new definition be adopted, based on the duration of hospitalization and the expected degree of disability.

Severity indicator (for accidents) The term 'severity indicator' expresses the proportion of fatal casualties and is calculated by dividing the number of deaths by total casualties.

Socio-economic classification Arrangement of persons into groups according to education, occupation, and income; the one most commonly used, that of the Registrar-General of England and Wales is based on occupation. It has six classes:

    I—professional occupations
    II—intermediate occupations
IIIN—non-manual skilled occupations
IIIM—manual skilled occupations
   IV—partly skilled occupations
    V—unskilled occupations

A list is available of all occupations with the corresponding classification for each. Skill may be required in eliciting the correct information about occupation before it can be correctly classified. More complicated classifications, for example those that take into account education and income, are more difficult to administer and analyse.

Soundex code A sequence of letters used for recording names phonetically, especially in record linkage.

Special surveillance programmes Programmes designed individually for the surveillance of a single disease or infection.

Statutory Required by law. Some notification systems are statutory.

Sudden death Death within 24 hours of some distinct changes in the patient's state of health providing that there were no history, ante-mortem physical findings or post-mortem evidence to suggest that coronary heart disease was not the primary cause of death.

Supplemental classifications Supplemental classifications are separate, additional classifications which exist without standard linkage capability.

Survey An investigation (finite rather than ongoing, unlike surveillance) in which information is systematically collected but in which the experimental method is not used.

Target The desired end-result of certain activities.

Tertiary health care Rehabilitative and long-term care.

Thrombolysis Any drug intervention that aims at a lysis of a presumed or existing thrombus in the circulation.

Time-trend studies Studies designed to determine long-term movement in an ordered sequence of time.

Validity The extent to which a particular measure reflects what it is supposed to measure.

Vital statistics Systematically tabulated information concerning births, marriages, divorces, separations, and deaths based on registrations of these vital events.

WHO collaborating centre for international drug monitoring In Uppsala (Sweden) since 1976, having grown out of an internationally staffed co-ordinating unit first located in Alexandria, Va, USA and called the Research Centre for International Monitoring for Adverse Reactions to Drugs of the WHO.

Author index

Subject index